PLAGUE AND CONTAGION IN THE ISLAMIC MEDITERRANEAN

BLACK SEA WORLD

PLAGUE AND CONTAGION IN THE ISLAMIC MEDITERRANEAN

Edited by
NÜKHET VARLIK

ARC HUMANITIES PRESS

Library of Congress Cataloging in Publication Data
A catalog record for this book is available from the Library of Congress

ISBN 9781942401155
e-ISBN 9781942401162

http://mip-archumanitiespress.org
Printed and bound in the United States of America

CONTENTS

LIST OF ILLUSTRATIONS

Figures

Maps

Tables

INTRODUCTION

OVER THE LAST decade or two, the field of Middle Eastern and Islamic studies has witnessed the convergence of new perspectives on the history of epidemic diseases. A proliferation of research projects since the early 2000s have yielded a number of publications that enables us to explore connections between Middle Eastern studies and the histories of medicine and health. This volume serves as a testament that the field has reached a certain level of maturity.

The purpose of this volume is to showcase recently produced work in this field with a view to opening it up to broader inquiry. Much like the emergent field of studies to which it contributes, this volume itself represents burgeoning work. The idea behind putting together this volume grew out of conversation in a roundtable discussion at the 2010 meeting of the Middle East Studies Association (MESA). In its embryonic form, this project had a more ambitious scope than its current form, both spatially and temporally. It aimed to bring together the works extending across the Islamic Mediterranean, from the Iberian Peninsula and North Africa to the Eastern Mediterranean and the Black Sea. However, along the way, the volume developed around a more defined focus—the Ottoman Empire. This definition also characterized the temporal range, bearing testimony to the challenge of disease and the responses of a pre-modern society to it. The articles in the volume largely cover the early modern period, touching upon, on one hand, the late medieval era, and on the other, the era of modernization.

Fortunately, the expertise of this volume's contributors made it possible to retain the focus on early modern Ottoman society while exploring its connections to the broader Middle Eastern, Mediterranean, and European contexts. Yet this has been also a humbling reminder that any sweeping generalization would have to face the immensity of its object of study: the Ottoman Empire and the historical reality it represents spanning temporally and spatially beyond any single scholar's area of expertise. Turning this very challenge into a source of strength, each of these essays works with different toolkits, as much in their selection of sources as in their use of interdisciplinary methodologies.

Despite their different individual focuses, the articles in the volume capture an essential characteristic that defines the larger field: the necessity of adopting an interdisciplinary approach. The essays here cut across disciplinary boundaries, drawing from history of medicine, animal studies, political history, disaster studies, and psychology. By straddling several fields, they remind us that we can no longer afford to study Ottoman history in a bubble. This effort is quite timely. In recent years, historians have been eager to explore the connections between history and other disciplines—a goal that each of us tries to achieve here in different ways. Collectively, this volume seeks to integrate the theme of disease into the larger texture of Ottoman history, while searching for its links to other areas of research, both within history and beyond it. In particular, we are at the cusp of a truly remarkable moment in the marriage of history and science, pregnant with new cross-disciplinary possibilities. To mention but one example, a provocative editorial recently published in *Nature*, titled "Geneticists and historians need to work together on using DNA to explore the past," cautioned historians sternly that they "will be left behind if they fail to incorporate genetics into their research."[1] The history of infectious diseases works exceptionally well with such cross-disciplinary endeavors.

As the essays in the volume show, this emergent field harbors a multitude of approaches and methodologies. At times, this plurality manifests itself as contradictory opinions between different contributors. To clarify, the goal here is by no means to offer the last word; this is a field of inquiry still very much in the making. On the contrary, the collective aspiration is to open up the field to further inquiries. In doing so, we experiment with a conceptual totality, the Islamic Mediterranean, which lends itself well to the study of health (or lack thereof) in past societies. The healthscape of the Islamic Mediterranean is under close scrutiny here with respect to its relations to the environment and climate, as well as to human and nonhuman agents of history. As the essays in the volume make clear, studying health and disease within the framework of the Islamic Mediterranean promises invaluable insights.

What remains to be reconsidered is whether there is compatibility between the subject matter (disease histories—epidemic or not) and the conventional fields of academic inquiry (such as the Islamic Mediterranean—one that is as much informed by cultural studies as environmental ones). If they are compatible, then one can only hope for the enrichment of the field in the future by the participation of scholars from a variety of disciplines. If not, then this is a learning moment about the need to continue seeking new definitions of terrain on which scholarship can be built. Diseases, as much in the past as in the present, defy human boundaries and force us to think in novel ways.

Another question to consider is whether the study of certain diseases fits into such conceptual totalities better than others. Among the diseases covered in the volume, one seems to be historiographically privileged: plague. On different occasions, the reader will encounter the ways in which the study of past plagues benefits from a well-developed tradition of scholarship, however controversial that may be. As regards the other diseases addressed here, such as smallpox, epilepsy,

1 "Source Material," *Nature* 533, no. 7604 (May 25, 2016): 437–38.

and cholera, as well as cattle epizootics, no comparable historiographical privilege is in place. This reminds us that an undertaking such as this one might also hope to serve as a road map for future scholarship.

The sources used by the contributors to the volume are as diverse as the questions they pursue and methodologies they engage. The essays in the volume utilize an impressive range and variety of archival, manuscript, and published sources. The archival repositories consulted in the preparation of this volume include the Prime Ministry's Ottoman Archive in Istanbul, Turkey (Başbakanlık Osmanlı Arşivi), Topkapı Palace Museum Archive (Topkapı Sarayı Müzesi Arşivi), the Bulgarian Historical Archive (Bŭlgarski Istoricheski Arkhiv), the State Archives of the Russian Federation (Gosudarstvennyi Arkhiv Rossiiskoi Federatsii), the Russian State Military History Archive (Rossiiskii Gosudarstvennyi Voenno-Istoricheskii Arkhiv), the Russian State Historical Archive (Rossiiskii Gosudarstvennyi Istoricheskii Arkhiv), the State Archives of Venice (Archivio di Stato di Venezia), the National Archives of Egypt in Cairo (Dār al-Wathā'iq al-Qawmiyya), National Archives of France (Archives Nationale de France), the Archive of the Chamber of Commerce and Industry in Marseille, France (Archives de la Chambre de Commerce et d'Industrie), the National Archives of the United Kingdom, and the archives of the American Philosophical Society, in Philadelphia, as well as a rich corpus of unpublished works preserved in the manuscript collections across the world.

The sources used by the contributors to this volume are also diverse linguistically. The authors use published and unpublished sources in several languages, including Ottoman Turkish, Arabic, French, Italian, Bulgarian, Russian, and others. The transliterations followed here for terminology, book titles, place names, and names of individuals loosely follow the conventions of the field, while preserving the preferences of each author. Place names and personal names in Ottoman Turkish have been simplified following modern Turkish spelling. Names and book titles in Arabic follow a simplified version of the *International Journal of Middle East Studies* transliteration conventions. Terms pertaining to the Islamicate culture that are already established in English are used in Anglicized form. Dates in the main text are given in the Common Era. In the notes, documents from Ottoman archives are cited in their original Hijri date, followed by the Gregorian calendar. Hijri months have been used in the following form: Muharrem, Safer, Rebiülevvel, Rebiülahir, Cemaziyelevvel, Cemaziyelahir, Receb, Şa'ban, Ramazan, Şevval, Zilkade, and Zilhicce.

* * *

The chapters in this volume largely fall in three different clusters, constituting the three parts of the volume. Even though there are occasional conceptual, regional, and chronological overlaps between individual essays, they have been arranged according to their primary area of emphasis and they loosely follow a basic chronological order. The first part of the volume, "Rethinking Historiography and Sources," is devoted to essays that address historiographical issues, introduce new sources, and revisit some older questions in the light of newer trends in the field. There are three essays in the first part. The first essay by Miri Shefer-Mossensohn captures the overall state-of-the-field of the scholarship on plague and epidemics in Ottoman and Islamic history. Shefer-Mossensohn charts the terrain in the historiography, by identifying major studies, trends, and methodologies, and offers a thorough reading of them in their proper historical context. The essay maps out the works, their authors, and the intellectual climate in which they produced, while discussing the production and consumption of knowledge about the history of epidemics in the pre-modern Islamic Mediterranean. It encapsulates the important turning points in the historiography, such as the "social turn" or the rise of new methodological approaches to the study of plague in the Islamic Mediterranean since the 2000s. In addition, it lays out the inner biases of the field (e.g., preferred or avoided subjects, linguistic limitations, and choice of sources) and how these formed the fault lines of the field. Shefer-Mossensohn presents an optimistic portrayal of the field, with a growing number of scholars, who expand their areas of interest (both spatially and temporally) and their access to more interdisciplinary toolkits (underlining the importance of bioarcheology, genetics, climate science, and so on). Overall, the essay would serve well as an introduction to the historiography for the uninitiated, as much as an essential reference work for the specialist.

John Curry's contribution to the volume reminds us that treasure troves about plague history occasionally appear in the least expected sources. In its analysis of Ottoman hagiographical texts as well as religious and legal works, the essay demonstrates how different types of sources can be tactfully used to approach Ottoman responses to plagues and epidemics. First, the essay traces the life and afterlife of a seventeenth-century legal treatise on plague, composed by a Hanbali jurist in Cairo, its acquisition by a Hanafi jurist in Istanbul and later by the Ottoman Chief Jurisprudent, offering additional evidence of copies owned by other Ottoman notables and possibly members of the dynastic family. Juxtaposing the different layers of production, circulation, and consumption of the treatise, the essay stitches together various interpretations of plague across time and space, as we catch glimpses of the diversity of beliefs entertained by the religious elite of the empire. The essay then moves on to introducing examples from another rich corpus to study the history of plague and epidemic diseases: the hagiographical accounts and personal writings of Ottoman sufi authors. Here, we hear the myriad stories of Ottoman mystics ranging from protecting their communities and offering treatment to plague victims to afflicting their enemies with plague.

Overall, this effort for exploring unusual sources to study the history of plague goes beyond the purpose of data mining. In so doing, Curry's work calls forth an important methodological endeavor: using different genres of sources in conjunction with each other can indeed offer novel insights.

Nükhet Varlık's essay calls for a reckoning with the legacy of plague in the early modern Mediterranean history and historiography. Situated at the intersection of historical epidemiology, history of public health, environmental history, and orientalism, the essay takes issue with the so-called "Oriental plague," a term used in post-Enlightenment Europe in reference to epidemics in the Ottoman Empire. Starting in the eighteenth century, as plague started to fade in the European memory, the Orient (read: the Ottoman Empire) came to be associated with the plague, owing to the continued presence of the disease there. The essay starts with nineteenth-century European imagination of the Ottoman Empire as a sickly, disease-ridden healthscape. This imagination both reflected and reinforced narratives of epidemiological boundaries—a historical artifact shaped by nineteenth-century European anxieties of public health, epidemiology, and internationalism. This fiction of boundaries not only informed European policy of border control but also the writing of history. Then the essay tackles the legacy of this vision in history writing that has prevailed into modern historiography. Next, it offers a close reading of the construction of "epidemiological orientalism" in the writings of the Europeans. Drawing from the notion "environmental imaginaries" used by environmental historians, it traces how the Orient came to be seen as the site of disease and made into Europe's epidemiological "Other."

After this first part devoted to discussions of historiography, sources, and methodologies, the next part of the volume delves into diseases and their environmental, social, political, and cultural contexts in the Islamic Mediterranean. There are four essays in this part that explore different diseases in early modern Ottoman history. Even though they have different emphases, each of these essays situates disease (cattle plague, smallpox, and epilepsy) at the center of inquiry and explores connections with its larger historical context. At the same time, they each set an example about how to pursue disease histories, as much in their selection of sources as in their attempts to explore novel connections and innovative methodologies.

Much like humans, non-human agents are also part of disease environments. A large majority of infectious diseases that affected humans since at least the Neolithic era have their origins in animals. The zoonotic transmission (from animal-to-human) indeed applies to many of the diseases discussed in this volume: plague, smallpox, and cholera are all zoonoses. Given that animals, much like humans, are subjected to many ecological pressures and larger historical changes, it becomes all the more important to understand the effects of zoonoses on human societies. Nonetheless, studying animal diseases is also important when animal diseases do not pose a direct health hazard for humans. Epizootics—diseases that spread among animal populations—that result in high levels of mortality could affect humans in several ways. Especially when these infections affected livestock, this set a serious crisis for human societies.

Two essays here deal with the question of epizootics of livestock, in particular, cattle. Sam White's essay focuses on the sheep and cattle plagues of the early modern era. Using Ottoman narrative and documentary evidence in conjunction with European sources, the chapter sheds light on the early modern panzootic of rinderpest—a viral infectious disease that affected cattle and sheep—that spread to a very large area across Eurasia. At first, White situates the environmental, climatic, and social circumstances that led to the break out of this pestilence among the livestock of Anatolia and the Balkans in the late sixteenth century. Reconstructing this particular ecological configuration is not only critical to understand the Ottoman case. It also serves as a model, as White demonstrates, for studying the rise of the eighteenth-century European panzootic. Contrary to what is sometimes assumed, the essay demonstrates that the pestilence did not arrive to Europe from the Ottoman lands. Instead, White identifies the conditions that contributed to its break out: the transport of livestock over longer distances, colder winters, and wars—very similar to the circumstances that caused the late sixteenth-century Ottoman panzootic. In this manner, the essay brings together scattered pieces of evidence to study a massive panzootic in a connected narrative. Furthermore, White considers the rise of veterinary medicine and theories of epizootics in eighteenth-century Europe, corresponding to the later stages of the panzootic. Finally, White's essay offers an important lesson learned from history: that livestock plagues are potential dangers in today's world as well, because of the intensification of animal production, climate change, and globalization.

Alan Mikhail's essay focuses on veterinary medicine in nineteenth-century Egypt. Offering a close-up analysis of how humans and animals interacted in the nineteenth-century Egyptian setting, Mikhail highlights two critical changes: the establishment of the Egyptian School of Veterinary Medicine in 1827 and the emergent global context of epizootics. Coinciding with wide-ranging transformations in the scientific study of animals and the Egyptian government's economic and military want for maintaining a healthy supply of animals, the school placed heavy emphasis on the question of epizootics and how to prevent them. New scientifically-driven procedures were implemented to regulate the bodies, working conditions, productivity of the animals, as well as how humans ought to engage with them. Mikhail traces the story of how this ambitious attempt that aimed to replace Egyptian peasants' deep-seated local knowledge by a biopolitical program failed quickly, with the closing down of the veterinary school twenty-two years later. Epizootics continued after that, perhaps even intensified in the second half of the nineteenth century, despite the myriad efforts to keep them under control. No longer products of their local Egyptian environmental contexts, these severe epizootics were intimately entangled with the global exchanges of the nineteenth century. Methods aimed at controlling animal diseases brought more changes, such as quarantines that further separated humans and animals, as Mikhail maintains, setting a complete break with the deep history of interspecies relationships in Egypt.

Günhan Börekçi's essay focuses on an outbreak of smallpox in early seventeenth-century Istanbul and its impact on the fate of the Ottoman imperial family. By situating the smallpox epidemic at the intersection of body politics, imperial power struggles, and succession crises at the Ottoman court, the essay captures a critical moment in the history of the dynastic family and unpacks the uncertainties about its perpetuation—perhaps even the fate of the empire. It is well known in the Ottoman historiography that during the first half of the seventeenth century, a series of underage and/or childless sultans ascended the Ottoman throne. This was a time that also witnessed relentless military rebellions in the capital, ongoing wars, and epidemics of plague and smallpox. Using evidence from Ottoman and Venetian sources, Börekçi's essay offers a corrective to this historiography. The essay focuses on a critical moment in this tumultuous state of affairs when both the newly enthroned young sultan Ahmed I (r. 1603–17), and his younger brother Prince Mustafa (the future Mustafa I, r. 1617–18; 1622–23) contracted smallpox and nearly died in March 1604. Hence it demonstrates that the first time the Ottoman dynasty faced the threat of genealogical extinction can be dated to the early years of the seventeenth century, and not to the early 1640s, as is commonly accepted. Offering a close reading of court factions and inner conflicts of the Ottoman imperial rule, as well as political and economic problems the empire faced at this time, Börekçi's essay underscores the anxiety epidemic diseases caused for all, but above all for the ruling family.

Özgen Felek's essay approaches the question of epidemic diseases and contagion from the unusual point of view offered by epilepsy. Situating epilepsy—an illness that is clearly not understood in modern medicine as contagious—at the center of historical inquiry, Felek questions the Islamic episteme of medical and religious healing about such diseases that were deemed incurable, hence often understood in spiritual and supernatural terms. The essay emphasizes the complex etiology of epilepsy and how this shaped different methods of prevention and treatment. Given the epistemic complexity of the illness, Felek rightfully turns to an assortment of sources. In addition to medical works, historical chronicles, and travelers' accounts, the essay utilizes Ottoman hagiographical narratives that include rich details about epileptic individuals and efforts to treat them. In doing so, Felek, like John Curry, reminds us how Ottoman hagiographies can be exploited for studying the history of diseases and healing. First, the essay surveys a selection of Ottoman medical texts to illustrate examples about the taxonomy, etiology, prophylaxis, and therapeutics of epilepsy. Next, it turns to the corpus of Islamic and prophetic medicine collections that informed Ottoman understanding of epilepsy and its treatment. The essay then turns to social perceptions of epilepsy and epileptic individuals and discusses the social stigma associated with it. In the end, it includes a brief discussion of the case of Sultan Murad III (r. 1574–95).

The third part of the volume focuses on responses to epidemic diseases in Ottoman society. Here the goal is to offer glimpses about the diversity of social, religious, and administrative responses in Ottoman society, rather than to establish formulaic patterns of conduct and generalities. The four essays here span a wide spatial extent: they take us from the Black Sea and the Balkans to Syria and Egypt, and to the Red Sea and beyond. In terms of temporal scope, they address the eighteenth and nineteenth centuries. Mostly on epidemics of plague and cholera, essays in the third part of the volume offer insights about individual and communal experiences of disease and the social ties that kept members of the Ottoman society together, or led them to flee, or, alas, held their remains together for eternity. Also in this section, we hear about the more organized and institutionalized forms of response, specifically in the form of Ottoman quarantines.

Yaron Ayalon's essay revisits the question of religion's role in responses to epidemics and other catastrophic events in Ottoman society. Drawing from Ottoman narrative and archival sources and European visitors' writings on the one hand, and from modern disaster studies and psychology, on the other, Ayalon examines common behaviors at times of plagues and motivations behind them. At first, the essay underscores the growing importance of interdisciplinary disaster studies in the last decade or so, and discusses how they can offer novel insights for historians in the study of past societies. The essay suggests that this approach is applicable to studying responses to plague epidemics in pre-modern Ottoman society. Then, it revisits the historiography that stressed the role of religion in Ottoman society in shaping responses to plague. Contrary to the conventional historiography, Ayalon suggests that religious belief was not the main factor that determined people's responses to plague. To illustrate the point, Ayalon reconsiders the question of flight at times of plague. Reviewing the evidence, the essay argues that flight was limited to small sections of the early modern Ottoman urban population; the vast majority simply did not leave. Further, the essay surveys the reasons for this behavior, drawing from historical sources and studies in psychology. In particular, Ayalon draws from "attachment theory" to explain why people chose to stay and care for their loved ones, instead of fleeing disease areas. The implications of this conclusion go beyond responses to plagues: religious boundaries in pre-modern Ottoman society were much more fluid than once assumed and religious identity, though important, was not everything.

Edna Bonhomme's essay questions the relationship between plague, death, and memory through a close reading of the 1791 plague epidemic in Egypt that caused massive numbers of deaths. Chroniclers of the time recorded the death of the elite carefully, while they noted—only in passing—that thousands of Cairo's urban poor were buried in mass graves. Bonhomme's essay seeks to commemorate the nameless plague victims, whose deaths were rendered invisible owing to an absence of spatial or physical markers of their graves. The essay takes issue with the erasure of the memory of plague deaths and explores the burial of thousands in large pits dug in Giza near a mosque. Following a brief reference in the work of the famous eighteenth-century Egyptian chronicler al-Jabartī, Bonhomme traces the location of the burial site, its meaning, and seeks to restore it to historical memory. The essay reminds us of the differentials of death in eighteenth-century Cairo, the inequalities that followed individuals to their graves, and how the materiality of graves (or its absence thereof) shapes historical memory: the elite victims of the plague with individualized tombs and tombstones found their way to historical memory, whereas the unnamed plague victims were erased from it. It was not the indiscriminate mortality caused by plague but the differentials of burials that shaped historical memory of plague and its victims.

Andrew Robarts's essay explores responses to epidemic diseases in the Ottoman Balkans in the late eighteenth and early nineteenth centuries, drawing from Ottoman, Bulgarian, and Russian archival sources, as well as from travelers' accounts. First, it surveys epidemics in the Ottoman Balkans in the eighteenth and early nineteenth centuries. Here the focus is on population movements that were generated as a response to epidemics. Second, it takes a closer look at beliefs and rituals used for protection from disease and death, commonly held among local populations. Full of rich details about popular beliefs and practices, this section is a treasure trove for the student of disease in the Ottoman Balkans. Third, it examines the Ottoman measures of quarantine, especially with respect to their use in border control and surveillance. The case study of the quarantine station in İzmir (Smyrna) is particularly helpful in developing a sense of the day-to-day functioning of such an institution. In particular, the essay challenges the common assumptions in the historiography that the Ottoman quarantine was primarily a response to control epidemic diseases. Instead, Robarts emphasizes the multifaceted functions of these quarantine stations in the nineteenth century and shows how they functioned as border control units that oversaw population movements, trade, customs, and intelligence-gathering, among other crucial functions. The essay demonstrates that the Ottoman state expanded quarantine measures in the 1830 and 1840s, not so much as a response to the threat of epidemics but rather to increase its control over the populations in the Balkans.

Like Robarts, the essay by Gülden Sarıyıldız and Oya Dağlar Macar deals with the question of quarantine. This essay focuses on an Ottoman quarantine station in the Red Sea in the context of trade, pilgrimage, and international politics of sanitation in the late nineteenth century. It explores the establishment, organization, and function of the Ottoman quarantine station at Kamaran island. Despite being the focus of international sanitary and political controversies in the late nineteenth and early twentieth centuries, Kamaran quarantine has curiously been neglected in the historiography. This essay is a close investigation of the quarantine on the basis of Ottoman and British archival sources. First, it reconstructs the historical significance of this quarantine station. Second, it traces the establishment, renovation, and structure of the quarantine complex, as well as the procedures that were followed, while carefully pointing out the different voices at each stage. Here, we learn about the operation of the quarantine more closely, about the problems encountered, and about the actors that made decisions on the ground. Then, the essay turns to criticisms of the Kamaran quarantine and offers a critical reading of those criticisms in historical context. Next, the essay reviews Kamaran as a site of conflicting international interests. Here, we read about the commercial and political interests of European states and how those conflicted with each other as well as with those of the Ottoman Empire. At the intersection of international politics, sanitation, pilgrimage, and disease, this essay reminds us about the complexity and messiness of historical inquiry through the untold story of the Kamaran quarantine.

* * *

I would like to express gratitude to several individuals and institutions that supported and helped improve this work. My greatest debt of gratitude is to my fellow contributors to the volume for their dedication and patience. Each has not only contributed to this joint effort but also to the field of Ottoman history of disease at large. I have benefitted from their work immensely as I collaborated with them at various conferences and other academic projects. At an early phase of conception of the project, I have benefitted from the guidance of Ann Carmichael, of Indiana University, who has not only offered generous encouragement but also the necessary vision about how it should be pitched to reach out to the non-Ottomanist audience. I would like to thank Justin Stearns, who was initially part of this project. Even though circumstances have not allowed us to include his contribution to the volume, he has remained an invaluable resource and kindly read and offered helpful suggestions to one of the essays here. In the later stages of writing and editing, Lori Jones, of the University of Ottowa has been extremely helpful. With her knowledge of early modern English plague literature, she offered help in many ways and saved me from many embarrassing mistakes. My special thanks go to Marta Hanson for her insightful comments on my own essay in this volume. I would also like to acknowledge Benjamin Hutchens for his helpful suggestions about the structure and organization of the volume. In addition, I would like to express my deepest gratitude to Ann Carmichael (again!), Monica Green, Lester Little, Uli Schamiloglu, George Sussman, and Michelle Ziegler, as well as the other members of the plague working group for their generous help in sharing with me their knowledge of the plague and epidemics. Stretched over many years, this project has benefited from the institutional support offered by Rutgers University-Newark. As always, I remain grateful to my institution and colleagues for their constant support and encouragement. In addition, I would like to acknowledge the assistance of Rutgers University Libraries personnel, in particular John Cotton Dana Library Interlibrary Loan staff for their hard work. Finally, I would like to thank Emily Yates, Senior Commissioning Editor and Michael Bourne, Editorial Administrator for Humanities at Ashgate, as well as Andrew Cunningham of the University of Cambridge and Ole Peter Grell of the Open University, editors of the "The History of Medicine in Context" series for their work in the earlier stages of this project. My sincere thanks go to Erin Thomas Dailey, Acquisitions Editor, Erika Gaffney, Senior Acquisitions Editor, and the anonymous reviewers for the Black Sea World series, as well as the production team at Arc Humanities Press.

Nükhet Varlık

PART ONE

RETHINKING HISTORIOGRAPHY AND SOURCES

A HISTORIOGRAPHY OF EPIDEMICS IN THE ISLAMIC MEDITERRANEAN

MIRI SHEFER-MOSSENSOHN*
Tel Aviv University

THIS ARTICLE IS a survey of the historiography of epidemics in the Islamic world written mainly in English and French, with some Turkish and German. My aim is to identify the main historiographical trends in studies concerning pre-modern epidemics (especially plague) in the Islamic world. The gist of my argument is as follows: earlier scholars of Islamic plague history obeyed the rules of the field of Islamic history / Islamic studies within which they operated. Current scholars, however, see themselves as operating within several fields of study rather than being restricted to Middle Eastern studies. Therefore, they are a part of the community of plague historians, of environmental historians, or historians of colonialism, to name but few possibilities. I intend to follow this shift and discuss the way in which the historiography of epidemics in the Middle East changed and its methodologies reformulated.

The chapter is organized as a discussion of themes, styles, norms and prejudices common in academic writing on epidemics in the pre-modern Middle East. I will point out to the common ground and discrepancies that molded individual studies into a corpus with a discourse. The article shows the similarities of questions and methodologies between Islamic plague historians and their colleagues specializing in other regions, yet highlighting the specific concerns, interests, aims, as well as problems that characterize this field. The chapter displays that although Islamic plague history evolved quite later than other themes in Islamic historiography – only in the last quarter of the twentieth century, the current generation of plague historians matured to form an independent academic discourse.

Long Delay in the Coming of Islamic Plague History

Islamic or Middle Eastern history is a well-established field. Since its modern inception around the turn of the twentieth century, Middle Eastern history diversified and covered numerous branches of enquiries, ranging from language to law, from architecture to politics. Plague was not one of them.

* I wish to thank the editor, Nükhet Varlık for long and insightful discussions of our field, and my research assistant, Ms. Sapir Sadon.

In European historiography, interest in the history of epidemics is evident in the nineteenth century.[1] The cholera pandemic of the 1830s seems to have been what inspired European historians to write about the history of plague. The 1890s, however, was the ultimate turning point because of the break out of the Third Plague Pandemic and cholera. The explosion of publications started from then onwards. In 1894, *The English Historical Review* (published by Oxford University Press) featured a book review by Augustus Jessopp on two books dealing with epidemics in the medieval period. Jessopp, who authored an essay on the plague himself,[2] opened his review with the statement that "[t]he story of the great pestilence in the fourteenth century has during the last twenty years incited the researches of students at home and abroad with a strong fascination."[3]

The interest among the historians of Europe in plague history continued throughout the twentieth century, diversified and intensified in terms of geography and range of studies. The *Annales* School, for instance, weighed the factors of medicine and disease in historical patterns, and its impact was felt well outside France from the 1930s onwards. William McNeill's 1976 *tour de force* of the historical roles of infectious diseases in *Plagues and Peoples* and its immediate success is another benchmark for the evolution of the field.[4] Indeed, McNeill regarded *Plagues and Peoples* as his principal contribution to historical learning.[5] Other major texts were authored by Alfred Crosby,[6] Emmanuel Le Roy Ladurie,[7] and more recently Jared Diamond[8]

1 See, for instance, J. F. C. Hecker, *Der schwarze Tod im vierzehnten Jahrhundert* (Berlin, 1832), and its translation into English, J. F. C. Hecker, *The Epidemics of the Middle Ages*, trans. B. G. Babington (London: Trübner, 1859).

2 Augustus Jessopp, "The Black Death in East Anglia," in *The Coming of the Friars and Other Historic Essays* (London: T. Fisher Unwin, 1906), 166–261.

3 Jessopp, "*A History of Epidemics in Britain, from A. D. 664 to the Extinction of the Plague* by Charles Creighton and *The Great Pestilence (1348–9), Now Commonly Known as the Black Death* by Francis Aidan Gasquet," *The English Historical Review* 9, no. 35 (1894): 567.

4 William H. McNeill, *Plagues and Peoples* (Garden City, NY: Anchor Press, 1976).

5 McNeill, *The Pursuit of Truth: A Historian's Memoir* (Lexington: University Press of Kentucky, 2005): 101–3.

6 Alfred W. Crosby, *The Columbian Exchange: Biological and Cultural Consequences of 1492* (Westport, CT: Greenwood Publishing Group, 1972); idem, *Ecological Imperialism: The Biological Expansion of Europe, 900–1900* (Cambridge: Cambridge University Press, 1986).

7 Emmanuel Le Roy Ladurie, *Histoire du climat depuis l'an mil* (Paris, 1967); idem, "Un concept: l'unification microbienne du monde (XIVe–XVIIe siècles)," *Revue suisse d'histoire* 23 (1973): 627–96.

8 Jared M. Diamond, *Guns, Germs, and Steel: The Fates of Human Societies* (London: W. W. Nor-

whose work indicates that the history of epidemics also caught the interest of scholars outside historical studies.

For historians of the pre-modern Islamic world, plagues and epidemics were not subject of academic interest until the late 1960s. There were occasional short papers on plague or a presentation in a conference even earlier,[9] with few articles,[10] but not more, let alone analytic monographs,[11] were dedicated to plague before 1970s. Particularly puzzling is the fact that plague history did not find an audience, despite the importance of history of medicine, a vibrant field with a respected history of its own in the discipline of Middle Eastern history. Already in the 1920s and 1930s, eminent scholars such as Max Meyerhof and Joseph Schacht wrote extensively about Islamic medicine. They studied medical theories and famous physicians, and edited manuscripts, but for reasons unknown to us, epidemics never generated interest.[12]

The next generation of scholars in Islamic studies, among which the towering figure of Franz Rosenthal, also studied medicine. Scholars of this generation added new aspects of medicine, but similar to their predecessors they did not treat epidemics as a topic of interest. For instance, Rosenthal dedicated many years to the

---

ton, 1998); idem, *Collapse: How Societies Choose to Fail or Succeed* (New York: Viking, 2005).

9 Ahmet Süheyl Ünver, "Sur l'histoire de la peste en Turquie," in *Neuvième Congrès international d'histoire de la médecine, București (România) 10-18 septembre 1932; comptes-rendus*, ed. Victor Gomoiu and Victoria Gomoiu (Bucharest, 1932), 479–83; idem, "About the History of the Leproseries in Turkey," in *Festschrift zum 80. Geburtstag Max Neuburgers*, ed. Emanuel Berghoff (Vienna: Maudrich, 1948), 447–50.

10 David Neustadt (Ayalon), "The Plague and Its Effects Upon the Mamluk Army," *Journal of the Royal Asiatic Society*, 66 (1946): 67–73; Gaston Wiet, "La grande peste noire en Syrie et en Égypt," in *Études d'Orientalisme dédiées à la mémoire de Lévi-Provençal* (Paris: Maisonneuve et Larose, 1962), 1 : 367–84.

11 Some descriptions of epidemics and quarantines include Bedi N. Şehsuvaroğlu, *Tarihi Kolera Salgınları ve Osmanlı Türkleri* (Istanbul: İsmail Akgün Matbaası, 1954); Ahmet Süheyl Ünver and Bedi N. Şehsuvaroğlu, *Türkiye'de Cüzam Tarihi Üzerine Araştırma* (Istanbul: İsmail Akgün Matbaası, 1961).

12 Some of their publications are: Max Meyerhof, *Studies in Medieval Arabic Medicine* (London: Variorum, 1984); Meyerhof, ed., *The Book of the Ten Treatises on the Eye Ascribed to Hunain ibn Ishaq (809–877 A.D.)* (Cairo: Government Press, 1928); Meyerhof, ed., *Sharḥ asmāʾ al-ʿuqqār (L'explication des noms de drogues): un glossaire de matière médicale* (Cairo: Imprimerie de l'Institut français, 1940); Joseph Schacht and Max Meyerhof, *The Medico-Philosophical Controversy between Ibn Butlan of Baghdad and Ibn Ridwan of Cairo: A Contribution to the History of Greek Learning among the Arabs* (Cairo: University of Chicago Press, 1937). Meyerhof and Schacht continued to publish books and papers concerning medical issues in later decades of the twentieth century, separately and together.

study of the concept of knowledge in medieval Arabic Muslim society and the classical heritage in Islam. His occupation with knowledge was wide ranged to include also non-philosophical bodies of knowledge as well as social, non-intellectual practices: he wrote about gambling and humor; in the context of the present article, his works on hashish and other narcotics, dentistry, and the medical profession are at the forefront of our interest. Rosenthal published his medical-related studies in professional journals for historians of medicine, for instance the *Bulletin of the History of Medicine*, one of the leading academic journals in history of medicine worldwide throughout the twentieth century. Thus, he opened the way for comparative work by engaging with historians of medicine and made possible a theoretical shift, which scholars fifty years later would fully embrace.[13]

Only with Michael W. Dols did plague history become the target of attention by an Arabist, shifting the context from medical history to social history. In 1967 Dols entered Princeton University's Near Eastern Studies doctoral program and met his future advisor, A. L. Udovitch who pursued social and economic history of medieval Islam. Under Udovitch's supervision, Dols picked the Black Death as his topic for a dissertation. He submitted it in 1971 and in 1977 this pioneering work was published as a book with Princeton University Press.[14] He then proceeded to study hospitals, leprosy, and lunacy in the Arabic medieval East.[15] In all cases, his works were the first systematic treatments of the subject. To compile his study, he needed to chase manuscripts and scattered evidence, thirty years later, his studies are still benchmarks in the scholarship.

A decade later, another dissertation was written in Princeton regarding the plague: again under Udovitch, Lawrence I. Conrad, dealt with the plague pandemic of late antiquity (known as the First Plague Pandemic or the Justinianic Plague, 541– ca. 750) in the Near East based on Arabic, Greek, and Syriac

13 Franz Rosenthal, "Isḥāq b. Ḥunayn's *Tāʾrīḫ al-aṭibbāʾ*," *Oriens* 7 (1954): 55–80; idem, "An Ancient Commentary on the Hippocratic Oath," *Bulletin of the History of Medicine* 30 (1956): 52–87; idem, "Bibliographical Notes on Medieval Muslim Dentistry," *Bulletin of the History of Medicine* 34 (1960): 52–60; idem, "'Life is short, the art is long': Arabic Commentaries on the First Hippocratic Aphorism," *Bulletin of the History of Medicine* 40 (1966): 226–45; idem, "The Defense of Medicine in the Medieval Muslim World," *Bulletin of the History of Medicine* 43 (1969): 519–32; idem, "ar-Rāzī on the Hidden Illness," *Bulletin of the History of Medicine* 52 (1978): 45–60; idem, "The Physician in Medieval Muslim Society," *Bulletin of the History of Medicine* 52 (1978): 475–91.

14 Michael W. Dols, *The Black Death in the Middle East* (Princeton, NJ: Princeton University Press, 1977).

15 Gary Leiser, "In Memoriam: Michael W. Dols," *Middle East Studies Association Bulletin* 24 (1990): 152–53.

sources.[16] Though it remained unpublished, the dissertation and the later works of Conrad—together with other recent scholarship—addressed early Islamic history in the context of the Justinianic Plague, and made a great contribution to the study of plague in the early medieval Near East.[17]

The First Phase: The Social Turn Combined with Partiality toward Arabic Texts

The late discovery of plague history by historians of Islam and its ascent in the context of social history set it apart from other, older fields within the scholarship on Islamic history with regard to methodology. The older, more traditional approach evolved from close ties to language and linguistics. The centrality of the philological skills led to partiality toward textual analysis over other research agendas, and favoring texts necessitated in turn philological excellence.[18]

The first generation of Islamic plague history, however, evolved in another intellectual climate, namely the Social Turn. Correspondingly, articles on plague appeared in journals, which advocated society and people. A good example is the *Journal of the Economic and Social History of the Orient* (*JESHO*). Since its establishment in 1957, the journal follows its mission of integrating cultural and intellectual history with economic, social, and political analysis. In 1979, *JESHO* published the first article on plague, which established the chronology of the plague recurrences in the Middle East from the middle of the fourteenth century until the end of the nineteenth century and described the character of the collective response to it; it was only appropriate that the author was none other than Dols.[19] Other publications on epidemics soon followed: William F. Tucker delineated the economic, psychological, and religious effects of natural disasters on the peasantry in

16 Lawrence I. Conrad, "The Plague in the Early Medieval Near East," PhD diss., Princeton University, 1981.

17 Michael G. Morony, "'For Whom Does the Writer Write?': The First Bubonic Plague Pandemic According to Syriac Sources," in *Plague and the End of Antiquity: The Pandemic of 541–750*, ed. Lester K. Little (Cambridge: Cambridge University Press, 2007), 59–86; Hugh N. Kennedy, "Justinianic Plague in Syria and the Archaeological Evidence," in *Plague and the End of Antiquity*, 87–95.

18 Zachary Lockman, *Contending Visions of the Middle East: The History and Politics of Orientalism* (Cambridge: Cambridge University Press, 2004); Suzanne L. Marchand, *German Orientalism in the Age of Empire: Religion, Race, and Scholarship* (Cambridge: Cambridge University Press, 2009); Ursula Wockoeck, *German Orientalism: The Study of the Middle East and Islam from 1800–1945* (London: Routledge, 2009).

19 Dols, "The Second Plague Pandemic and Its Recurrences in the Middle East: 1347–1894," *Journal of the Economic and Social History of the Orient* 22 (1979): 162–89.

Mamluk Egypt,[20] and Conrad explained the concepts associated with epidemics in the seventh and eighth centuries.[21]

Over the following decades, plague was picked up in *JESHO* articles in which epidemics were treated as an obvious aspect of various social and economic phenomena, be it population estimates of medieval Islamic lands,[22] childhood in the medieval Islamic world,[23] pious foundations in early modern Ottoman Trabzon on the shore of the Black Sea,[24] eighteenth-century Alexandria as an Ottoman commercial hub yet a backwater town,[25] early Islamic economy and its relation to Antiquity,[26] and economic performance and growth in the early Islamic world.[27]

Despite the gestation of Islamic plague history under the umbrella of the social turn, the field also exposes the traditional preference toward texts and philological questions. Dols himself integrated issues of terminology into his social and medical study of plague (and later of madness). His *The Black Death in the Middle East* surveys medieval observations and interpretations of the plague, demographic effects, urban communal behavior, and economic consequences. The appendices, notwithstanding, include a discussion of the Arabic terminology of plague, a list of plague occurrences in texts from the middle of the fourteenth century to the early sixteenth century (late Mamluk period), and a synopsis of the Arabic manuscript sources for late medieval Islamic plague history.

In the context of the first systematic book-length study of plague in the Islamic world, the discussion of the terminology and the primary sources was a service of paramount importance for the scholarly community. At the same time, this type of

---

20 William F. Tucker, "Natural Disasters and the Peasantry in Mamlûk Egypt," *Journal of the Economic and Social History of the Orient* 24 (1981): 215–22.

21 Conrad, "*Ṭāʿūn* and *Wabāʾ*: Conceptions of Plague and Pestilence in Early Islam," *Journal of the Economic and Social History of the Orient* 25 (1982): 268–307.

22 David Ayalon, "Regarding Population Estimates in the Countries of Medieval Islam," *Journal of the Economic and Social History of the Orient* 28 (1985): 1–19.

23 Avner Giladi, "Concepts of Childhood and Attitudes towards Children in Medieval Islam," *Journal of the Economic and Social History of the Orient* 32 (1989): 121–52.

24 Ronald C. Jennings, "Pious Foundations in the Society and Economy of Ottoman Trabzon, 1565–1640," *Journal of the Economic and Social History of the Orient* 33 (1990): 271–336.

25 Michael J. Reimer, "Ottoman Alexandria: The Paradox of Decline and the Reconfiguration of Power in Eighteenth-Century Arab Provinces," *Journal of the Economic and Social History of the Orient* 37 (1994): 107–46.

26 Michael G. Morony, "Economic Boundaries? Late Antiquity and Early Islam," *Journal of the Economic and Social History of the Orient* 47 (2004): 166–94.

27 Maya Shatzmiller, "Economic Performance and Economic Growth in the Early Islamic World," *Journal of the Economic and Social History of the Orient* 54 (2011): 132–84.

research on Dols's part showed that while being a social historian of medicine, he was not divorced from the professional skills that were the traditional entrance ticket to the field: Arabic language and textual analysis.

The importance of linguistic competence as an aim in itself, much more than a mandatory basic research tool, continued as a preference of the scholar when showing one's Arabic was no longer a prerequisite to justify the field or legitimate a new scholar. Conrad is such an example. His writings about early medieval Islamic plague and its social and cultural consequences were in addition to other, medical and non-medical history topics.[28] His scholarship on medical history reveals a tight link between superb lingual skill, literary studies, and social context of medicine. In one article, for instance, he discussed the literary genre of early Islamic plague treatises.[29] In a later article, he relied on Arabic poetry to reconstruct the fragmented knowledge about late sixth-century epidemic in Syria.[30] In a third article, however, Conrad was sensitive to the ways in which epidemics were interpreted in early Islamic sources and thus threw light on the ideologies and mentalities of the Arab-Muslim community up to the middle of the ninth century.[31] Likewise, in a fourth article Conrad analyzed an especially volatile quarrel between two eleventh-century physicians in Egypt as a competition over professional and social recognition and not just a scientific learned dispute. His article was a revisit to a topic already studied by Meyerhof and Schacht. According to Conrad, the strict philological approach of these scholars prevented them from understanding the social background to a debate over medical authority.[32] In yet a fifth article, he identified the social milieu in which ninth-century Ibn Qutayba, an Arab bureaucrat and scholar, moved—a circle that included humoral medical thinking alongside theological debates about the omnipotent Muslim God.[33]

28 See, for instance, Albrecht Noth and Lawrence I. Conrad, *The Early Arabic Historical Tradition: A Source-Critical Study* (Princeton, NJ: American Oriental Society, 1994).

29 Conrad, "Arabic Plague Chronologies and Treatises: Social and Historical Factors in the Formation of a Literary Genre," *Studia Islamica* 54 (1981): 51–93.

30 Conrad, "Epidemic Disease in Central Syria in the Late Sixth Century: Some New Insights from the Verse of Ḥassān ibn Thābit," *Byzantine and Modern Greek Studies* 18 (1994): 12–58.

31 Conrad, "Epidemic Disease in Formal and Popular Thought in Early Islamic Society," in *Epidemics and Ideas: Essays on the Historical Perception of Pestilence*, ed. Terence Ranger and Paul Slack (Cambridge: Cambridge University Press, 1992), 77–99.

32 Conrad, "Scholarship and Social Context in the Near East," in *Knowledge and the Scholarly Medical Traditions*, ed. Don Bates (Cambridge: Cambridge University Press, 1995), 81–101.

33 Conrad, "A Ninth-Century Muslim Scholar's Discussion of Contagion," in *Contagion: Perspectives from Pre-modern Societies*, ed. Lawrence I. Conrad and Dominik Wujastyk (Aldershot: Ashgate, 2000), 163–77.

This thread of history of medicine and history of plague as philological enquiry lingers. For example, Josef van Ess analyzed early Arabic texts about the seventh-century plague in Syria that affected the Arab army. He explained that the real heroes of the texts are not the plague or its victims, but rather the theological reflections about the meaning of the plague and God's intent (some were idealistic while others were more pragmatic and realistic).[34] This was van Ess's contribution to the 1999 Giorgio Levi Della Vida conference, convened in his honor (together with André Raymond) upon their receiving the Giorgio Levi Della Vida award. In the opening remarks he called to bring philology back into the mainstream of Islamic studies.

Josef van Ess is a scholar of Islamic theology rather than a historian of Islamic medicine. His education and career is the product of the German academic system from the 1950s onwards, where Islamic studies evolved from Semitic linguistics and put much emphasis on linguistic skills and textual analysis. He taught in UCLA and the American University of Beirut, but his main service to academia was done in Germany and in German (he retired from Tübingen in 1999).[35] He advocates that one cannot separate philology from history, and meaningful methodology (and contextualization) is only possible on the basis of satisfactorily mastering the languages and understanding the text in a preliminary way.

Indeed, van Ess's methodological position fits the intellectual world that bred him. However, many younger scholars who grew in a very different intellectual climate still exhibit similar preferences toward texts. These scholars may investigate literary devices and stylistic patterns rather than philology per se, but they again go back to the manuscripts themselves, producing modern editions and translations alongside textual criticism. This was the aim of *Epidemics in Context: Greek Commentaries on Hippocrates in the Arabic Tradition*, a collection of essays published in 2012. The authors that make up the collection engage with the influential Hippocratic and Galenic theoretical and clinical medical texts in their Arabic versions.[36] They are established but younger scholars, in their early to middle stages

34 Josef van Ess, "Texts and Contexts: Heroes of the Plague," in *Text and Context in Islamic Societies*, ed. Irene A. Bierman and Afaf Lutfi Al-Sayyid Marsot (Reading: Ithaca, 2004), 13–22. See also idem, *Der Fehltritt des Gelehrten: die "Pest von Emmaus" und ihre theologischen Nachspiele* (Heidelberg: Universitätsverlag, 2001).

35 On van Ess: *Katalog des Deutschen Nationalbibliotek* (http://d-nb.info/gnd/115444149; accessed Sept. 20, 2014).

36 Peter E. Pormann, ed., *Epidemics in Contexts: Greek Commentaries on Hippocrates in the Arabic Tradition* (Berlin: de Gruyter, 2012). See also Cristina Álvarez Millán, "Graeco-Roman Case Histories and Their Influence on Medieval Islamic Clinical Accounts," *Social History of Medicine* 12 (1999): 19–43; Pormann, "Case Notes and Clinicians: Galen's *Commentary* on

of their career (save Gotthard Strohmaier),[37] implementing the older methodology that values philology as their main theme, maybe influenced by the New Philology. Other scholars of their generation, such as Justin Stearns (on whom more detail below) and Nahyan Fancy,[38] reflect the spirit of Dols and Conrad: their works include a crucial linguistic analysis, but the social context is not a by-product of a philological enquiry but the aim served by philology.

Regional and Temporal Biases

The methodological bias toward Arabic philology went hand in hand with preferences over regional and temporal scope. During most of the twentieth century, research on epidemics in the Islamic world concentrated on the central lands of the Arabic-speaking Middle East; whereas Muslim Spain and North Africa (also Arabic-speaking but further to the west) or the Turkish- and Persian-speaking areas, were more or less excluded. As many scholars of Islamic epidemics were Arabists in training and preferences, their focus on Arab lands and Arab historical periods makes sense. Yet this meant the scholarly marginalization of other periods and regions. Indeed, one major shift in the conception of current studies is the realization that the elites during the late medieval and early modern periods did not necessarily speak or write Arabic, and even if they did, it was not their only language of literary, scientific, and administrative output.

In addition to the geographic focus favoring Egypt and the Levant, the chronological preference was toward either the medieval period or to the nineteenth century and onwards. The medieval period enjoyed the reputation of being the glory of Islam. Epidemics allowed scholars who focused on the medieval period to explain the spread and evolution and consolidation of Islam as a religion and as a political entity. The nineteenth century interested scholars since it allowed them to deal with Islamic responses to European intervention in the Islamic world as the driving force for modernization and westernization. The study of epidemics fits this research program very well: anti-disease measures (education, quarantines, etc.) were regarded as the yardstick of the introduction of western scientific medicine into the Islamic world and the ability (or lack thereof) of Islamic states

---

the Hippocratic *Epidemics* in the Arabic Tradition," *Arabic Sciences and Philosophy* 18 (2008): 247–84.

37 Save Gotthard Strohmaier: Peter E. Pormann, editor and contributor, and contributors Robert Alessi, Leigh Chipman, Philip J. van der Eijk, Bink Hallum, Brooke Holmes, N. Peter Joosse, Grigory Kessel, Oliver Overwien, Simor Swain, and Uwe Vagelpohl.

38 Nahyan Fancy, *Science and Religion in Mamluk Egypt: Ibn al-Nafis, Pulmonary Transit and Bodily Resurrection* (London: Routledge, 2013).

to control borders and populations. Hence anti-epidemic policies were assumed to be a sign of power and modernization.

Nancy Gallagher and LaVerne Kuhnke's works from the 1970s to the 1990s are prominent outcomes of this historiographical period and agenda.[39] Gallagher and Kuhnke dealt with the importation of Western medicine and public health during the long nineteenth century and the evolution of public health in a nation state. They analyzed how local experts and elites confronted epidemics and the European political, economic, and scientific penetration. During most of the nineteenth century there was still no inherent scientific supremacy of European medicine, but the political and medical elite identified Western medicine with superiority, prestige, and power, and shifted toward it. Kuhnke and Gallagher (in her book dedicated to Egyptian public health, less so in the book about Tunisia) also framed the medical dangers confronted by the local population: epidemic diseases like cholera, typhus, smallpox or plague, fatal as they were, generally burdened the population less than endemic diseases like trachoma or parasitic infections of hookworm and schistosomiasis (bilharzia).

Their monographs were unique when they came out and attracted the attention of review sections in high-profile scholarly journals. Reviewers were not blind to problems and limitations, but overall praised these studies as unusual and contributing to the historical understanding of the political situation in crucial moments in Middle Eastern history.[40] These fine studies, rich with information that generated much interest and offered long overdue rebuttal to common Orientalistic misconceptions such as fatalism, were nevertheless limited both spatially and chronologically.

There were however some noted exceptions—scholars who did take interest in the interim period between the late medieval and modern periods. Dols himself wrote an article on the continued visitations of the plague in the early modern

39 Nancy Gallagher, *Medicine and Power in Tunisia, 1780–1900* (Cambridge: Cambridge University Press, 1983); idem, *Egypt's Other Wars: Epidemics and the Politics of Public Health* (Syracuse, NY: Syracuse University Press, 1990); LaVerne Kuhnke, *Lives at Risk: Public Health in Nineteenth Century Egypt* (Berkeley: University of California Press, 1990).

40 Review on Gallagher's *Medicine and Power in Tunisia, 1780–1900*: K. David Patterson, *American Historical Review* 90 (1985): 197. Reviews on Gallagher's *Egypt's Other Wars:* Lawrence I. Conrad, *Medical History* 37 (1993): 213–14; Ghada Karmi, *Bulletin of the School of Oriental and African Studies* 56 (1993): 368–69; Soheir A. Morsy, *Medical Anthropology Quarterly* 7 (1993): 101–7. Reviews on Kuhnke's *Lives at Risk: Public Health in Nineteenth-Century Egypt*: Nancy E. Gallagher, *International Journal of Middle East Studies* 24 (1992): 147–48; Lawrence I. Conrad, *The Middle East Journal* 47 (1993): 145; Morsy, *Medical Anthropology Quarterly*; John W. Livingston, *Journal of the American Oriental Society* 115 (1995): 329–31; Roger Owen, *Harvard Middle Eastern and Islamic Review* 3 (1996): 172–73.

period.[41] Yet for Dols, this was a side story to his main interest, which was medieval Arabic Islamic plague and medicine. Another plague historian, Daniel Panzac, made plague in the eighteenth and nineteenth centuries his main research focus. He was very much rooted in the French tradition, interested in society, demography, and the Mediterranean. He wrote extensively on plague, sanitation, and quarantines in order to explain the changing realities of the Ottoman Empire as a political and commercial power during that period.[42]

A New Historiographical Generation in the 2000s

Since Dols and Conrad, the community has moved rather quickly. The Islamic plague experience that was rendered invisible to the scholarship until then has become much more noticeable as new scholars insisted on shifting the temporal and spatial discussion so as to include non-European considerations.[43] There is now a plethora of studies and new scholars, as this volume reveals, who regard epidemics and plagues as their major academic project, not just a sideline.

The main shift in Islamic plague historiography, however, occurred in the 2000s. The change had several articulations: the histories of new regions and periods started to receive scholars' attention, but more importantly, new types of questions are set forward. These questions connect Islamic history with broader and updated trends in the historiography of plague. In other words, scholars engaging with plague and dissemination and control of diseases, no longer work strictly within the confines of Middle Eastern studies, but make use of a wide range of theories derived from histories of different regions or disciplines.

A region that was now scrutinized for the first time by Islamic plague historians is North Africa and Islamic Spain. Similar to Michael Dols, Justin Stearns analyzed theological, legal, and medical perceptions of disease in the late medieval Mediterranean and the social realities thereof. But Stearns went further. First, he expanded the geographical scope to the western parts of the Mediterranean world. Second and more important, he challenged Dols's thesis of community divisions between Christians and Muslims on the basis of religious difference; the Chris-

41 Dols, "The Second Plague Pandemic."

42 A sample of his work includes: Daniel Panzac, *La peste dans l'empire ottoman 1700–1850* (Leuven: Peeters, 1985); idem, "Politique sanitaire et fixation des frontières: l'exemple Ottoman (XVIIIe–XIXe siècles)," *Turcica* 31 (1999): 87–108; idem, "La peste dans les possessions insulaires du Grand Seigneur (XVIIe–XIXe siècles)," in *Insularités Ottomanes*, ed. Nicolas Vatin and Gilles Veinstein (Paris: Maisonneuve & Larose, 2004), 223–40.

43 Nükhet Varlık, "New Science and Old Sources: Why the Ottoman Experience of Plague Matters," *The Medieval Globe* 1 (2014): 193–227, especially 196–201.

tians combating actively with disease whereas Muslims were fatalistic and passive (this kind of argument becomes more acceptable as more scholars share the view of the Middle East as made of fluid inter-faith borders, with contrasting interests to keep them shifting or rather stable.) Stearns contrasted the clear-cut dichotomy with a much more complex reality of practical and theoretical inter-faith sharing. In so doing, he demonstrated how rich the range of responses in each community could be, on the basis of religious and legal thought as well as empirical evidence.[44]

Stearns was not alone to challenge Dols. In fact, Stuart Borsch undertook a comparative approach to the study of plague in his 2005 book, in which he explained the opposing outcomes of the mid-fourteenth century Black Death in Europe and the Middle East: recovery in the west and long social and economic decline in the east. Whereas Dols differentiated between Europe and the Middle East along religious and cultural lines (comparing "Christianity" and "Islamic societies"), Borsch compared the economic systems of Egypt and England (both were based on agriculture) in the aftermath of the Black Death. Based on analysis of economic data, Borsch proposed that Egypt's centralized and urban landholding system was unable to adapt to massive depopulation, whereas England's localized and rural system could recover much more quickly.[45]

Another symptom of the historiographical change, one that also drove the revision forward, was that the Ottomanists entered the field. This started already with Panzac's work in the 1980s, and then continued in a "drizzle" in the 1990s in the form of Ronald Jennings's unfolding social and economic realities in Trabzon based on the local Muslim judicial registers, and the persistence of plague as a factor in these realities.[46] Heath Lowry continued in this direction by trac-

44 Justin Stearns, *Infectious Ideas: Contagion in Premodern Islamic and Christian Thought in the Western Mediterranean* (Baltimore: Johns Hopkins University Press, 2011); idem, "New Directions in the Study of Religious Responses to the Black Death," *History Compass* 7 (2009): 1–13; idem, "Enduring the Plague: Ethical Behavior in the Fatwas of an 8th/14th Century Mufti and Theologian," in *Muslim Medical Ethics: From Theory to Practice*, ed. Jonathan Brockopp and Thomas Eich (Columbia: University of South Carolina Press, 2008), 38–54; idem, "Contagion in Theology and Law: Ethical Considerations in the Writings of Two 14th Century Scholars of Nasrid Granada," *Islamic Law and Society* 14 (2007): 109–29. Even though it is in the context of leprosy, Russell Hopley too discussed contagion and responses to it in the western Mediterranean. Russell Hopley, "Contagion in Islamic Lands: Responses from Medieval Andalusia and North Africa," *Journal for Early Modern Cultural Studies* 10 (2010): 45–64.

45 Stuart J. Borsch, *The Black Death in Egypt and England: A Comparative Analysis* (Austin: University of Texas Press, 2005). And more recently, idem, "Plague Depopulation and Irrigation Decay in Medieval Egypt," *The Medieval Globe* 1 (2014): 125–56.

46 Jennings, "Pious Foundations in the Society and Economy of Ottoman Trabzon"; idem,

ing outbreaks of plague in the early Ottoman centuries (fifteenth and sixteenth centuries). His goal was to provide an explanation of the impact of pestilence on Ottoman urban life and population in general and in Istanbul in particular. Additionally, he made an attempt at analyzing and discerning possible changes in the official Ottoman views on plague following the conquest of the Arab, older Islamic, lands.[47] Uli Schamiloglu, on his part, found it inexplicable that the Black Death was absent from the pages of history of the Ottoman Empire. He suggests that the plague had a direct impact on the rise of the Ottoman state, even though early Ottoman sources do not mention it: on the one hand the catastrophic epidemic weakened the Byzantine Empire and the rival Turkish principalities, while on the other, the nomadic Ottomans suffered less. Furthermore, there was a cultural shift among Anatolian Muslim Turks in the form of a rise in religiosity and "Turkishness" which supplied identity and ideology for the burgeoning state.[48]

Panzac, Jennings, Lowry, and Schamiloglu opened the door to several young Ottomanists who in the 2000s made plague the focal point of their research agenda, bringing about a turning point in both Ottoman and Islamic plague historiographies in several ways. They combined traditional Ottoman plague history with current trends in the larger field, and introduced new agendas and methodologies to the Ottoman historiography that went beyond the commonly used social, cultural, and political analysis. In particular, these works include discussions of health, environment, natural disasters, and the interaction between human and non-human factors.

In my own work, plague was featured as related to medicine and health. I discussed medical theories and clinical realities in the Arabic and Turkish-speaking regions of the Ottoman Empire. I refrained from discussing early modern medicine against the backdrop of other medical systems (Christian or European), as such comparisons conjure images of dependence, simplicity, and crudeness. Instead, I consider them as hermeneutic wholes. I showed the continuation of concepts and ideas from medieval Islamic medicine regarding the etiology of plague, its

---

"Plague in Trabzon and Reactions to It According to Local Judicial Registers," in *Humanist and Scholar: Essays in Honor of Andreas Tietze*, ed. Heath W. Lowry and Donald Quataert (Istanbul: Isis Press, 1993), 27–36.

47 Health Lowry, "Pushing the Stone Uphill: The Impact of Bubonic Plague on Ottoman Urban Society in the Fifteenth and Sixteenth Centuries," *Journal of Ottoman Studies* 23 (2003): 93–132.

48 Uli Schamiloglu, "The Rise of the Ottoman Empire: The Black Death in Medieval Anatolia and Its Turkish Civilization," in *Views from the Edge: Essays in Honor of Richard W. Bulliet*, ed. Neguin Yavari, Lawrence G. Porter, and Jean-Marc Ran Oppenheim (New York: Columbia University Press, 2004), 255–79.

transmission through miasma or contagion, but also deviations from it, in terms of both theory and everyday practice. Such an analysis allowed me to clearly argue that pre-modern Ottoman conceptions of medicine and health were very far from being "passive" or "fatalistic." When this is our starting point, it is easy to see that medicine among Ottomans was not that different from that of Christians around the Mediterranean.[49]

Other scholars contextualize Ottoman plague history in very new and different manners. Nükhet Varlık goes back to earlier Ottoman period (1347–1600), a period that has been understudied thus far, and integrates new kinds of sources (e.g., Ottoman plague treatises). She challenges Daniel Panzac's earlier claim that the Ottoman Empire was the ultimate source of outbreaks of plague in Europe. Instead, she demonstrates how epidemics were introduced into Ottoman domains from the west through port cities and from them, toward the inland. She further argues that the emergence of new commercial networks integrated the Ottoman regions into the Mediterranean world and into Europe. This, in turn, led to the intensification of outbreaks of plague in Ottoman lands and demanded the investment of more resources from medical scholars and from the political and legal apparatus. She also questions the assumption of quarantines as a uniquely European and especially Italian public health measure. Her conclusion of the sources underscores the importance of shared-knowledge and debates among Mediterranean communities and interaction between east and west.[50]

An important contribution to the field was offered by Sam White and Alan Mikhail who introduced the "Environmental Turn" to Ottoman studies. White and Mikhail opened up the analysis of the impact of environmental factors on the economic and political trajectory of the Ottoman Empire. Within this framework, they explore epidemics as an important force forming and transforming state-society relations and in creating, evading, and transgressing political, economic, and cultural loci of power. Both scholars tackle the issue of the "imperial ecology": resource extraction and provisioning systems. White explained how climatic changes and disease in humans and non-humans around 1600 altered this system, leading to long lasting political, social, and demographic consequences.[51] Mikhail

49 Miri Shefer-Mossensohn, *Ottoman Medicine: Healing and Medical Institutions 1500–1700* (Albany, NY: State University of New York Press, 2009); idem, "Communicable Disease in Ottoman Palestine: Local Thoughts and Actions," *Korot* 21 (2011–2012): 19–49.

50 Varlık, *Plague and Empire in the Early Modern Mediterranean World: The Ottoman Experience, 1347–1600* (Cambridge: Cambridge University Press, 2015); idem, "Conquest, Urbanization and Plague Networks in the Ottoman Empire, 1453–1600," in *The Ottoman World*, ed. Christine Woodhead (London: Routledge, 2012), 251–63.

51 Sam White, *The Climate of Rebellion in the Early Modern Ottoman Empire* (Cambridge:

showed how natural resources in Ottoman Egypt, such as water and animals, shaped the nature and the legitimacy of power and rule in the pre-modern Ottoman world by connecting and dividing localities and imperial centers, peasants and urban elites, humans and non-humans.[52] White and Mikhail both emphasized the symbolic and material meanings of plague in that complex.

Yaron Ayalon also belongs to this historiographical phase. He frames plagues as part of history of all sorts of calamities, which nature summons upon humanity, and hence contributes to the environmental discourse of epidemics by focusing on human psychological and social behavior patterns that determine resilience and recovery. His other contribution is the integration of Muslim and non-Muslim communities into the same theoretical framework.[53]

Quarantines continuously attracted the attention of many scholars. The focus on quarantines seems to have overshadowed other anti-disease measures that were highly important at the time for all players in the epidemic scene. These were an assortment of public health policies like vaccinations, hospitals, municipal regulations, personal hygiene regimen, etc. Some of the more recent studies on quarantines appear to tread in known territory. While they supply fresh evidence, they preserve previous discourses, concerning the delay in the Ottoman application of quarantines until the nineteenth century and the intellectual and political climate that allowed for the introduction of proactive anti-disease measures in that century. Some differ from previous scholars in trying to prove that quarantines were not a western imposition on the Ottoman Empire, but all are still rooted in the context of struggle between the Ottomans and various European powers, and the outcome of European interventions.[54] Anne-Marie Moulin, for instance, discusses how

Cambridge University Press, 2011); idem, "Rethinking Disease in Ottoman Society," *International Journal of Middle East Studies* 42 (2010): 549–67.

52 Alan Mikhail, *Nature and Empire in Ottoman Egypt: An Environmental History* (Cambridge: Cambridge University Press, 2011); idem, *The Animal in Ottoman Egypt* (New York: Oxford University Press, 2013); idem, "The Nature of Plague in Late Eighteenth-Century Egypt," *Bulletin of the History of Medicine* 82 (2008): 249–75.

53 Yaron Ayalon, *Natural Disasters in the Ottoman Empire: Plague, Famine, and Other Misfortunes* (Cambridge: Cambridge University Press, 2014); idem, "Ottoman Urban Privacy in Light of Disaster Recovery," *International Journal of Middle East Studies* 43 (2011): 513–28.

54 Compare Birsen Bulmuş, *Plague, Quarantines and Geopolitics in the Ottoman Empire* (Edinburgh: Edinburgh University Press, 2012); Nuran Yıldırım and Hakan Ertin, "European Physicians / Specialists during the Cholera Epidemic in Istanbul 1893–1895 and their Contribution to the Modernization of Healthcare in the Ottoman State," in *Health, Culture and the Human Body: Epidemiology, Ethics and History of Medicine; Perspectives from Turkey and Central Europe*, ed. İlhan İlkılıç, Hakan Ertin, Rainer Brömer, and Hajo Zeeb (Istanbul: BETIM Center Press, 2014), 189–215.

anticontagionist ideas disseminated in Mehmet ʿAli Pasha's Egypt by being shared by different players. Foreign physicians and local administrators alike partook in the discourse of modernization and reform, but understood it in very different and diverging ways. For Clot-Bey, the famous French expert brought to Egypt, anti-plague theories and policies were about science and secularism. For the Egyptian governor, anti-plague measures, were a political idea of social control.[55]

More studies with reference to quarantine implement new methodologies and reach original insights. As mentioned above, Nükhet Varlık challenged the concept that quarantine was a European practice in the context of the early modern Mediterranean and Ottoman worlds.[56] Other scholars demonstrate it with the sources for the later Ottoman periods. Andrew Robarts, for instance, investigates the Ottoman-Russian Black Sea frontier from the late eighteenth century to the early nineteenth century by looking at population movement and the spread of plague and cholera. He looks at quarantines as part of world history, and situates this discussion in "the Imperial Turn" that deals with comparative history of empires. Contrasting Ottoman and Russian migration and settlement policies and the implementation of quarantine regulations, Robarts demonstrates that both empires identified epidemic diseases (plague and cholera) as the primary "security threats" to their subject populations, and how the accelerated human mobility resulted in the empires' commitment to implement restrictions to that mobility by border controls in the forms of documents and quarantines. His argument is that in the Black Sea region, the empires communicated and coordinated in all levels regarding epidemic disease across their mutual frontier, alongside geo-strategic and ideological confrontation between them.[57]

Certainly, the British Empire too was very relevant to the Middle East. Michael Christopher Low investigates the inter-imperial competition between the Ottomans

---

55 Anne Marie Moulin, "The Construction of Disease Transmission in Nineteenth-Century Egypt and the Dialectics of Modernity," in *The Development of Modern Medicine in Non-Western Countries: Historical Perspectives*, ed. Hormoz Ebrahimnejad (London: Routledge, 2009), 42–58.

56 Varlık, "Disease and Empire: A History of Plague Epidemics in the Early Modern Ottoman Empire (1453–1600)," PhD diss., University of Chicago, 2008.

57 Andrew Robarts, "A Plague on Both Houses: Population Movements and the Spread of Disease across the Ottoman-Russian Black Sea Frontier, 1768–1830s," PhD diss., Georgetown University, 2010; idem, *Migration and Disease in the Black Sea Region: Ottoman-Russian Relations in the Late Eighteenth and Early Nineteenth Centuries* (London: Bloomsbury, 2017); idem, "Imperial Confrontations or Regional Cooperation? Bulgarian Migration and Ottoman-Russian Relations in the Black Sea Region, 1768–1830s," *Turkish Historical Review* 3 (2012): 149–67.

and British India in the second half of the nineteenth century, over the Arabian Peninsula, the Red Sea, and the Indian Ocean. He further explores the importance of the pilgrimage to Mecca and how it served as a special arena for the opponents to play out their rivalry. For the Hamidian-era Ottoman Empire (1876–1909), Muslim pilgrimage was a mandatory scene in its pan-Islamic claims, while for the British, it posed a dual danger of both health and security.[58] Likewise, Valeska Huber and Patrick Zylbermann connect Ottoman and British realities, but from a different angle. They examine the ways in which Britain and Western Europe as a whole tried to control the Middle East and safeguard Europe in faraway shores by means of a unified action promoted by medical anti-epidemic discourse and actions.[59]

There are three recurrent themes to the studies that deal with the imperial context of epidemics in the Islamic world. One is that imperial history brings in global and colonial facets. During the nineteenth century, modern medicine emerged simultaneously with the ideology and the political and administrative institutions of colonialism. It was not the only context of the diffusion of western medicine in other regions globally, but especially in one of the more important and influential settings.[60] Accordingly, it has become quite common for historians of Islamic medicine of the nineteenth and twentieth centuries to consider this phenomenon. Their work was influenced by analysis of medicine and disease in other world regions, most notably colonial India. Here it is important to note David Arnold, one of the founding fathers of Subaltern studies in the 1970s, who explored in the 1990s the vital role of the state in medical and public health activities. He argued that western medicine became a battleground between the colonized and the colonizers. He focused on smallpox, cholera, and plague to show the ways western medicine was transferred to India by transformations shaped by

58 Michael Christopher Low, "Empire and the Hajj: Pilgrims, Plagues, and Pan-Islam under British Surveillance, 1865-1908," *International Journal of Middle East Studies* 40 (2008): 269–90.

59 Valeska Huber, "The Unification of the Globe by Disease? The International Sanitary Conferences on Cholera, 1851–1894," *The Historical Journal* 49 (2006): 453–76; Patrick Zylberman, "Civilizing the State: Borders, Weak States and International Health in Modern Europe," in *Medicine at the Border: Disease, Globalization and Security, 1850 to the Present*, ed. Alison Bashford (New York: Palgrave Macmillan, 2006), 21–40. See also: Cornelia Essner, "Cholera der Mekkapilger und Internationale Sanitätspolitik in Ägypten (1866–1938)," *Die Welt des Islams* 32 (1992): 41–82 and Zeinab Abul-Magd, "A Crisis of Images: The French, Jihad, and the Plague in Upper Egypt, 1798–1801," *Journal of World History* 23 (2012): 315–43.

60 Hormoz Ebrahimnejad, "Introduction: For a History of Modern Medicine in Non-Western Countries," in *The Development of Modern Medicine in Non-Western Countries: Historical Perspectives*, ed. Hormoz Ebrahimnejad (London: Routledge, 2009), 1–22.

Indian needs and conditions. He thus demonstrated how medicine, epidemics, and the human body were central to the British colonial rule in India.[61]

A second common thread in the scholarship is tracing the movement, in space and time, of human and non-human actors. The technological transformations of the nineteenth century with the advent of trains and steamships intensified the volume of people on the road, shortened the length of their travels, and changed the speed they negotiated distances. These transformations affected the communicability of diseases dramatically.

As a matter of fact, the movement of humans and disease in space also destined epidemics to be a challenge to borders, which is another theme that appears in current epidemic scholarship dealing with the modern period. Epidemics defy boundaries and test sovereignty. At the same time, they offered opportunities for states and rulers to devise mental borders and to draw concrete lines on maps. The ensuing boundaries in the scholarship tend to reproduce these earlier divisions. Firoozeh Kashani-Sabet showed that cholera both necessitated and facilitated the precise drawing of the Ottoman-Iranian border in Iraq, in a way that was neither needed nor possible before the advent of the modern state and national identities.[62] Likewise, Sandra Sufian argued that Zionist malariologists used the science of malariology to uphold the geographic borders that had been newly created by the British and French mandates and communal borders between Palestinian Arabs and Jewish Zionists.[63]

Malaria and mosquitos, newer subjects of the scholarship, allowed scholars to use yet another epidemic as a means to scrutinize the emerging social, economic, and political institutions as well as the new expertise that made modernization in the Middle East. Timothy Mitchell's work was the first in the Middle Eastern context to connect parasites and the profound technological, political, and industrial transformations that made modern states. His case study was Egypt and its political economy.[64] Since Mitchell's study, social historians and historical geographers of Turkey[65] and

---

61 David Arnold, *Colonizing the Body: State Medicine and Epidemic Disease in Nineteenth-Century India* (Berkeley: University of California Press, 1993).

62 Firoozeh Kashani-Sabet, "'City of the Dead': The Frontier Polemics of Quarantines in the Ottoman Empire and Iran," *Comparative Studies of South Asia, Africa and the Middle East* 18 (1998): 51–58.

63 Sandra Sufian, "Colonial Malariology, Medical Borders, and Sharing Scientific Knowledge in Mandatory Palestine," *Science in Context* 19 (2006): 381–400.

64 Timothy Mitchell, *Rule of Experts: Egypt, Techno-Politics, Modernity* (Berkeley: The University of California Press, 2002).

65 Kyle T. Evered and Emine Ö. Evered, "State, Peasant, Mosquito: The Biopolitics of Public Health Education and Malaria in Early Republican Turkey," *Political Geography* 31 (2012):

medical historians of mandate Palestine[66] have investigated how civilizational agendas of modernization were articulated through landscape in which malaria epidemics raised both medical and political concerns. In addition, they have demonstrated how anti-malaria campaigns were used to promote newer levels of effective governance.

The study of malaria epidemics is an especially fertile ground, as it allows scholars of different Islamic regions to ask similar questions, and thus reach together a more nuanced awareness that may explain the longer and subtler patterns of the spread of disease. This advantage may continue with new projects on sexually-transmitted diseases, like syphilis or now HIV. They sketch how state-led campaigns meant to collect information on citizens, order sexualities, and lead to the expansion of the state and its regulation.[67]

Here we also see the theme of women's role as defenders of health and vectors of disease and hence targets of state's attention that runs through many studies. This issue has attracted scholars of late Ottoman and early Turkish republic as well as of other Middle Eastern regions, like Egypt[68] or Iran. Women's function and action in health and disease, however, is part of a larger process that historians investigate with regard to the national period of the Middle East, namely the historical moment of state formation and the rise of nationalism. For example, Kashani-Sabet considered plague as part of hygiene campaigns that targeted women in Qajar Iran. These were part of debates about demography, reproductive politics, and women's role in a modern state and society. The final goal was to bring about social change in the form of creating new Iranian maternalism as part of modern Iranian citizenship.[69]

311–23; idem, "Governing Population, Public Health, and Malaria in the Early Turkish Republic," *Journal of Historical Geography* 37 (2011): 470–82.

66 Sandra M. Sufian, *Healing the Land and the Nation: Malaria and the Zionist Project in Palestine, 1920–1947* (Chicago: University of Chicago Press, 2007).

67 Emine Ö. Evered and Kyle T. Evered, "Sex and the Capital City: The Political Framing of Syphilis and Prostitution in Early Republican Ankara," *Journal of the History of Medicine and Allied Sciences* 68 (2013): 266–99; Kyle T. Evered and Emine Ö. Evered, "Syphilis and Prostitution in the Socio-Medical Geographies of Turkey's Early Republican Provinces," *Health and Place* 18 (2012): 528–35; Ebru Boyar, "'An Inconsequential Boil' or a 'Terrible Disease'? Social Perceptions of and State Responses to Syphilis in the Late Ottoman Empire," *Turkish Historical Review* 2 (2011): 101–24; Palmira Brummett, "Dogs, Women, Cholera, and Other Menaces in the Streets: Cartoon Satire in the Ottoman Revolutionary Press, 1908–11," *International Journal of Middle East Studies* 2 (1995): 433–60.

68 Khaled Fahmy, "Women, Medicine, and Power in Nineteenth-Century Egypt," in *Remaking Women: Feminism and Modernity in the Middle East*, ed. Lila Abu-Lughod (Princeton, NJ: Princeton University Press, 1998), 43–45.

69 Kashani-Sabet, *Conceiving Citizens: Women and the Politics of Motherhood in Iran* (Oxford:

Abundance of Methodologies but No Bioarcheology (Yet)

Islamic plague historiography has evolved and continues to expand in new and multiple methodological contexts. One venue that has yet to be explored is the mobilization of material and laboratory evidence into historical research. The field of historical plague studies must be redefined in various dimensions, one of which has to be the methodological registers used to investigate, says Monica Green, one of the most influential historians of pre-modern medicine of this decade. Today, with new methods of ancient DNA (aDNA) retrieval, we have made genetic identification of pathogens, the gold standard of identifying past diseases. Instead of relying only on symptoms that are revealed in written texts and visual materials that historians are so adept at analyzing (and is by definition interpretive and open to errors), we have now the added advantage of using physical evidence that is analyzed under the microscope. If medicine was revolutionized by the laboratory in the nineteenth century and never stopped, it is now the history of medicine—at least with regard to epidemics—that has followed suit since the 1990s. The question, however, is much more than the identification of which disease was involved in a past epidemic, but rather opening new questions regarding long-distance spread of disease and the varied-range of species that carried it. This is where historians can contribute by analyzing ways of transmission across Eurasia and long-lasting effects on human individuals and communities.[70]

Hence, after being sidelined in the debates about global plagues, historians join again the discussion about plagues in history and address the methodological problems involving retrospective diagnosis. By bringing in contexts and meanings, they contribute to the knowledge of disease vectors, the impact of climate on epidemics, and venture into reconstructing disease ecologies. Many topics are addressed, including comparisons between different outbreaks of epidemics, analysis of mortality and demography, living conditions, the patterns of epidemic spread, and the interaction of plague with other disasters. The pursuit of such a wide range of threads opens up new opportunities for collaboration with geneticists, biologists, and archeologists to better understand continuities and diversi-

---

Oxford University Press, 2011). See also R. M. Burrell, "The 1904 Epidemic of Cholera in Persia: Some Aspects of Qājār Society," *Bulletin of the School of Oriental and African Studies* 51 (1988): 258–70; Amir Arsalan Afkhami, "Defending the Guarded Domain: Epidemics and the Emergence of an International Sanitary Policy in Iran," *Comparative Studies of South Asia, Africa and the Middle East* 19 (1999): 122–36.

70 Monica H. Green, "Editor's Introduction to *Pandemic Disease in the Medieval World: Rethinking the Black Death*," *The Medieval Globe* 1 (2014): 9–25; idem, "Taking 'Pandemic' Seriously: Making the Black Death Global," *The Medieval Globe* 1 (2014): 27–61.

ties across time and space and the means of dissemination of diseases and the human experience of epidemics.[71]

This picture of archeologists, anthropologists, and historians of epidemics joining hands is applicable mostly for Europe and Eurasia. As Lester Little pointed out in 2011, it is still a major task for historians to devote more attention to the Middle East and the Islamic world in connection to epidemiology.[72] Although some recent studies include a call for bioarcheology and other types of collaborative inquiry,[73] further research is sorely needed.

Another lacuna in the historiography of epidemics in the Islamic world is the paucity of scholars who deal with the Islamic-Mongol link. Owing to unique lingual needs, there are only a handful of scholars who investigate disease and epidemics in this region. Uli Schamiloglu's earlier work situates plague history in the Central Asian steppe context. He argues, for instance, that fourteenth-century plague outbreaks brought about population movements, fragmentation of centralized authority in the Golden Horde, and setbacks in the development of Turkic literature and literacy.[74] While Schamiloglu connects Islamic Central Asia to global outbreaks of plague, Paul Buell points to the unique plague experience in Mongol Asia, where there was no enormous plague epidemic in the magnitude of the Middle East or the West. Buell maintains that the local disease and physical environments, together with specific historical realities related to the nomadic Mongols that favored oceanic contacts rather than overland, isolated the eastern parts of Asia even from "sister" Central Asian Muslim Mongol dynasties and thus protected them from major outbreaks of disease.[75] The latest on this topic is Robert Hymes's hypothesis that ties plague in East and Central Asia with the Mongol expansion. He sees in the Mongols' repeated assaults and eventual highly destructive conquests a critical moment in the spread of plague outside its origin. His proposition places the deep history of the Black Death in the middle of the thirteenth century, that is, a century earlier than is conventionally accepted.[76]

---

71 Based on Lester K. Little, "Plague Historians in Lab Coats," *Past and Present* 213 (2011): 267–90.

72 Ibid., 286–87.

73 Borsch, "Plague Depopulation and Irrigation Decay in Medieval Egypt," *The Medieval Globe* 1 (2014): 125–56; Varlık, "New Science and Old Sources."

74 Schamiloglu, "Preliminary Remarks on the Role of Disease in the History of the Golden Horde," *Central Asian Survey* 12 (1993): 447–57.

75 Paul D. Buell, "Qubilai and the Rats," *Sudhoffs Archiv* 96 (2012): 127–44.

76 Robert Hymes, "Epilogue: A Hypothesis on the East Asian Beginnings of the *Yersinia pestis* Polytomy," *The Medieval Globe* 1 (2014): 285–308.

The small number of studies investigating the interplay of war and epidemics is puzzling. Throughout history, one of the principal disasters of war has been epidemics. This well-known historical lesson is under-investigated in Middle Eastern and Islamic contexts. Several scholars have mentioned, if briefly, but rarely problematized the interconnected nature of war and disease in this particular historical context. Khaled Fahmy, for instance, mentions the spread of syphilis among the soldiers of the Egyptian army in Syria in 1831 as a source of concern for doctors, military officers, and the political elites. It is one of the pieces of evidence Fahmy brings to explain anti-prostitution measures and regulation of women's health in general in order to minimize sexually transmitted diseases in the army of Mehmet ʿAli Pasha and the population at large.[77] Few studies focusing on World War I, in which epidemics are brought sometimes to the forefront, are an exception to the rule. Some scholars discuss how epidemics weakened armies' combat abilities;[78] others discuss the effects of epidemics on the civilian population.[79] One hopes that with the centennial of WWI, we may see more studies on major wars and epidemiology which would help explain the war itself as much as the reformatting of the region in the post-Ottoman period in the aftermath of the war.

In addition to filling the three lacunae outlined above, a further task that is just being picked up by plague historians is to integrate the studies of Jewish experiences of epidemics in the Middle East and epidemics in Israel/Palestine with Islamic and Middle Eastern scholarship (these questions are not of historical value alone, but are relevant to current agreements between Israel and its neighbors). Scholars of Jewish or Israeli history, to a large extent, rely mainly on Jewish and European sources. Additionally, the main volume of their publications is in Hebrew thus less accessible to non-Hebrew readers.[80] The works of scholars such as Justin Stearns or Yaron Ayalon, and more recently Nükhet Varlık, which deal with both Muslim and non-Muslim communities should be more common.[81]

77 Fahmy, "Women, Medicine, and Power in Nineteenth-Century Egypt."

78 Hikmet Özdemir, *The Ottoman Army 1914–1918: Disease and Death on the Battlefield*, trans. Saban Kardaş (Salt Lake City: University of Utah Press, 2008); Eran Dolev, "'I Am Campaigning Against Mosquitoes': General Allenby's Campaign against Malaria, Palestine 1918," *Korot* 21 (2011): 75–88.

79 Oya Dağlar, *War, Epidemics, and Medicine in the Late Ottoman Empire (1912–1918)* (Haarlem: Sota, 2008).

80 Some examples are Dan Barel, *An Ill Wind: Cholera Epidemics and Medical Development in Palestine in the Late Ottoman Period* (Jerusalem: Mosad Bialik, 2010) [in Hebrew]; Yael Buchman, "Life in the Shadow of the Plague," *Jerusalem and Eretz-Israel*, 2 (2004): 51–75 [in Hebrew].

81 Varlık, "Plague, Conflict, and Negotiation: The Jewish Broadcloth Weavers of Salonica

Islamic plague historiography has now evolved to be an interdisciplinary endeavor. This promises the field to be especially dynamic and at the cutting edge of historical research.[82] The question remains whether plague history will form a sub-field of its own within Middle Eastern and Islamic history. Currently, it is in-between several disciplines: language-based, area studies, social history, environmental history, history of science, medicine, technology, and political history. But to which particular research field do plague historians belong? Who is willing to acknowledge them as part of their academic discipline? Do they need to belong? With whom are they in communication? Who are their audiences? These questions are answered partly by the studies of the authors contributing to this volume, and partly by the readers of this volume who shall evaluate how the unique point of view of plagues furthers their own studies.

Miri Shefer-Mossensohn (shefer@post.tau.ac.il) is an Associate Professor of Ottoman history in Middle Eastern and African History at Tel Aviv University. She studies early modern Muslim medicines, health, and wellbeing in the Turkish- and Arabic-speaking worlds. Her books include *Ottoman Medicine: Healing and Medical Institutions 1500–1700* (State University of New York Press, 2009) and *Science among the Ottomans: The Cultural Creation and Exchange of Knowledge* (University of Texas Press, 2015).

---

and the Ottoman Central Administration in the Late Sixteenth Century," *Jewish History* 28 (2014): 261–88.

82 New studies continue to be produced in this field. For recent dissertations on the history of disease, environment, and medicine in the Middle East, see, for example: Christopher Gratien, "The Mountains are Ours: Ecology and Settlement in Late Ottoman and Early Republican Cilicia, 1856–1956," PhD diss., Georgetown University, 2015; Seçil Yılmaz, "Love in the Time of Syphilis: Medicine and Sex in the Ottoman Empire, 1860–1922," PhD diss., City University of New York, 2016; Graham A. Pitts, "Fallow Fields: Famine and the Making of Lebanon, 1914–1948," PhD diss., Georgetown University, 2016.

SCHOLARS, SUFIS, AND DISEASE: CAN MUSLIM RELIGIOUS WORKS OFFER US NOVEL INSIGHTS ON PLAGUES AND EPIDEMICS AMONG THE MEDIEVAL AND EARLY MODERN OTTOMANS?

JOHN J. CURRY*
University of Nevada, Las Vegas

RESEARCHERS FACE A number of obstacles when seeking to understand how the Muslim populations of the medieval and early modern period of Ottoman times coped with plagues and other epidemic diseases. Among these difficulties is that fact that information is often scattered across a wide variety of sources, many of which do not treat the topic directly. Utilizing these sources, which have not been addressed in the historiography to date, can yield interesting results. My contribution to this volume aims to demonstrate the potential usefulness of specific types of early modern Ottoman religious writings, which can illuminate how various segments of the Ottoman population viewed plagues, diseases, and possible remedies for them in the pre-modern era.

Specifically, the religious literature examined here will encompass two types of sub-genre. First, I will focus on a legal text compiled in the early seventeenth century, written by an Ottoman Hanbali jurisprudent named Marʿī b. Yūsuf b. Abu Bakr Zayn al-Dīn al-Karmī (d. 1624), and entitled *Taḥqīq al-ẓunūn bi-akhbār al-ṭāʿūn* ("Verification of Suppositions via the Accounts of Plagues").[1] The work subsequently gained popularity among a substantial segment of the Ottoman religious elite in the centuries that followed, despite its author being a member of the Hanbali law school. While texts of a similar type have been treated in the existing scholarly literature, such as the sixteenth-century works of İdris-i Bidlisi, *Risālat al-ʿibāʾ ʿan mawāqiʿ al-wabāʾ* ("Treatise on Turning Away from the Locations of Epidemics"); Kemalpaşazade, *Risālah fī al-ṭāʿūn* ("Treatise on the Plague"); and

* I would like to thank Prof. Justin Stearns for reading and commenting on an earlier draft of this chapter, and saving me from potential errors in the process. I would also like to thank Prof. Nükhet Varlık for a number of useful comments made on the chapter during the course of its evolution, and to Prof. Irfana Hashmi for directing me to helpful material contained in her dissertation. That being said, any remaining errors are solely my own.

1 The best surviving copy of this text is Marʿī b. Yūsuf b. Abu Bakr Zayn al-Dīn al-Karmī (d. 1033/1624), *Taḥqīq al-ẓunūn bi-akhbār al-ṭāʿūn* (Istanbul, Süleymaniye Library, ms. Hacı Ahmed Paşa 115); additional texts also survive and will be treated subsequently.

Taşköprüzade's *Risālah al-shifā' li-adwā' al-wabā'* ("Treatise on the Cure for Epidemic Disease"); this particular example has not been treated in sufficient detail.[2] Marʿī's contents deserve greater scrutiny because his text emerges out of a period in Ottoman history that came to be marked by an "ethos of verification." This was an early modern intellectual movement among some Muslim thinkers whereby they sought not merely to explain the content of earlier works, but also to give various kinds of evidentiary proofs to further develop their interpretations, and thereby take a more critical spirit toward the topics under investigation.[3] This background is important, because previous scholarship has suggested that the Ottoman thinkers of the sixteenth century gradually moved away from the mythical conceptions of the plague in earlier eras toward one more harmonized with ideas of preventing contagion, and attempting to avoid or control disease.[4] Texts like Marʿī b. Yūsuf's, as we shall see, suggest that this intellectual trajectory could generate a wide range of responses and literary approaches to the plague that might have reached alternative conclusions. They clearly addressed an important debate among Ottoman subjects over these issues, and are therefore included in the wider narrative on this topic. By examining his writings in more detail, we can

2 Leaving aside encyclopedic references, the only three references to the text of which I am aware are brief notices in Michael W. Dols, *The Black Death in the Middle East* (Princeton: Princeton University Press, 1977), 334; Jacqueline Sublet, "La peste prise aux rêts de la jurisprudence: le traité d'Ibn Ḥağar al-ʿAsqalānī sur la peste," *Studia Islamica* 33 (1971), 148; and Christopher Melchert, "Marʿī b. Yūsuf," *Essays in Arabic Literary Biography 1350–1850*, ed. Joseph E. Lowry and Devin J. Stewart (Wiesbaden: Harrassowitz Verlag, 2009), 290. In all cases, it is mentioned only in passing. For a still-serviceable bibliographical essay of the medieval and Ottoman manuscript literature on the plague, see Dols, *Black Death*, 320–35, which should be complemented with the more detailed coverage for the Ottoman literature in Nükhet Varlık, *"Disease and Empire: A History of Plague Epidemics in the Early Modern Ottoman Empire (1453–1600),"* PhD diss., University of Chicago, 2008, 172–204 and 264–65 and Birsen Bulmuş, *Plague, Quarantines, and Geopolitics in the Ottoman Empire* (Edinburgh: Edinburgh University Press, 2012), 40–48 and 68–75. For manuscript copies of the noted works, see Kemalpaşazade, *Risālah fī al-ṭāʿūn* (Istanbul: Süleymaniye Library, ms. Esad Efendi 3567/4), 60a-64a; and Taşköprüzade's *Risālah al-shifā' li-adwā' al-wabā'* (Istanbul: Atatürk Kitaplığı, ms. Osman Ergin 736), 42b-88b.

3 For more on the seventeenth- and eighteenth-century movement toward the creation of a "verification" (*taḥqīq*) literature, see Khaled El-Rouayheb, "Opening the Gate of Verification: The Forgotten Arab-Islamic Florescence of the 17th Century," *International Journal of Middle East Studies* 38 (2006), 263–65.

4 In addition to the aforementioned dissertation reference in n. 2 previous, these ideas are developed further in Nükhet Varlık, "From '*Bête Noire*' to '*le Mal de* Constantinople': Plagues, Medicine, and the Early Modern Ottoman State," *Journal of World History* 24: 4 (2013): 741–70.

shed some light on these alternative intellectual reactions to the topic of plague and epidemic disease from the religio-legal perspective he employed.

Second, I will examine the writings of noted Ottoman Sufi authors, in the form of both hagiographical accounts and personal writings. Many Ottoman Sufi shaykhs were noted for their ability to cure sicknesses or deflect catastrophic events, such as plagues and epidemic diseases, from the wider community. However, just as in the religio-legal literature, the relationship between shaykhdom and disease was a contested one. Furthermore, some Sufis seem to have addressed the legal debates over proper responses to the plague. As Justin Stearns has noted, references to these events as recorded in the writings of various Sufi figures, or the hagiographical literature about them, can offer historians additional clues about the ways that pre-modern Muslim thinkers reacted to plague and disease events.[5] While Ottoman Sufi writings require careful analysis due to their otherworldly elements, historians can use them to evaluate the social and political contexts that intersect with the outbreaks of plague and disease, and the responses to these events.

Combined together, these two genres of religious source material offer possible windows of insight on how the topics of epidemic disease, sickness, and remedies were perceived by Ottoman thinkers during the transition from the medieval to early modern period of world history. While I make no claims to comprehensive coverage in this short chapter, the sources utilized here nevertheless enrich our knowledge of the complex intellectual range of Muslim responses to issues of disease and public health.

Religio-Legal Texts Dealing with Plague and Disease

On 28 April 1619, the Hanbali jurisprudent Marʿī b. Yūsuf b. Abu Bakr Zayn al-Dīn al-Karmī finished dictating a lengthy text addressing the issue of plague to one of his noted students, Muḥammad b. Mūsa b. Muḥammad al-Sharīf, who would later go on to serve as the chief *qadi* in Cairo.[6] Compiling this response was a matter

---

5 See, for example, the discussion of the Moroccan Sufis Muḥammad b. al-Ḥasan al-Banānī and Aḥmad b. ʿAjība in Justin K. Stearns, *Infectious Ideas: Contagion in Premodern Islamic and Christian Thought in the Western Mediterranean* (Baltimore: Johns Hopkins University Press, 2011), 149–50.

6 His *laqab* "al-Madanī al-Mālikī" suggests that he may have been a Maliki jurist from Medina; see Marʿī b. Yūsuf b. Abu Bakr Zayn al-Dīn al-Karmī (d. 1033/1624), *Taḥqīq al-ẓunūn bi-akhbār al-ṭāʿūn* (Istanbul: Süleymaniye Library, ms. Laleli 1344), 38a; Muḥammad b. Mūsa is noted as Marʿī b. Yūsuf's student in Kasım Kırbıyık, "Merʿî b. Yûsuf," *Türkiye Diyanet Vakfı İslâm Ansiklopedisi* (Istanbul: Türkiye Diyanet Vakfı İslâm Araştırmaları Merkezi, 2004), v. 29, 185.

of urgency at the time, since another source reported that a plague outbreak was decimating Cairo's population during that year.[7] As a result, despite the possibility that he adhered to a different school of law, Muḥammad was keen to acquire these teachings. Furthermore, Marʿī was a well-regarded jurist by this point in his career and Muḥammad probably saw his opportunity to acquire this text as an honor and a privilege.

As for Marʿī, he was born in the town of Tulkarem in Palestine, and began studying at a young age with Hanbali scholars in Jerusalem. He subsequently moved to Cairo to continue his studies at the prestigious al-Azhar university with various prominent Egyptian jurists just prior to the turn of the century.[8] Marʿī went on to hold prestigious positions at some of the most prestigious mosque complexes in Cairo, such as those of Ibn Tūlūn and Sultan Hasan. During the course of his career, he authored at least 46 works about various religious topics, including his manuscript on the plague, and this corpus does not include a number of texts that have not survived.[9] Furthermore, his student Muḥammad was not the only copyist to record this text. A second copyist, Muḥammad b. Khalīl b. İbrāhīm al-Sawāfī al-Khalīlī al-Maqdisī, also added the text into a *mecmua* that includes works on the plague from al-Baylūnī, Kemalpaşazade and Zakariyya al-Ansārī that date from sometime between 1620 and 1626. This period following the first promulgation of Marʿī's text would culminate in the death of approximately 300,000 Egyptians.[10] The text later proved sadly relevant for Muḥammad b. Khalīl, as a subsequent folio contains marginalia informing us that both he and his brother ʿAbd al-Rahman lost sons to a later recurrence of the plague many years later in the spring of 1643.[11] In

---

7 As noted in an addendum to a copy of Zakariyya al-Ansārī, *Tuḥfat al-rāghibīn fī bayān amr al-ṭawāʿīn* (Istanbul: Süleymaniye Library, ms. Esad Efendi 3567), 74a.

8 See the brief biographical sketches in Melchert, "Marʿī b. Yūsuf," 287; and Kırbıyık, "Merʿî b. Yûsuf," 185.

9 For an extensive list of all his known works, both extant and lost, see Melchert, "Marʿī b. Yūsuf," 284–87.

10 Marʿī b. Yūsuf b. Abu Bakr Zayn al-Dīn al-Karmī (d. 1033/1624), *Taḥqīq al-ẓunūn bi-akhbār al-ṭāʿūn* (Istanbul: Süleymaniye Library, ms. Esad Efendi 3567), 21a-59a; Muḥammad b. Khalīl began copying the *mecmua* in 1029/1620 (18b-19a); subsequently, appended texts were added up to 1035/1626 (74a). For the impact of the plagues of the 1620s, see André Raymond, "Les Grands épidémies de peste au Caire aux XVIIe et XVIIIe siècles," *Bulletin d'études orientales* 25 (1972): 204–5; interestingly, to acquire this background information, Raymond seems to have consulted some kind of addendum to Marʿī's work *Kitāb nuzhat al-nāzirīn*, which was ostensibly completed over twenty years earlier, cf. Melchert, "Marʿī b. Yūsuf," 288.

11 Ibid., 39a; corroborating the observations of Raymond, 205.

addition to the two Muḥammads, three additional copies of the text are known to exist in various libraries around the world, suggesting that the text received at least a modest degree of circulation in Ottoman domains.[12]

The original autograph manuscript that Muḥammad b. Mūsa had prepared later found its way from Cairo to Istanbul, where it ended up in the hands of a Hanafi jurist named Süleyman b. Ahmed b. Yūsuf b. ʿAbdullah b. al-Shaykh Muḥammad al-Madanī al-Hanafī, who had been appointed as the prayer-caller for the Rüstem Pasha Mosque in Eminönü. It is not clear how Süleyman came by the manuscript, though the implied Medinese origin in the *laqab* of both the earlier copyist and the prayer-caller might provide a clue. Süleyman had the highest praise for the manuscript, claiming it had no equal on the subject, and praising its thoroughness in laying out the various critical perspectives. Given that the handwriting of the original was somewhat difficult to read, Süleyman prepared a clearer and fully voweled Arabic text of the manuscript for his own use, completing the job in 1703. It is also possible that the original manuscript was loaned to him by someone with links to the Ottoman royal family, since stamps in the work identify it as having been donated to the Laleli Mosque's manuscript collection as *waqf* by Sultan Selim III upon his founding of a library collection there in 1802.[13] We do not know when Süleyman passed away, but we do know the fate of his beautifully copied manuscript. Multiple stamps in the work indicate that it came into the possession of the future *şeyhülislâm* Ebü'l-Hayr Ahmed Efendi (d. 1741), a descendant of the notable Köprülü family of grand viziers who dominated later seventeenth-century Ottoman politics.[14]

The esteem that these Ottoman notables held for a Hanbali jurist such as Marʿī may require some explanation. After all, the Ottoman Empire and its learned hierarchies had deeply invested themselves in the promotion of the Hanafi school of law, and tended to discourage recourse to the representatives of other legal schools to some extent.[15] The answer likely lies in other works that Marʿī wrote which offered high praise for the Ottoman rulers of Egypt that attracted the atten-

---

12 Additional copies of the work that could not be consulted for this study have been catalogued in Riyadh, Berlin, and Paris; see Kırbıyık, 186.

13 Marʿī b. Yūsuf, *Taḥqīq al-ẓunūn bi-akhbār al-ṭāʿūn* (Istanbul: Süleymaniye Library, ms. Laleli 1344), 38b; as for a summary of the library's history, see İsmail E. Erünsal, "Lâleli Kütüphanesi," *Türkiye Diyanet Vakfı İslâm Ansiklopedisi* (Istanbul: Türkiye Diyanet Vakfı İslâm Araştırmaları Merkezi, 2003), v. 27, 89.

14 Marʿī b. Yūsuf, *Taḥqīq al-ẓunūn* (Süleymaniye Library, ms. Hacı Ahmed Paşa 115), 1a and 130b.

15 For a detailed account of the Ottoman relationship with the Hanafi school of law, see Guy Burak, *The Second Formation of Islamic Law: The Hanafī School in the Early Modern Ottoman Empire* (New York: Cambridge University Press, 2015).

tion of Ottoman readers.[16] As Irfana Hashmi points out in her recent dissertation, Marʿī most likely did this in conjunction with his attempts to reform the system of *waqf* administration in Egypt and restore his own position, for conflicts over resources with other scholars had caused him personal hardship.[17] Nevertheless, among subsequent generations of Ottoman officials and scholars, gratitude for Marʿī's strong backing of their rule likely reduced any reservations they might have had over his adherence to a different law school. By tracking the evolution of the text, therefore, we can establish that Muslim thinkers adhering to multiple law schools, and including notable Ottoman religious elites, developed a high regard for Marʿī's work. This alone makes an evaluation of the contents of his treatise on the plague a worthwhile endeavor.

Given the fact that plague was raging in Cairo at the time of its composition, it is perhaps not surprising that Marʿī arranged the text as a response to twenty questions that had been asked of previous generations of Hanbalite scholars, and likely also addressed questions being addressed to him by various contemporaries. As previous studies of Islamic jurisprudence have noted, the questions can be just as interesting as the answers, since they represent a mixture of historically rooted and contemporary issues of concern to Muslim communities. Interestingly, Marʿī's text seems to reflect a mixture of both the formal and more abstract models of textual jurisprudence that marked Islamic law in later periods, and the more immediate voices of contemporary questioners who sought to expand the discussion.[18] In compiling his responses to these queries, Marʿī ultimately structured a contemporary document aimed at addressing the latest of a series of recurrent waves of plague that had hit Egypt since the fourteenth century.[19]

---

16 One of these works was discussed by Michael Winter, "A Seventeenth-Century Arabic Panegyric of the Ottoman Dynasty," *Asian and African Studies* 13 (1979): 130–56.

17 See the remarks in Irfana Hashmi, "Patronage, Legal Practice, and Space in al-Azhar, 1500–1650," PhD diss., New York University, 2014, 226–28.

18 See, for example, Setrag Manoukian, "Fatvas as Asymmetrical Dialogues: Muḥammad Karim Khan Kirmani and his Questioners," *Islamic Legal Interpretation: Muftis and their Fatwas*, ed. Muḥammad Khalid Masud, Brinkley Messick, and David S. Powers (Cambridge: Harvard College, 1996), 162–72; and Brinkley Messick, *The Calligraphic State: Textual Domination and History in a Muslim Society* (Berkeley: University of California Press, 1993), 135–51, for more on these issues.

19 For the recurrent nature of the plague in Egypt, see Dols, *Black Death*, 305–14; Stuart J. Borsch, *The Black Death in Egypt and England: A Comparative Study* (Austin: University of Texas Press, 2005); idem, "Plague Depopulation and Irrigation Decay in Medieval Egypt," *The Medieval Globe* 1 (2014): 125–56; and Alan Mikhail, *Nature and Empire in Ottoman Egypt: An Environmental History* (Cambridge: Cambridge University Pres, 2011), 214–30.

The dialogue begins with Marʿī's response to a long-standing question: "When the plague occurred among the people, was it a punishment from God (*rijz*) and chastisement in all cases, or is it a chastisement in the exoteric (*zāhir*) sense but not in the esoteric (*bātin*) one, or is it aimed at the unbelievers and a kindness toward the Muslims?" Marʿī responded by listing the first known advent of the plague, which was unleashed upon Pharaoh due to his unwillingness to accept Moses's demands. In this case, he argues, the plague represents a chastisement of the unbelievers and a kindness toward Muslims. He corroborates this interpretation by citing other reports illustrating that the Israelites were punished for fornication and injustices that they committed. He then goes on to cite Prophetic traditions from the various canonical collections that indicate that the plague was a remnant of the punishments of the past, coming and going as it pleased, that had been inflicted by God upon the various unbelieving or sinning communities. He also introduces a standard view from the Prophetic traditions, which argues that if the plague occurs in the place where you are, you should not leave, and if you were to hear of it in a place where you had not yet gone, you should not travel there. He concludes with a tradition drawn from Abu Dawūd confirming that divine punishment for Muslims only occurs in the manifest world, and not in the afterlife. Oddly, in this tradition, the punishment in the manifest world takes the form of civil strife (*fitna*), earthquakes, and warfare (*qatl*), suggesting that these events were analogous to the appearance of plague.[20]

In terms of how Muslim thinkers viewed plague and epidemics, the second question Marʿī was asked is more interesting for our purposes: "What is the cause of the plague, and from what does it emanate? Is its cause putridity of the content of the air, as the physicians say, and if you say no, then what is the proof of the falseness of their doctrine in light of rational and transmitted proofs? Is the plague different from epidemic disease (*wabāʾ*), or is it the same thing?" To this question, Marʿī b. Yūsuf begins by responding with a fairly good summary of the state of Muslim medical knowledge on the topic—but then goes on to reject those conclusions:

> The doctors say the plague is a poisonous substance giving rise to a fatal tumor, and if its cause is putridity of the substance of the air, then Ibn Sīnā said that infectious disease is putridity of the substance of the air, which is the very component of human life and its support, and henceforth, life is not possible among living things without breathing. And corollary to

---

20 Marʿī b. Yūsuf, *Taḥqīq al-ẓunūn* (Süleymaniye Library, ms. Hacı Ahmed Paşa 115), 8b-14a; in staking out these positions, Marʿī closely follows the views of Ibn Ḥajar al-ʿAsqalānī, see Dols, *Black Death*, 110–13 and Stearns, *Infectious Ideas*, 27–28.

> that is the doctrine of some of them that infectious disease is composed of putridity occurring in the substance of the air via malignant, heavenly, or terrestrial causes, such as shooting stars and meteorites at the end of summer, and brackish water, and numerous decaying corpses. [But] whatever the physicians say about this being the cause of the plague, it is a falsehood. Those who adhere to the Law among the Traditionists and jurisprudents do not approve.[21]

Deferring the transmitted proofs part of the question to later chapters, Marʿī drew on the famed Hanbali jurist Ibn al-Qayyim al-Jawziyya (d. 1350),[22] an author of several books on medical topics, for the rational proofs arguing for the rejection of the physicians. In Marʿī's view, Ibn al-Qayyim had argued that if plague came from some kind of putridity in the air, then its spread among people and animals should be universal, and furthermore, plague occurs even in lands that have the healthiest air and water—a point which he reiterated multiple times in the text.[23] In addition, he pointed out that the plague did not spread evenly throughout the body, but that its effects were concentrated in certain parts of it. Moreover, since the doctors could find no effective cure for it, then it must be something caused by God, and concludes with the classic formulation that every plague is a form of infectious disease, but not every infectious disease is a plague. However, when Marʿī's presentation is compared to Ibn al-Qayyim's *al-Ṭibb al-nabawī*, it suggests that Marʿī was either misrepresenting, or unaware of a significant part of the Hanbali master's views on the subject. Ibn al-Qayyim did note the lesser incidence of disease in the springtime, but he did not categorically deny the importance of putrefaction as a cause of plague despite its ultimate spiritual causes.[24] This section therefore raises an interesting question—might some elements of the Ottoman religious elite have acquired a misleading idea of Ibn al-Qayyim's views on the subject via Marʿī's work?

Additional evidence appears in the subsequent ninth chapter of the work, which tackled the question of whether flight from the plague and avoidance of

---

21 Ibid., 14b-15a.

22 For a full biography and works, see Livnat Holtzman, "Ibn Qayyim al-Jawziyyah (1292–1350)," *Essays in Arabic Literary Biography 1350–1850*, ed. Joseph E. Lowry and Devin J. Stewart (Wiesbaden: Harrassowitz Verlag, 2009), 202–23.

23 See, for example, Marʿī b. Yūsuf, *Taḥqīq al-ẓunūn* (Süleymaniye Library, ms. Hacı Ahmed Paşa 115), 15b and 19a.

24 Compare the remarks in Ibn Qayyim al-Jawziyya, *Medicine of the Prophet*, trans. Penelope Johnstone (Cambridge: The Islamic Texts Society, 2004), 27–32 and esp. 29–32 with ibid., 15a-16b.

places where it was present was categorically prohibited or not. In a lengthy discussion of the sources that ruled on the topic, Marʿī again invoked Ibn al-Qayyim's discussion of the subject and presented his views as follows: "The Prophet combined the full range of precautionary measures for his community in his prohibition of entering into it [i.e., plague-ridden areas] and fleeing from it. Verily in going to a land that has [plague] in it, there is an exposure to calamity while coming to it in the place of its ascendancy, and acting against one's interests, and this is contrary to sacred law and reason. On the contrary, it is his avoidance of entering its land via a well-defended entrance, which God has shown to him. And it is a defense against dangerous places and climes."[25] However, Marʿī did not include the subsequent advice of Ibn al-Qayyim that avoiding polluted places during a time of plague and restricting one's activity while it was occurring was the best strategy to cope with it.[26] Instead, he stressed multiple narratives that suggested that those who fled never came to any good end, and that caliphal exemplars such as ʿUmar b. al-Khattāb and ʿUmar b. ʿAbd al-ʿAzīz had set precedents rejecting the idea of either entering plague-stricken areas or fleeing from them. In other words, while Ibn al-Qayyim's discussion of the plague suggested that potential victims could engage in behaviors that might help to avoid the worst dangers of the plague, a reader of Marʿī's plague text would instead absorb a message that there was no way to avoid the will of God, and resignation to his will was the only logical response. Ultimately, in the way he constructed his responses to these questions, Marʿī seems to be following more the argumentation laid down in scholars like Ibn Ḥajar or his Hanbali predecessor Muḥammad al-Manbijī (d. 1383), rather than following Ibn al-Qayyim.[27]

Moving on to the third question, Marʿī was asked to distinguish between the explanations of the plague given by the physicians and the jurisprudents. He began by citing Ibn Sīnā's description of the symptoms of the plague in detail, including the location of the buboes and the fact that their color often indicated whether recovery was possible or not. He then concluded by noting that "some of them

25 The remarks are roughly quoted from Ibn Qayyim, *Medicine of the Prophet*, 30–31; compare with ibid., 44a–b.

26 Ibn Qayyim, *Medicine of the Prophet*, 31–32.

27 See, for example, the close parallels in Ibn Ḥajar's work that are described in Lawrence I. Conrad, "Review of *Badhl al-Māʿūn fī fadl al-ṭāʿūn*," *Medical History* 39: 3 (1995), 391–3; and Dols, "Al-Manbiji's Report of the Plague: A Treatise on the Plague of 764–5/1362–4 in the Middle East," *The Black Death: The Impact of the Fourteenth-Century Plague*, ed. Daniel Williman (Binghamton, NY: Medieval and Renaissance Texts and Studies, 1982), 65–76. The discussion of various sources pointing in this direction takes up nearly one-tenth of the text; see Marʿī b. Yūsuf, *Taḥqīq al-ẓunūn* (Süleymaniye Library, ms. Hacı Ahmed Paşa 115), 44b–54a.

explain that the plague is from a rushing of the blood to one of the limbs, and most of them say that it is an agitation (*hayajān*) of the blood and its swelling up (*intifākh*)."[28] In Marʿī's view, however, this posed no serious contradiction to the explanations given by Muslim jurisprudence. The physicians accurately reported the external manifestations of the problem; what they lacked was the understanding of the hidden meaning behind them, and this was where the jurisprudent had the superior position. There was no contradiction between the observations of the physicians and the causes argued by Hanbali jurisprudence, which is that the plague is caused by the stabbing of the victim by unseen *jinn*—thus the inflammation and bloody, pus-filled discharges from within the body.

However much Marʿī disparaged the views of the physicians on the causes of the plague, he reserved special condemnation for astrologers who claimed to have knowledge about the plague in a later chapter, comparing their work to that of pre-Islamic soothsayers (*kāhin*) and diviners (*ʿarrāf*).[29] He even cited the Abbasid caliph al-Mansūr's use of astrologers in founding the city of Baghdad in the year 763, under the presumption that no caliph would ever perish in the city. While al-Mansūr himself would die while traveling on the road to Mecca, eventually the caliph al-Amīn died under siege in the city some fifty years later, and subsequent caliphs did as well. This ultimately proved the falsity of the astrologers' claims about anything, much less the causes of the plague.[30]

Moving on to the fourth question, Marʿī's audience predictably asked what the cause of this assault of the *jinn* upon humankind would be. Marʿī responded by citing multiple sources to prove that the reason for the plague is the outbreak of widespread fornication (*fāḥisha*) and sinful behavior. Ultimately, since fornication takes place largely in secret, the secret attacks of the *jinn* on humankind are the result.[31] However, those who were asking for the opinions were perhaps not so quick to buy into these explanations, as they demanded a clarification via a subsequent fifth question: "So you said that its cause was fornication. So what is the frame of reference of whoever dies from it, but has no incidence of fornication, such as children, among whom it is no more preponderant than the perpetrators of fornication? And how did it occur frequently in the early period of Islam, given the limited nature of their fornication ... and its rule that it be lessened with a decline in fornication, and increasing when it increases?"[32]

28 Ibid., 17b-18b.

29 Ibid., 97a; see also Stearns, *Infectious Ideas*, 25.

30 Ibid., 100a–b.

31 Ibid., 26a–b.

32 Ibid., 3b–4a.

Here, Marʿī b. Yūsuf's questioners were touching on age-old debates from the formative years of Islamic theology about predestination. According to tradition, the Muslim scholar Abu al-Hasan al-Ashʿarī (d. 936) had in fact broken with the Muʿtazilite movement over this very point, as a sinner allowed to grow old enough to commit sins would end up suffering God's punishment, whereas a child who died young was given the grace of not being allowed to reach such a stage.[33] Not surprisingly, Marʿī followed the line of al-Ashʿarī by arguing that God had predestined such a thing for children as a form of good fortune, in that it gave them the status of martyrs. The lack of ability to engage in sexual intercourse only increased their righteousness in this regard. He also cites a tradition from Ibn Ḥibbān to the effect that God assigns all human beings a rank which they attain by their actions, and thereafter he would tempt them with detestable things until they attained that rank. As for the early and most pious generations of Islam, Marʿī fell back on the argument that due to the level of their piety, they would receive God's censure for even the least of sins, since their example was the one upon which the subsequent generations of the Islamic community would draw.[34]

The topic apparently had a strong resonance with Marʿī's audience, however, as the issue came up in the final two questions that his treatise addressed. The nineteenth question focused on the issue of people who had lost at least three sons to disease, and confirmed the understanding that people who had suffered in this manner would be guaranteed a place in Paradise. Drawing on multiple traditions from various sources across the canonical spectrum, Marʿī tells of how a woman approached the Prophet Muḥammad with a sick infant son and beseeched him to intercede with God on his behalf, since she had already buried three prior to him. In good concordance with the Muslim views on God's predestination, the Prophet could only promise her that she would never enter Hell, as an impenetrable barrier would be erected to prevent her from ever going there. He also cites another tradition upon which God questions His angels in regard to having seized a son from one of his servants. When asked "what did my servant say?" the angels replied that he had praised him and uttered the traditional Muslim acceptance of God's will in such matters. God responded by commanding the building of a house for his servant in Paradise as a reward.[35] In a subsequent tradition, it is even

33 For more on al-Ashʿari's break with the Muʿtazilites, see W. Montgomery Watt, *The Formative Period of Islamic Thought* (Oxford: Oneworld, 2007), 304–6; which builds on ideas first advanced in idem, *Free Will and Predestination in Early Islam* (London: Luzac & Company, 1948), 136–37.

34 Marʿī b. Yūsuf, *Taḥqīq al-ẓunūn* (Süleymaniye Library, ms. Hacı Ahmed Paşa 115), 31a–b.

35 Ibid., 110b-111a.

recounted that the dead children have the power to intercede on behalf of their bereaved parents on the Day of Judgment, suggesting the degree to which comfort needed to be provided for those who had lost so much.[36]

As if to underscore the worries of the Muslim community in regard to this matter, it came up again in the final twentieth chapter, which asked about the requirements for finding consolation and forbearance in the face of losing loved ones, but also tacked on a final addition "and where is the dwelling place of infants which are the sensory organs of the heart (*ḥussāsat al-qalb*) and light of the eyes?"[37] Marʿī responded by stressing once again that the consensus opinion among both the Hanbali and Shafiʿi schools of law was that infants would go to heaven, and ended his work with two traditions. The first stated that the souls of the children of Muslims were among the small birds dwelling in the tree of Paradise, with the Prophet İbrāhīm acting as their guardian, and the second tradition concluded by noting that all infants are born into Islam, so they are properly fed and given sufficient drink in Paradise while saying "O Lord, bring my father to me."[38] Both traditions reflect a historical context where sufficient food, drink, and protection for children had become heightened concerns, and underscored the appeal to Ottoman thinkers still recovering from the ravages of the seventeenth century.[39]

Even in sections of the text where, at least in theory, the question of children's ultimate fate was not at issue, remarks about it were inserted into the text. As shall be noted shortly, when listing all of the plagues that had afflicted the Muslim community since its inception, Marʿī made a note of the numerous sons born to members of the early generations of Islam among the Companions and others who perished during the plague. Citing clearly hyperbolic numbers, in the plague of al-Jārif, the famed Companion Anas b. Mālik supposedly lost 33 children, and Abu Bakr lost 40. In another plague thirty years later, another Companion, Ibn Sīrīn, supposedly buried 30 children in his own right.[40] While these asides are not directly linked to the chapters involving the fate of children killed by the plague,

36 Ibid., 112b-113a.

37 Ibid., 8a.

38 Ibid., 128a-b.

39 For more on the difficult and often food-insecure conditions of the late sixteenth and early seventeenth century, see Sam White, *The Climate of Rebellion in the Early Modern Ottoman Empire* (Cambridge: Cambridge University Press, 2011); and Geoffrey Parker, *Global Crisis: War, Climate Change and Catastrophe in the Seventeenth Century* (New Haven: Yale University Press, 2013).

40 Marʿī b. Yūsuf, *Taḥqīq al-ẓunūn* (Süleymaniye Library, ms. Hacı Ahmed Paşa 115), 94b–95a.

they served to offer comfort to Marʿī's audience by underscoring the price paid by even the most pious members of the community.

Additional comfort could be offered to the victims of plague as well, in the form of a guaranteed marker of martyrdom for those who died from it. This idea was not a novel one in earlier religious literature, and Marʿī offered up a lengthy list of corroborating traditions from various sources that likened plague victims to those who had fallen on the battlefield in the cause of Islam, as long as they followed the aforementioned religious injunctions to not flee from the plague. As a result, plague victims would be exempt from the tribulations of the grave. This could even extend to sinners and perpetrators of great crimes, although Marʿī cited discussions from Ibn Ḥajar that suggested that people who fell into this category were not necessarily at the same level as their more pious counterparts.[41] However, this simple fact then led into another discussion where Marʿī had to deal with additional questions about how to classify the nature of martyrdom when it occurred in different contexts—how did dying from the plague compare to other possible forms of martyrdom? After all, Marʿī noted, there were some twenty-three different recorded possibilities for martyrdom that were mentioned in the various Muslim sources of which he was aware, ranging from dying due to gastric ailments, tuberculosis, pneumonia, or strokes.[42]

This careful categorization of the possibilities of martyrdom ultimately required that martyrdom be divided into three separate types: 1) martyrdom in both this world and the afterlife; 2) martyrdom in this world only; and 3) martyrdom only in the afterlife. This basic categorization was not new, and Marʿī was likely following the lead of the aforementioned Hanbalite jurist al-Manbijī, who had first laid out these comforting ideas in a series of works following the first waves of plague in the fourteenth century.[43] The first group is the easiest to identify, in that they die striving in the way of God, often in battle with enemies of the faith, and the proof of their martyrdom can be attested to by both the people of this world and the denizens of the unseen world. However, the martyrs of this world represent people who go out to strive in the way of God, but do so in such a way that they are not pure in their intentions. For example, a person may go off to battle with an enemy of the Muslims out of hypocrisy, or solely to maintain their

---

41 Ibid., 54a–60a.

42 Ibid., 60a–b.

43 Anna Akasoy, "Islamic Attitudes to Disasters in the Middle Ages: A Comparison of Earthquakes and Plagues," *The Medieval History Journal* 10: 1–2 (2007): 398–99; for a brief description of al-Manbijī's intersection with the plague, see Dols, "Al-Manbiji's *Report of the Plague*," 65–76.

good name, or simply to win a share of the wealth. Others might die fleeing from an advancing enemy, rather than obeying God's injunctions to have courage in the face of danger. As a result, their martyrdom only applies to this world, and God and his angels may well accuse them of malfeasance in his actions in the afterlife, leading to their consignment to the Fire. Plague victims, on the other hand, belong to the most exalted rank of the third group, who are the martyrs of the afterlife only. In this case, since their death cannot be witnessed in this world, the witnesses to their martyrdom will be found only in the afterlife in the form of God and his angels, who will then direct those who have been afflicted to their place in Paradise. The analogy to those who have fallen in combat with the enemy proved apt in this case, because Marʿī's text had already characterized plague as an internal, unseen stabbing of a person's inside by malevolent *jinn*. His audience was left with the comfort that since the people of this world were only capable of seeing the effects of these internal wounds rather than their cause, they could not bear witness to the actual process of martyrdom; that could be undertaken only by God and his angels.[44]

Given Marʿī's rejection of putrefaction as a cause of plague, it is not surprising that he argued against the tactic of avoiding contamination. When asked about the permissibility of paying visits to sick people, Marʿī promptly presented a tradition that said that not only was it considered a permissible practice, but one of five duties that a Muslim had toward other Muslims, which also included returning a greeting, participating in funerals, and the like.[45] In terms of the plague, he cited a tradition from Mālik b. Dīnār to the effect that times of plague offered no better time to acquire benefit via the burial of the dead, the praying of funeral prayers, and the consolation of the bereaved.[46] However, such visitations could not include prayers aimed at prolonging the life of the afflicted person, for such prayers were pointless attempts to deny the predetermined will of God on such matters. For those who might argue that there were examples of the Prophet Muḥammad beseeching God for an end to sickness, Marʿī argued that in this case, the prayer included the understanding that there could be no cure for sickness save the power of God himself.[47]

---

44 The discussion of this various cases is laid out as a conclusion to the sections on martyrdom in Marʿī's text; see Marʿī b. Yūsuf, *Taḥqīq al-ẓunūn* (Süleymaniye Library, ms. Hacı Ahmed Paşa 115), 63b–66b.

45 Ibid., 107a.

46 Ibid., 109a.

47 Ibid., 102a and 108b.

The question of whether or not it was permissible to pray for the remission of the plague was a much more fraught question. After all, the Prophet had prayed for his community to be afflicted by affliction and plague, which Marʿī confirmed in his response to the twelfth question about the ramifications of such a statement. Would it really be acceptable to pray for the remission of something which the Prophet himself had sanctioned? Interestingly, Marʿī hedged on the question when asked whether this act was legitimate. On the one hand, he claimed that he could not find any evidence of any pious figure engaging in such an act until after the tenth century—explicitly locating it as an innovation brought to bear in a later time frame in Islamic history. On the other hand, he also could not find anyone explicitly declaring it forbidden. In the end, drawing on figures like Ibn Ḥajar (d. 1449) and al-Suyūṭī (d. 1505), he suggested there were certain distinctions that had to be drawn. Some argued that since plague was a special category of disease, it was not permissible to pray for its lifting, as opposed to more mundane forms of infectious disease. Others argued that there was no harm in praying for its remission at an individual level, but just as with prayers for rain, it was an innovation to gather large numbers of the community for public prayers for its lifting. Marʿī himself sided with this point of view, which would have put him and his followers in conflict with common Ottoman practice.[48] Furthermore, in a subsequent chapter, Marʿī denied any efficacy of the attempts of physicians to prevent or cure the plague, likening such actions to attempting to cure old age or intellectual disabilities.[49]

By way of conclusion, historians will find Marʿī's discussion of the Prophet's well-sourced statement that "my community is not destroyed save by conflict (*taʿn*) and plague (*ṭāʿūn*)" of interest. Given the more extensive inquiry into topics that marked his era, Marʿī was not content to simply rely on the obvious soundness of the Prophetic traditions on the matter here, and proceeded to comb through all of the historical works at his disposal to further document his case. Following the lead of earlier authorities on the subject, Marʿī began by focusing primarily on the victims of intra-Muslim conflict, rather than just generalizing the Prophet's remarks toward all Muslims engaged in any kind of conflict, and then listed all the examples of conflict or civil strife (*fitna*) that occurred, starting from the assassination of the caliph ʿUthmān and the outbreak of civil war thereafter and carrying

48 Ibid., 72b–76a (noting that fol. 74 was accidentally skipped by the archivist). In contrast to Marʿī's presentation, Ibn Ḥajar may have given contradictory statements in regard to public prayers on the plague; see the remarks in Stearns, *Infectious Ideas*, 164; idem, "New Directions in the Study of Religious Responses to the Black Death," *History Compass* 7, no. 5 (2009): 1363–75. See also Dols, *Black Death*, 246–51.

49 Ibid., 77a.

on the list all the way up to the seventeenth century with strife among the tribes of the Arabian Peninsula, Egypt and Syria.[50] He then commences with a similar list seeking to document the casualties caused by various plagues since the inception of the Muslim community:

Table 1. List of Outbreaks in Islamic Lands and Estimated Mortality, According to Marʿī b. Yūsuf. Source: *Taḥqīq al-ẓunūn bi-akhbār al-ṭāʿūn*, Istanbul, Süleymaniye Library, ms. Hacı Ahmed Paşa 115.

Event and year of occurrence	Reported number of casualties
Plague of ʿAmwās (639)	25,000–30,000
Plague of al-Jārif (690)[51]	over 214,000
Plague of al-Fityān (date unknown)	not given
Plague of al-Ashrāf (ca. 702–714)	not given
Plague of ʿAdī b. Artān (719)	not given
Plague of Abbasid Revolution (ca. 750)	not given
Great Plague from Hind, al-ʿAjam (1032)	4,000 (in Mosul alone)
Plague in Mosul, al-Jazīra, Baghdad (1047)	400,000
Ten-month plague in Egypt (1063)	not given
Plague in Damascus (1076)	496,500
The Black Death / "Universal Plague" (1348)	half the population; 20,000 per day in Cairo
Second "Universal Plague" (1430)	not given
Plague in Egypt (1449)	5,000 per day in Cairo
Widespread Plague (1601)	not given
Second Widespread Plague (1611)	3,000 per day in Cairo

The list assembled by Marʿī suggests that in his historical investigation, the plague had occurred in four waves. The first struck the early Muslim community and the Umayyads and waned with the coming of the Abbasids; the second occurred in the eleventh century in conjunction with the invasion of the Seljuks and other groups into the Middle East; the third was that of the Black Death and its recurrences; and the last were the plagues of the seventeenth century that marked Marʿī's own

50 Ibid., 86b–93b.

51 Literally, "the plague that swept away many in torrents," so named because of the number of people it carried off; see ibid., 94a.

time.[52] In particular, the inclusion of the eleventh-century wave of plagues corresponds to historical discussions of waves of epidemic disease that followed in the wake of famine and ecological crisis in the region.[53] Underscoring the challenge that the plagues posed to Marʿī and his contemporaries, another compilation of texts on the plague that includes a copy of Marʿī's work ended with its copyist adding that plagues had also occurred in 1619, the date that Marʿī finished his text, followed by two more outbreaks in 1622 and 1626. Another text recorded an additional outbreak in the spring of 1643.[54]

Ultimately, the interest that Marʿī b. Yūsuf's text on the plague generated may be indicative of a more conservative intellectual trend among some members of the Ottoman elite during the seventeenth and eighteenth century. Marʿī's text represented a selective compilation of Hanbalite jurisprudence that reinforced a fatalistic approach to the plague grounded in obedience to divine authority. From this perspective, human agency in confronting outbreaks of plague was sharply limited, and an acceptance of God's will was the only proper response. In return, God would reserve special rewards and comforts for His suffering and afflicted community in the afterlife. Since the ultimate cause of the plague was grounded primarily in human immorality and its chastisement, taking any action to flee the plague or neglect one's basic human obligations to others who were ill could not have a good outcome. Questions still remain as to why Marʿī's various Ottoman followers found this vision compelling even a century later, in contrast to some of the alternative Ottoman responses that had developed during this time frame. It is possible that Ottoman elites wanted to shore up declining tax resource bases negatively affected by flight from various locales, or to prevent the continued swelling of overcrowded urban centers, but for the time being, this can only remain a point of speculation.[55]

52 Ibid., 93b-97b. This model diverges from a Eurocentric periodization of historical plague pandemics. For further discussion, see Varlık, "New Science and Old Sources: Why the Ottoman Experience of Plague Matters," *The Medieval Globe* 1 (2014): 193–227.

53 As detailed in the recent work of Ronnie Ellenbaum, *The Collapse of the Eastern Mediterranean: Climate Change and the Decline of the East, 950–1072* (Cambridge: Cambridge University Press, 2012), 100–2.

54 See remarks added to end of Zakariyyā al-Ansārī, *Tuḥfat al-rāghibīn*, 74a; and Marʿī b. Yūsuf, *Taḥqīq al-ẓunūn* (Istanbul: Süleymaniye Library, ms. Esad Efendi 3567), 39a. As noted in n. 10 above, these dates are corroborated by Raymond, 204–5.

55 See, for example, the remarks of Sam White, "Rethinking Disease in Ottoman History," *International Journal of Middle East Studies* 42: 4 (2010): 553–61.

Hagiographical and Sufism-Based Accounts of Disease and Public Health

From the fifteenth century onward, Ottoman Sufi leaders and devotees, building on earlier traditions, began to record anecdotal narratives about key religious figures in increasing numbers.[56] While the otherworldly elements in these texts force us to use caution in drawing conclusions from them, they often allow for an evaluation of the social and political contexts for Sufi responses to outbreaks of disease via hagiographical narratives, or even the personal papers of Sufi leaders. This section will focus on works produced by the devotees of the Halveti order, for while the patterns of their writings may not necessarily be representative of the whole of Ottoman Sufi thinking about these issue, they represent a useful test case against which other Sufi orders might be compared because of the order's extensive range and influence during the early modern Ottoman period.[57]

Since the advent of the Enlightenment tradition, the appearance of supernatural or divine phenomena in the writings of medieval and early modern religious figures, Muslim or otherwise, led to their marginalization as sources for historical inquiry. However, recent scholars have advocated for a more sophisticated approach to these types of sources as they seek to reinterpret their contents in a way that does not require that they be taken as literal representations of past events. Instead, these scholars advance the proposition that hagiographical sources act as a reflection of the changing ideas and didactic strategies employed by mystical thinkers in the times and places they were constructed, and therefore have potential utility in interpreting various intersections between Sufi writings and their social contexts.[58] Furthermore, as we shall see below, overlaps between different kinds of sources increasingly suggest that these narratives may have actual historical foundations that undergird the didactic or miraculous elements inserted by subsequent authors.

Multiple accounts describing Ottoman Halveti responses to disease occur in sources dating from the sixteenth through the eighteenth centuries. Of course,

---

56 For a brief overview of this phenomenon, see John J. Curry, "The Growth of a Turkish-Language Hagiographical Literature Within the Halveti Order of the 16th and 17th Centuries," *The Turks*, edited by Hasan Celal Güzel et al. (Ankara: Yeni Türkiye Press, 2002), v. 3, 912–20.

57 For more on the origins and spread of the Halveti order in Ottoman domains, see John J. Curry, *The Transformation of Muslim Mystical Thought in the Ottoman Empire: The Rise of the Halveti Order 1350–1650* (Edinburgh: Edinburgh University Press, 2010).

58 See, for example, the introduction and articles in John J. Curry and Erik S. Ohlander, eds., *Sufism and Society: Arrangements of the Mystical in the Muslim World, 1200–1800* (London: Routledge Press, 2012).

many of these narratives were marked by *topoi* grounded in earlier models of Muslim sainthood that the Halveti had inherited from their past. As a result, confirmation of sainthood could be found in relation to the incidence of epidemic disease in two basic forms. The first was that of "community protectors," who traded security from the afflictions of the natural world in return for their personal intercession with the Divine, which sometimes required self-sacrifice. The second was that of the "director," based on the idea that saints could control whether natural calamities would afflict people. For example, they could channel various forms of natural affliction as a means to punish wayward or disrespectful members of the Muslim community, or alternatively, rescue them from it.

In the earliest Halveti sources, the "protector" model appeared more frequently. The most notable example was the Cemal el-Halveti (d. 1499).[59] A descendant of the prominent Aksarayî family of the Karaman region which would also produce Sultan Selim I's grand vizier Pirî Pasha (d. 1532) and *şeyhülislam* Zenbilli Ali Efendi (d. 1525), Cemal took a different path by becoming a wandering devotee of various Halveti shaykhs sometime after 1461. However, he re-emerged in Ottoman political circles a decade and a half later in conjunction with the court of Şehzade Bayezid II (d. 1512) in Amasya. After supporting Bayezid in his struggle with his brother Cem to claim the Ottoman throne in 1481, he was invited to the Ottoman capital to establish himself and his following at the Koca Mustafa Pasha Mosque.[60]

However, for our purposes, it was the end of his life that is most illuminating. Near the end of the fifteenth century, Istanbul was stricken by a deadly earthquake and a recurrence of plague (*ṭāʿūn*) that had swept across Afro-Eurasia since the Black Death. While dealing with one such event was terrifying enough to a premodern Ottoman society, to have both strike the population at the same time was especially unnerving and a potential portent of the Day of Judgment, and a great fear settled over the capital.[61] According to the hagiography of Sinaneddin Yusuf b. Ya'kub el-Germiyanî (d. 1581), Bayezid II gathered the religious dignitaries of the capital together to discuss the situation, and they concluded that a prominent

59 Some studies claim Cemal el-Halveti's death date as 900/1494; however, given the suspicious correlation with the end of the Muslim ninth century, the latter, more frequently mentioned date is probably a better guess.

60 For a more thorough discussion of Cemal el-Halveti's life and career, see John J. Curry, "The Intersection of Past and Present in the Genesis of an Ottoman Sufi Order: The Life of Cemal el-Halveti (d. 900/1494 or 905/1499) and the Origins of the Halveti *Tarîqa*," *Journal of Turkish Studies (In Memoriam Şinasi Tekin III)* 32 (2008): 121–41.

61 For the linkage between earthquakes, plague, and Muslim eschatology and apocalyptic thought, see Akasoy, "Islamic Attitudes to Disasters," 391–96.

religious figure needed to be sent to the Prophet's tomb to offer prayers on behalf of the suffering population. Citing Cemal's ostensible line of descent from the first caliph Abu Bakr, the gathering nominated him for the task. The degree of importance attached to the project was symbolized by the 40,000 silver coins sent to Cemal, along with 50 gold coins sent to each of the forty followers who would accompany him on the journey. After the men of state ferried Cemal's entourage across the Bosphorus, the earthquake aftershocks ceased and the plague immediately went into remission. Bayezid responded by trying to recall Cemal, but this came to naught when Cemal informed him that "our life has come to an end; the pilgrimage garb has not yet been guided to us, the implements of residence have been exchanged for the implements of the journey." He subsequently died while on the pilgrimage route several stages south of Damascus.[62]

This narrative established Cemal as a "protector" of the Ottoman capital who sacrificed himself to save the population from natural calamity. However, tensions over Cemal's role surface in other hagio-biographical accounts dealing with his life in the form of variant readings. In the earliest known account of these events recorded by Lâmiʿî Çelebi (d. 1532), the affliction of the capital city is described as "epidemic disease" (*wabāʾ*), not plague, although the account corroborates the narrative about Cemal being sent by the Sultan to pray for intercession in the Holy Cities, and claims he died at a staging point known as Barʾiyya without accomplishing that aim. Nevertheless, Istanbul was free of disease for many years thereafter.[63]

A subsequent account from Mahmud Helvacıbaşızade Ḥulvî (d. 1654), writing in the early seventeenth-century, drew on Sinaneddin Yusuf's account as a source, but transformed the narrative yet again. The focus for the disaster was placed on earthquakes rather than the plague, and described Istanbul as having been transformed into a city of tents. While a major earthquake could certainly have contributed to the outbreak of disease via disruptions in sanitation and food and water supplies, it is still interesting that the narrative omitted mention of disease. However, this source may also be the least reliable, as it dated these events as taking place in the year 1504–05, at least five years after the most generally accepted death date for Cemal el-Halveti.[64] Given that a major wave of plague afflicted the

62 Sinaneddin Yusuf b. Yaʾkub (d. 989/1581), *Tezkiretü'l-Halvetiyye* (Istanbul: Süleymaniye Library, ms. Esad Efendi 1372/1), 13a-14a.

63 Mahmud b. ʿOsman b. ʿAli Nakkaş b. İlyas Lâmiʿî Çelebi (d. 938/1532), *Nefehâtü'l-Üns: Evliyâ Menkıbeleri*, eds. Süleyman Uludağ and Mustafa Kara (Istanbul: Marifet Yayınları, 1998), 708–9.

64 Mahmud Helvacıbaşızade Ḥulvî (d. 1064/1654), *Lemezât-ı Hulviyye ez-Lamaʿât-ı ʿUlviyye* (Istanbul: Süleymaniye Library, ms. Halet Efendi 281), 211a–b. However, Ḥulvî's work, though valuable, was not always noted for its historical accuracy with dates; see the remarks

Ottoman Empire between 1491 and 1503, and Istanbul specifically between 1497 and 1502, the sources are hardly irreconcilable.[65]

Whatever the case, all of the narratives carry a strong overtone of Cemal undertaking an act of self-sacrifice to ensure the health and safety of the Muslim community. According to Ḥulvî, Cemal was not the only figure to have done this, as his own Sufi master, Muḥammad el-Erzincanî (d. 1474), died under similar circumstances when he suddenly began engaging in ascetic and intercessory prayers in the central mosque at a time of year when such things were not normally undertaken. When asked about it, he responded that God was angry with them, and planned to punish them with an earthquake. His activity was meant to deflect God's wrath from them, seeing as the community had always been kind to him and his following. When the earthquake came, the community of Erzincan was spared, but the mosque's roof caved in and killed Muḥammad and several of his followers. Like his successor Cemal, Muḥammad protected his community from natural calamity, be it epidemic disease or earthquake. However, the account also mentions that Muḥammad's sacrifice was immediately questioned by certain "hypocrites" who argued that a true shaykh would never have died this way. The debate was abruptly cut short by a loud call from the heavens: "O ye who claim to be all-knowing, speak not of things that ye know not lest you be held responsible." This epilogue indicates that by Ḥulvî's time, hostility or suspicion had developed toward ideas of Sufis' intercessory powers.[66]

Other Halveti shaykhs also reflected this role. İbrahim-i Gülşenî (d. 1534), a leader of one of the Halveti sub-branches in Egypt, was also presented as having sacrificed himself in a similar way. Muḥyi-yi Gülşenî (d. 1606), his hagiographer, related that Egypt was struck by a terrible plague in the month of Ramadan that took a heavy toll on the population. The pace of the disease was so rapid that many who left their homes for temporary business in other parts of the region took to placing their names and dwelling locations on scraps of paper inside of their turbans so their loved ones could be informed if they died. The speed with which the epidemic spread indicates one of the multiple and periodic recurrences of plague that took place between the fourteenth and nineteenth century.[67] In contrast to the

of Curry, *Transformation*, 22–23.

65 As noted in Varlık, *Plague and Empire in the Early Modern Mediterranean World: The Ottoman Experience, 1347–1600* (Cambridge: Cambridge University Press, 2015), 145–49.

66 Ḥulvî, *Lemezât-ı Hulviyye*, 201b-202a.

67 For a detailed study of various waves of plague following the initial fourteenth-century outbreak, see n. 19 above. In addition, see William H. McNeill, *Plagues and Peoples* (Garden City, NY: Anchor Press, 1976); Varlık, *Plague and Empire*. Recurrences of the plague in Egypt

later prohibition issued by figures like Marʿī b. Yūsuf, the religious and political notables made three attempts to pray for relief outside of Cairo. When they failed to obtain any result, they came to İbrahim and asked him to try.

İbrahim warned them that the will of God was not something he had control over, but told them to return on the eighth day of the month of Shawwal, after the Eid al-Fitr. When they did, İbrahim shocked the assembly by turning to his followers and bidding them farewell, saying "let my soul be a ransom and exchange for all of you." After an all-night vigil spent in prayer, he crumpled to the floor while trying to perform the prayers, and died.[68]

İbrahim's hagiographer Muḥyi was so invested in this idea that he invoked it a second time when discussing a recurrence of the plague that was sweeping through Egypt in 1602. By his account, after listening to his colleagues complaining about the plague, and realizing that the end of Ramadan was near, Muḥyi publicly prayed that his own soul be sacrificed in exchange for that of his friends, following the model of İbrahim. He nearly got his wish when he injured his leg while getting on his horse an hour later. While watching the injured area swell up, he wrote to himself in the manuscript, "I don't know, will it pass, or won't it?" Although Muḥyi would go on to live four more years, proving premature in his wish, he still claimed that Egypt's casualties during the epidemic were far smaller than in other regions of the Ottoman domains, implying that his gesture counted for something.[69]

Yet leaving aside these otherworldly interventions, Muḥyi also recorded that İbrahim had addressed the topic directly in this world. When the Akkoyunlu collapsed at the end of the fifteenth century, and their capital Tabriz fell to the Safavid troops, it was afflicted simultaneously with an outbreak of plague. In response, the people of the city went to İbrahim and asked for a *fatwa* allowing them to flee. As we have seen previously with Marʿī b. Yūsuf, this was a contentious issue: some Muslim thinkers rejected the legitimacy of flight from plague.[70] However, İbrahim and a colleague, Molla Muḥammad Nakhçıvanî, countered this view by stating that people should flee. They offered as proof that the Prophet Muḥammad

---

up to the mid-nineteenth century are also catalogued in Daniel Panzac, *La peste dans l'empire ottoman, 1700–1850* (Leuven: E. Peeters, 1985), 622; and in Dols, "The Second Plague Pandemic and Its Recurrences in the Middle East: 1347–1894," *Journal of the Economic and Social History of the Orient* 22: 2 (1979): 162–89.

68 Muḥyi-yi Gülşeni (d. 1014/1606), *Menâkıb-i İbrâhîm-i Gülşeni ve Şemlelizâde Ahmed Efendi, Şîve-i Tarikat-ı Gülşeni*, ed. Tahsin Yazıcı (Ankara: Türk Tarih Kurumu Basımevi, 1982), 449–50 and 463.

69 Ibid., 269–70.

70 See, for example, Stearns, *Infectious Ideas*, 162–63.

had avoided a winter pasture ground where a plague had occurred, along with the tradition "flee from the leper just like you flee from a lion." In citing these traditions, İbrahim took a firm position on a controversy that had been raging since at least the ninth century about the potential contradictions in the narratives related to the Prophet's views on contagion.[71] He also added, in reference to his own reaction to the growing Safavid threat, the fact that the Prophet had fled the danger in Mecca and gone to Medina, saying "flight is from whoever does not obey the laws of the messengers."[72] They continued by citing a narrative of the second caliph ʿUmar turning back from Syria because of the plague, and upon being criticized for avoiding God's judgment, replies that he was fleeing from His judgment to His will.[73] The two also noted that the Prophet neither condemned the people of Medina for fleeing an outbreak of disease there, nor did he choose to enter while it raged there, referencing Qur'an 2:195: "Do not throw yourself into destruction by your own hand." Their decision, however, recognized the complexity of the issue by stressing that one should not flee with the intent of avoiding death, since that contradicted the spirit of the Qur'an 4:78: "Even if you be in towers of lofty construction, death will overtake you," and 10:49: "When their time comes, they shall not remain an hour earlier or later." They qualified their judgment by noting it was not permissible to flee if it meant leaving behind the dead unwashed and unprepared for burial. But otherwise, the plague was like a fire—it was the duty of the believer to escape it. In the end, the shaykh's family fled the city along with many others, and was able to deflect the plague's impact on his own followers, which included his son and successor Ahmed el-Hiyālī (d. 1571), who by his own account recovered only when his father offered prayers on his behalf.[74]

However, the narratives that followed those of the sixteenth and early seventeenth century began shifting away from the "community protector" motif in favor of a more individualized relationship with their followers. Instead, an emphasis on a culture of secrecy and one-on-one experience with spiritual power, already present in Sufi ideology, came to the fore. Ḥulvî's complaints about "hypocrites" doubting the power of saints reflected growing pressure from puritanical move-

71 Following the remarks of Akasoy, "Islamic Attitudes to Disasters," 396–97.

72 Muḥyi-yi Gülşeni, *Menâkıb*, 250.

73 For the origins of this narrative, see Stearns, *Infectious Ideas*, 27–28.

74 Muḥyi-yi Gülşeni, *Menâkıb*, 251–52 and 256–59. In the telling of Ahmed el-Hiyālī, he witnessed a black dog chasing him down in a dream and biting him, with his father in hot pursuit. When his father struck the dog with a staff of light, it exploded into fire, and Ahmed awoke with fever and affliction with the plague. He was saved when his father arrived from Tabriz to the village where he was and recited the Qur'anic chapter of Ikhlās over him.

ments such as the Kadızadeli movement that sought to purge aspects of Ottoman Sufism they saw as dubious or overstepping the bounds of divine authority.[75] This led to a second type of narrative structure where hostility aimed at Halveti shaykhs resulted in a deadly illness or affliction being unleashed upon their opponents. Divine vengeance against opponents was hardly a novel addition to hagiographical convention; after all, the aforementioned Sinaneddin Yusuf had also told of how his father miraculously predicted the demise of an especially puritanical scholar, who had been persecuting Sufis in Egypt, in a shipwreck.[76] Nevertheless, the individual-focused nature of these narratives becomes more pronounced.

The phenomenon can be noted in a comparison between two hagiographies from the Şaʿbaniyye branch of the Halveti order: Şaʿban-ı Veli (d. 1569) and Ünsî Hasan (d. 1723). According to his hagiographer, ʿÖmer el-Fuʾadî (d. 1636), the founder of the order, Şaʿban-ı Veli, was criticized by a Muslim scholar hostile to Sufism. However, when the scholar fell terminally ill and sent a messenger to ask for forgiveness, Şaʿban went to him anyway. The narrative served a didactic purpose, with ʿÖmer el-Fuʾadî arguing that the lesson Şaʿban was teaching was that retaliation was not a meritorious Sufi act.[77]

But not all Şaʿbaniyye shaykhs shared this view. In the eighteenth century, an outbreak of disease appeared in a hagiography documenting the life of Aʿrec Ünsî Hasan Efendi, whose activities contrasted sharply with Şaʿban's. Although Ünsî Hasan's hagiographer, İbrahim el-Has, made a point of his shaykh's refusal to engage in any high-profile miraculous activity that might raise his public profile, that compunction dropped when Ünsî Hasan found himself being physically threatened by a group of students who had adopted the views of the puritanical Kadızadeli movement.[78] When Ünsî Hasan's attempts to reason with his attackers failed, he yelled at them, "how many negative words you say about us and our path! You censure the order and are cruel to the people of the path! And you say, 'Let's kill,' well then, we won't protect you!" Within a week, all of the students

---

75 For more on the Kadızadeli movement, see Madeline C. Zilfi, "The Kadizadelis: Discordant Revivalism in Seventeenth-Century Istanbul," *Journal of Near Eastern Studies* 45:4 (1986): 251–69 and *The Politics of Piety: The Ottoman Ulema in the Postclassical Age (1600–1800)* (Minneapolis: Bibliotheca Islamica, 1988); Semiramis Çavusoğlu, "The Kadızadeli Movement: An Attempt of Şerîʿat-Minded Reform in the Ottoman Empire," PhD diss., Princeton University, 1990; and Curry, *Transformation*, ch. 8.

76 Sinaneddin Yusuf, *Tezkiretü'l-Halvetiyye*, 35a–b.

77 ʿÖmer el-Fuʾadî (d. 1045/1636), *Menâkıb-ı şerîf-i pîr-i Halveti Hazret-i Şaʿbân-ı Veli* (Istanbul: Süleymaniye Library, ms. Hacı Mahmud Efendi 4598), 67–68; see also the analysis of Curry, *Transformation*, 131–33.

78 See n. 75 above.

were dying of a fatal disease that struck them down on the spot. When one of Ünsî Hasan's followers requested that he offer a benedictory prayer for a dying student, the shaykh shocked him by angrily responding that he should mind his own business. "Let them die!" he exclaimed.[79]

Nevertheless, miraculous acts involving disease also took on positive forms. In another interesting anecdote, we learn of Ünsî Hasan's surprisingly symbiotic relationship with a non-Muslim doctor in Gülhane:

> Across from the door of the ... [Halveti] lodge was a Christian doctor. They called him Miykal. He was a skilled expert in the science of medicine. His custom was that whenever a sick person came to him, if he were unable to cure him, or if a remedy for him was not possible, he would say to that person, "the remedy for this illness is in that lodge. Go into the lodge...The doctor for this illness is the shaykh."

One day a sick man who had come from Anatolia arrived at the lodge, and when he removed his headgear, the group saw that he had horrible boils all over his head. When the man told the shaykh that Miykal had sent him, saying that the cure would be found at his hands, Ünsî Hasan praised his Christian neighbor and assured the sick man that he had been well-advised. The shaykh then spit into his hands and rubbed them on the man's head. Within two days the man returned, completely cured, but the shaykh quickly swore all those who witnessed the act to secrecy.[80]

Whereas a standard expectation of Muslim hagiography might assume that this episode would conclude with the conversion of the Christian doctor to Islam as proof of the saint's irresistible power, no such event occurred in this case. The narrative describes a world in which various forms of treatment could transcend confessional boundaries. While this is no surprise from the secular standpoint, as seeking treatment from non-Muslim physicians had numerous precedents in the history of Islamic civilization, the degree of interconfessional religious acceptance seems more unusual. The most convincing explanation may lie with the cultural makeup of Istanbul by the early eighteenth century, which had become a fairly cosmopolitan place where even devout Muslims may have taken the diversity in their communities for granted.

To bring things full circle, we conclude by looking at the case of Muḥammad Nasuhî (d. 1718), a founder of an influential branch of the Halveti order in the

79 İbrahim el-Has (d. 1175/1761), *Risâle-i Menâkıb-ı Ünsî* (Istanbul: Süleymaniye Library, ms. Hacı Mahmud Efendi 4607), 22a-25a.

80 İbrahim el-Has, *Risâle-i Menâkıb-ı Ünsî*, 87b–90a.

Istanbul suburb of Üsküdar.[81] According to his hagiography, the daughter of a prominent religious dignitary, ʿİsa Efendi, was afflicted by plague. ʿİsa Efendi and his wife eventually despaired of her returning to life, and so he sent his follower Zakir Ahmed Efendi to Muḥammad Nasuhî to ask for his prayers and entreat him for some kind of miraculous intercession. Nasuhî responded by telling Ahmed Efendi that they should not grieve. Upon returning to give the news, Ahmed found that ʿİsa Efendi and his following were rejoicing, as his daughter had risen, drank some soup and was recovering from her illness. But the joy was tempered by the subsequent realization that Nasuhî's own teenaged daughter had subsequently fallen ill with the plague herself, and passed away shortly thereafter, as her father had warned her that she would shortly be confronting the afterlife.[82]

The story bears the hallmarks of a number of Sufi hagiographical *topoi*, such as the divinely inspired foreknowledge of the shaykh of future events, along with the ability to reward those who showed faith. However, the previous motif of self-sacrifice also recurs in the narrative, as Nasuhî sacrifices his own daughter so that his friend would not suffer a heartbreaking loss. However, Nasuhî was not defending the entire community from the plague; rather, he was acting in conjunction with a personal relationship with a devoted follower.

Once the narrative is interpreted in the light of Halveti didactic teachings, we could conclude that the narrative tells us little about plague or disease save that devout Muslims so afflicted sought intercession from Sufi leaders in a pre-modern context. However, a chance discovery in another source illuminates this narrative further. In the Nasuhî family library, preserved at least in part in Üsküdar, Muḥammad Nasuhî and his descendants recorded elements of their family history on various folios in their personal copy of Radī al-Dīn al-Sāghānī's *Kitāb Mashārīq al-anwār fī siḥaḥ al-akhbār*.[83] In his own hand, Muḥammad Nasuhî first recorded

81 The Nasuhî branch of the Halveti order has not received much scholarly attention outside of Turkey; for an overview, see Kemal Edib Kürkçüoğlu, *Şeyh Muhammed Nasûhî: Hayatı, Eserleri, Dîvânı, Mektupları* (Istanbul: Alem Ticaret Yayıncılık, 1996) and Mustafa Tatcı, *Üsküdarlı Muhammed Nasûhî ve Divanı* (Istanbul: Kaknüs Yayınları, 2004).

82 This narrative appears in multiple overlapping texts discussing the life of Muḥammad Nasuhî that ultimately derive from one of his devoted followers; see Hasan Efendizade Senayî (d. after 1153/1741), *Menâkıb-i Şeyh Muḥammad Nasûhî* (Istanbul: Süleymaniye Library, ms. Ali Emiri Şeriyye 1104), 14b-15a. The narrative also appears in Süleymaniye Library, ms. Hacı Mahmud Efendi 4573/1, 8a–b and mss. Hazreti Nasuhi Dergahı 165, 13b-14a and Hazreti Nasuhi Dergahı 273, 90a–91a.

83 This was an influential work of commentary on Prophetic tradition commonly used as a foundational teaching text for aspiring *ʿulamāʾ* well into the Ottoman period; for more on its background, see Mehmet Görmez, "Sâgânî, Radıyyüddîn," *Türkiye Diyanet Vakfı İslâm Ansiklopedisi* (Istanbul: Türkiye Diyanet Vakfı İslâm Araştırmaları Merkezi, 2008), v. 35, 488.

the birth of a daughter, Fatima, on 25 February 1694, followed many years later by a second, smaller entry stating that "the aforementioned daughter Fatima died at the end of Dhu'l-Qaʿda Thursday night at midnight ... [in the year] 1118" (a date which equates to 3 March 1707).[84] This additional finding corroborates the narrative further, and allows us to accurately date an outbreak of plague in Istanbul during the year 1707.[85]

Furthermore, the personal notebooks and papers of Muḥammad Nasuhî and his descendants preserved in Üsküdar suggest that the curative powers of Sufi shaykhs may not have been limited to divine intervention alone. For example, a recipe for a pharmaceutical potion aimed at curing stomach problems and impotence credited to Nasuhî by one of his descendants appears in one manuscript.[86] Subsequent notebooks that found their way into the order's library also recorded recipes for various illnesses such as fever and shortness of breath, although most do not seem to be aimed specifically at plague.[87] While admittedly an unusually well-sourced case study, Muḥammad Nasuhî and his ill-fated daughter raise interesting questions about the role Sufi shaykhs might play in this field.

Ultimately, the activities of Ottoman Sufi shaykhs strike an interesting counterpoint to the arguments of Marʿī b. Yūsuf. They did not accept that fleeing from the plague was invariably discouraged, nor did they reject the idea that non-Muslim medicine was without its uses, even if God, via the intercession of the Sufi shaykh, was the only true remedy for the worst of cases. The more diverse views of the Ottoman Sufi figures seemed to intersect with the idea that their spiritual power was deemed effective in coping with the plague, as opposed to Marʿī's view that the plague was merely an expression of God's will, for which Muslims had little

84 See the marginal notes found in the aforementioned work of al-Sāghānī mistakenly catalogued in the collection as ʿAbd al-Latīf b. Abd al-ʿAzīz b. Malik, *Kitāb Mashāriq al-anwār fī siḥaḥ al-akhbār* (Istanbul: Süleymaniye Library, ms. Hazreti Nasuhi Dergahı 34), 1b.

85 Further corroboration of the plague outbreak can be found in Panzac, *La peste*, 622.

86 See marginal notes found in the opening folios of a *mecmua* that commences with a copy of Şemseddin-i Sivasî, *Athbāt al-wājib fī māhiyyat al-wujūd* (Istanbul: Süleymaniye Library, ms. Hazreti Nasuhi Dergahı 40), 1a.

87 See, for example, notes found in the personal notebook of the Nasuhî shaykh Şemseddin Efendi, *Mecmua* (Istanbul: Süleymaniye Library, ms. Hazreti Nasuhi Dergahı 273), 226b, 228a-230a, along with instructions for curative talismans and prayers on 199a-201a; additional notes are also found in another *mecmua* (Istanbul: Süleymaniye Library, ms. Hazreti Nasuhi Dergahı 295), 45b–46a and 126a as well. A notable exception is the instructions for creating protective talismans for the plague, "to be given free of charge to the brothers," that appear in an addendum to Aʿrec Ünsî Hasan (d. 1136/1723), *Fī beyān-ı atvār el-ṣāba* (Istanbul: Atatürk Kitaplığı, ms. Osman Ergin 1508), 13b.

recourse. Furthermore, these findings suggest regional variation, in that Moroccan Sufi figures from a contemporary period were much closer to Marʿī's logic than those of their Ottoman counterparts, which suggest that the order a Sufi belonged to, or the regional environment from which they came, influenced the way they thought about these questions.[88] Ultimately, given the growing pressure of more puritanical strains of Islam over the course of Ottoman history, Ottoman Sufi activities came to take on a more personalized and secret nature, rather than the grand public gestures of an earlier era.

Conclusion

While this chapter cannot do comprehensive justice to the still largely unexplored Ottoman textual corpus on plague and disease in the early modern period, the various sources that I have explored nevertheless suggest alternative patterns of thought that evolved in various Ottoman elite and intellectual circles during the early modern period. In the case of the Muslim scholars and intellectuals who found Marʿī b. Yūsuf's work compelling, they may have moved away from the more flexible approaches advocated by fifteenth- and sixteenth-century Ottoman authors, and instead reinforced a strict view of causality that viewed the plague as a product of religious and moral forces that human agency could not combat. Stressing historical sources from the Muslim tradition that rejected the explanations of physicians about the plague, they set it apart from other forms of disease and argued that the Muslim community could only bear its impacts with equanimity.

Likewise, the reasons for this shift in emphasis in Sufi sources may have its origins in the processes of historical change that marked the transition from the medieval to the early modern Islamic world. The disruptions in Ottoman life over the course of the "seventeenth-century crisis" had weakened public belief in the idea of mystical saviors who could come to their rescue, and thus the ideological positions of Sufi leaders came to reflect a downplaying of miraculous occurrences in contemporary contexts. However, early modern society was full of various afflictions and calamities, and the idea of plague, disease, or other forms of catastrophe as divine punishment for sins remained a possibility. In one case, it even proved useful as a threat and deterrent against hostile activity directed at an order's membership. Thus, the channeling of divine punishment through the figure of a prominent Sufi remained in place as a key hagiographical element in the narratives of the time.

---

88 Noting the aforementioned discussion of al-Banānī and Ibn ʿAjība in n. 5 above from Stearns, *Infectious Ideas*, 149–50.

However, external causes were not the sole reason for the change, whatever role they may have played in encouraging it. Within Ottoman Sufi orders such as the Halveti, intellectual forces were at work that downplayed the physical use of spiritual power for grand gestures aimed at this-worldly salvation, in favor of a more inward-directed Sufism that encouraged followers to take up the mystical path for its own sake. As a result, individual Sufis were not as quick to present themselves as a cure for the diseases, afflictions and calamities of this world, especially in the public sphere. Their followers did not, however, decouple their presentation entirely from the motif of affliction and disease, for these potential catastrophes could still await those who failed to respect the spiritual power of Ottoman mystical leadership.

Nevertheless, in contrast to the writings of Marʿī b. Yūsuf, elements in some of the Ottoman Sufi sources over the course of this period suggests that the devotees of the Halveti order lacked the rigid conception of plague as a predestined force that humans lacked any agency to confront. This underscores the fact that religious thought about the plague, disease, and other calamities did not share a unified point of view, and continued to be contested long after the scholarly voices of the medieval period had laid down their various perspectives on the topic. The duty of subsequent scholarship is thus to situate the various references to plague and epidemics into their proper contexts, and thus to create a more thorough picture of how Ottoman intellectuals responded to these catastrophic events in an important transitional period of their history.

John J. Curry (john.curry@unlv.edu) graduated from The Ohio State University with a dual MA in History and Arabic Language (1998) and PhD in History (2005). He specializes in the history of the early modern Ottoman Empire in particular, and in the history of the Islamic world and global history more generally. He is the author of *The Transformation of Muslim Mystical Thought in the Ottoman Empire: The Rise of the Halveti Order, 1350-1650* with Edinburgh University Press (2010), a study of a major Ottoman religio-mystical brotherhood with branches throughout the Islamic world, in addition to a number of journal articles on various topics. He has also published an edited volume of studies on Sufism in the medieval and early modern Islamic world entitled *Sufism and Society: Arrangements of the Mystical in the Muslim World 1200-1800*, co-edited with Erik S. Ohlander of Indiana-Purdue University, Fort Wayne, to which he contributed both the introductory chapter and one of the twelve articles in the volume. He is presently an Associate Professor in the Department of History at the University of Nevada, Las Vegas, where he has taught since 2006.

"ORIENTAL PLAGUE" OR EPIDEMIOLOGICAL ORIENTALISM? REVISITING THE PLAGUE EPISTEME OF THE EARLY MODERN MEDITERRANEAN

NÜKHET VARLIK
Rutgers University—Newark

> "I saw the Ottoman's fortress—austere, and darkly impending high over the vale of the Danube—historic Belgrade. I had come, as it were, to the end of this wheel-going Europe, and now my eyes would see the Splendour and Havoc of The East."[1]

With these words, the nineteenth-century English historian and travel writer Alexander William Kinglake opens his famous *Eothen, or, Traces of Travel Brought Home from the East*. When the young Cambridge-educated Kinglake began his journey to the Ottoman Empire in 1834, he could not have known that his account of this journey would become a classic in Oriental travel writings. Indeed, the travelogue was an immediately successful publication, going through numerous editions as well as translations into German, French, and Italian.[2] It is generally acknowledged that the book's fame is owed not to the accuracy of Kinglake's narrative or the eruditeness of his literary style; rather, it is admired for its commanding ability to convey intriguing impressions and share engaging experiences, as though Kinglake was actually conversing with his target audience: European armchair travelers to the Orient.

Kinglake knew well how to speak to the sensibilities of his audience. He also knew how to season his narrative to offer his readers a taste of the exotic. After all, he was taking them on an adventure that demanded courage, determination, and a touch of imagination. Right from the outset of his travelogue, as he is about to cross the Ottoman border and step into uncharted territory, he prepares his reader for the dramatic transition from Europe to the East. "The two frontier towns," he writes, "are less than a gun-shot apart, yet their people hold no communion ... [they] are as much asunder as though there were fifty broad provinces that lay in the path between them ... [no] one had ever gone down to look upon the stranger

---

1 Alexander William Kinglake, *Kinglake's Eothen* (London: Clarendon Press, 1906), 7.

2 First published in 1844, *Eothen* went through several editions and translations. For a biography of Kinglake, see William Tuckwell, *A.W. Kinglake: A Biographical and Literary Study* (London: G. Bell and Sons, 1902).

race dwelling under the walls of that opposite castle."[3] Kinglake sketches the difference between what was familiar and what was about to be encountered—an unfamiliar lifestyle, veiled women, but most importantly a different healthscape. In unambiguous terms, he draws the line: "It is *the Plague*, and the *dread of the Plague*, that *divide* the one people from the other."[4]

How did the plague come to be imagined as something that divided two bordering towns when the disease was notorious for its spread across continents? How did it become a boundary marker between Europe and the Orient in the nineteenth century? And, how did the narrative of epidemiological boundaries create a legacy that has continued to influence the modern historical imagination? These questions and others call for an inquiry that is situated at the nexus of historical epidemiology, history of public health, environmental history, and orientalism. This essay will first position nineteenth-century narratives of epidemiological fronts in the context of epidemiology, internationalism, and orientalism. Then, taking this narrative as a critical moment in the formation of policy and history, it will trace its residual influence on modern historiography, with a view to identifying how it has obscured the epidemiological histories of the pre-nineteenth century Mediterranean world. Lastly, it will explore the rise of the Western gaze on the Oriental healthscape, and the manner in which the Orient was constructed as the site of sickness in the writings of early modern European travelers to the Ottoman Empire. In particular, it will examine how plague came to be anchored in a particular space outside of Europe and how this anchoring was subsequently used to articulate narratives of binaries, of "us" and "them." This involves exploring how Europeans viewed, experienced, imagined, reproduced, and represented the Ottoman healthscape in both visual and written form, the sum of which is called here "epidemiological orientalism."

The Narrative of Epidemiological Fronts

Kinglake's account articulated a discourse that used the plague as the marker of spatial demarcation between Europe and the Orient.[5] According to this model, the

3 Kinglake, *Eothen*, 7.

4 Kinglake, *Eothen*, 7, emphasis mine.

5 Here, it would be helpful to construe the term Orient broadly as "lands of non-Western 'civilizations'," since its meaning changed as Europe's global connections expanded. For a very insightful discussion of the geographical ambiguity of the Orient in the context of spatial and cultural constructs of East and West, see Martin W. Lewis and Kären E. Wigen, *The Myth of Continents: A Critique of Metageography* (Berkeley: University of California Press, 1997), especially 47–103. I thank Marta Hanson for bringing this work to my attention.

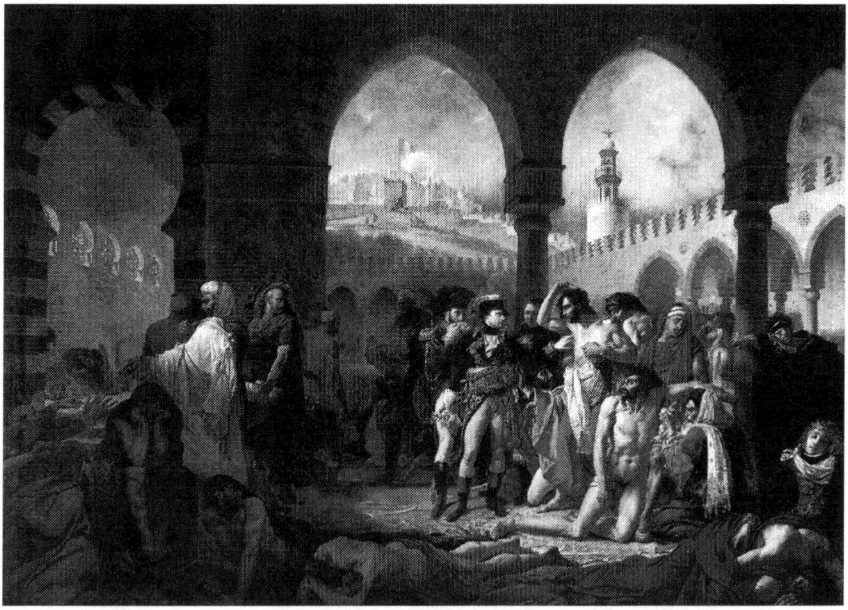

Figure 1. Antoine-Jean Gros, Bonaparte visitant les pestiférés de Jaffa (*Bonaparte Visits the Plague-Stricken in Jaffa*), 1804. Louvre, Paris.

absence of plague was what differentiated "civilized West" from the "sickly East." Rooted in nineteenth-century European anxieties that regarded public health as a measure of civilization, this particular vision helped to define the European difference, especially in contrast to the Orient. This contrast was perhaps best expressed in art. For example, Antoine-Jean Gros's 1804 painting *Bonaparte Visits the Plague-Stricken in Jaffa*, commissioned by Napoleon himself, depicts the dichotomy between civilized, healthy, European bodies and the sick, dying, and dehumanized Eastern bodies in an Oriental setting.[6]

Kinglake was neither the first nor the last to articulate the vision of a disease-ridden Ottoman Empire, which in the nineteenth-century was seen as the embodiment of illness. In the broader sweep of European history, this articulation came at a time when the Ottomans were no longer viewed as an immediate military threat to Europe: the empire had long lost the political and military supremacy it once enjoyed, and came to be regarded as a dead or dying body in broader European

6 For an analysis of the painting *Bonaparte visitant les pestiférés de Jaffa*, see, for example, Christine M. Boeckl, *Images of Plague and Pestilence: Iconography and Iconology* (Kirksville, MO: Truman State University Press, 2000), 138–41.

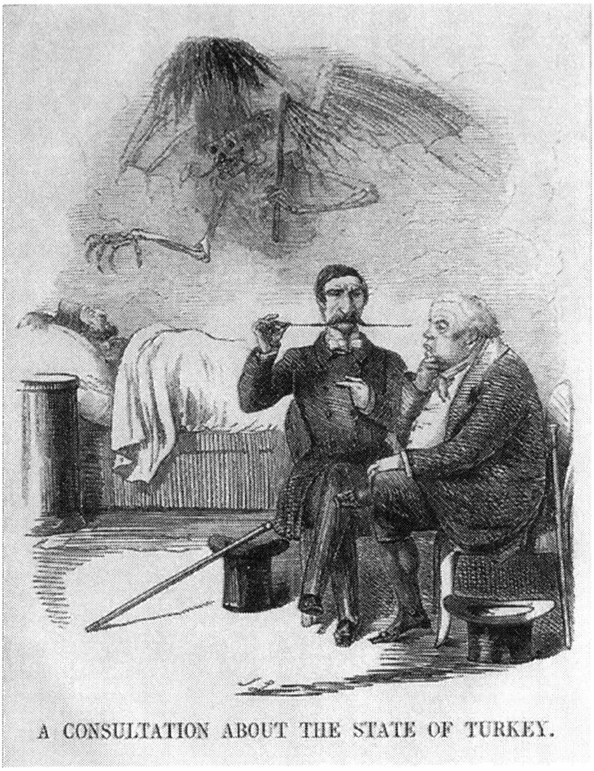

Figure 2. Turkey "The Sick Man of Europe," by John Leech, *Punch*, September 17, 1853.

geopolitics. Indeed, it did not take long for the empire to be framed as the "sick man of Europe."[7]

However, this particular narrative of epidemiological fronts was not owed to the weakening of Ottoman power alone. The discourse of the sickly Orient also responded to nineteenth-century European anxieties about how to maintain public health and keep infectious diseases in check, while still moving toward interna-

7 For a discussion of the Ottoman Empire as the "sick man of Europe" in the context of changing perceptions of the "Turks" in Europe, see Aslı Çırakman, *From the "Terror of the World" to the "Sick Man of Europe": European Images of Ottoman Empire and Society from the Sixteenth Century to the Nineteenth* (New York: Peter Lang, 2002), especially 164–72. The metaphor of the "sick man" has been used in other contexts, as well. For a discussion of the "sick man of the East" used in reference to China in the late nineteenth and early twentieth centuries, for example, see Yi Hu, *Rural Health Care Delivery: Modern China from the Perspective of Disease Politics* (Berlin: Springer, 2013), especially chapter 1: "The Double Meaning of 'the Sick Man of East Asia' and China's Politics," 3–9. I am grateful to Marta Hanson for her comments on the "sick man of the East."

tionalism.[8] Central to these endeavors was the new science of epidemiology and border control policies that it informed, which often clashed sharply with mercantile and trade interests in increasing connectedness with the world. In the words of Valeska Huber, there was an effort to figure out "how borders could be secured without resorting to traditional barriers; like semipermeable membranes they should be open for some kinds of communication but closed for others."[9]

Epidemiology can hardly be isolated from the nineteenth-century context in which it developed, and epidemiological epistemologies were heavily imbued with orientalism. In fact, orientalism, as an academic enterprise to study the Orient, and epidemiology are more closely intertwined than may be expected. Beginning in the mid-nineteenth century, the International Sanitary Conference series generated an explosion of literature, terminology, and matters of policy development that involved orientalist epistemologies.[10] Even before the sanitary conferences, there were many channels for the flow of information about epidemics experienced in the Orient, such as diplomatic exchanges, travelogues, and medical literature. Yet the best articulation of this entwinement is perhaps encapsulated in the terminology (and nosology) of the era, as evidenced in the creation of a new disease category: "Oriental plague."

The Making of Oriental Plague

After the initial blow of the Black Death pandemic (1346–53), outbreaks of plague continued to recur in the Mediterranean world into the early modern era.[11] Starting in the late seventeenth century, large-scale epidemics of plague gradually lessened in Western Europe. The Great Plague of London in 1665 and the Plague of Marseille in 1720–21 have been generally regarded as the last major

---

8 It might be helpful to remember that Kinglake's travels and subsequent writings came on the heels of the first great cholera outbreak in Europe in the 1830s, which had come from the East.

9 Valeska Huber, "The Unification of the Globe by Disease? The International Sanitary Conferences on Cholera, 1851–1894," *The Historical Journal* 49, no. 2 (2006): 453–76, quote on 453.

10 Fourteen International Sanitary Conferences were held between 1851 and 1938. See http://ocp.hul.harvard.edu/contagion/sanitaryconferences.html (accessed January 11, 2017). For an analysis of cholera in this context, see Huber, "The Unification of the Globe by Disease?"

11 For the most recent comprehensive reassessment of the Black Death, see Monica H. Green, ed., *Pandemic Disease in the Medieval World: Rethinking the Black Death," The Medieval Globe* 1 (2014).

historic eruptions of the disease in Western Europe, while sporadic outbreaks continued to affect Southern and Eastern Europe, as in Messina in 1743 and Bari in 1815. While plague was disappearing from Europe, repeated outbreaks ravaged the Russian and Ottoman lands through the eighteenth century. Moreover, in some parts of the Eastern Mediterranean, plague lingered throughout the nineteenth century.[12]

The divergence in epidemiological experience between Europe and the "Orient" makes for a complex historical and historiographical problem. This divergence marked a turning point in the European episteme about the locus of plague. After the Plague of Marseille and through the rest of the eighteenth century, Europeans identified the Eastern Mediterranean ports of the Ottoman Empire as the places from where the infection came.[13] This realization resulted in concerted effort to implement protective measures, first locally, then regionally and internationally. Quarantines established in port cities and *cordons sanitaires* set up along land borders served as the custodians of European public health. These physical restrictions in turn helped to construct the boundaries of the European healthscape—real or imagined. At the same time, the eighteenth-century European episteme of plague abounded with information about Oriental experiences with the disease. News about mortality, duration, and virulence of each outbreak traveled from Eastern Mediterranean port cities, such as Smyrna (İzmir), Alexandria, and from Constantinople (Istanbul), as much in popular accounts as in scholarly observations. It is possible to find such annotations in the reports of Levant Com-

12 For the Baltic plague of 1709–13, see Karl-Erik Frandsen, *The Last Plague in the Baltic Region, 1709–1713* (Copenhagen: Museum Tusculanum Press, 2010); for eighteenth-century plagues in Russia, see John T. Alexander, *Bubonic Plague in Early Modern Russia: Public Health and Urban Disaster* (Baltimore: Johns Hopkins University Press, 1980); for plagues in the Ottoman Empire, see Daniel Panzac, *La peste dans l'empire ottoman, 1700–1850* (Leuven: Peeters, 1985); Andrew Robarts, "A Plague on Both Houses? Population Movements and the Spread of Disease across the Ottoman-Russian Black Sea Frontier, 1768–1830s," PhD diss., Georgetown University, 2010; Robarts, *Migration and Disease in the Black Sea Region: Ottoman-Russian Relations in the Late Eighteenth and Early Nineteenth Centuries* (London: Bloomsbury, 2017). For a discussion of these outbreaks as recurrent waves of the Second Pandemic, see, for example, Lars Walløe, "Medieval and Modern Bubonic Plague: Some Clinical Continuities," in *Pestilential Complexities: Understanding Medieval Plague*, ed. Vivian Nutton (London: Wellcome Trust Centre for the History of Medicine at University College London, 2008), 59–73; for a critical assessment of the perodization of plague pandemics, see Nükhet Varlık, "New Science and Old Sources: Why the Ottoman Experience of Plague Matters," *The Medieval Globe* 1 (2014): 193–227.

13 Junko Thérèse Takeda, *Between Crown and Commerce: Marseille and the Early Modern Mediterranean* (Baltimore: Johns Hopkins University Press, 2011); Panzac, *La peste*.

pany representatives, of Venetian physicians participating in diplomatic missions, in merchants' letters, and the like.[14] In this manner, both infectious disease-control policy and epidemiological knowledge contributed to the making of a particular historical narrative.

According to this narrative, plague came from the Orient. Even though there were contradictory opinions about the exact origin and cause of this disease, why it was more prevalent in Oriental cities, and how local populations engaged with it, Europeans generally agreed that they received the infection from Eastern Mediterranean ports. As we shall see below, the roots of this narrative can be traced back to the European travel literature of the early modern era. Yet the conviction that plague came from the Orient was only fully validated in the authority of Enlightenment authors. The *Encyclopédie* of Diderot and D'Alembert, composed in the second half of the eighteenth century, offered a theoretical framework and scientific precision to widespread European opinions about Oriental origins of this disease. Louis de Jaucourt, a prolific writer of the *Encyclopédie*, wrote as follows in the entry on "*Peste*": "Plague comes to us from Asia, and for two thousand years all the plagues that have appeared in Europe have been transmitted through the communication of the Saracens, Arabs, Moors or Turks with us, and none of our plagues had any other source."[15] Interestingly enough, Jaucourt used the term *peste d'Orient*, but reserved it exclusively to his discussion of the First Pandemic, i.e., the Plague of Justinian in the sixth century.

Whether or not the mid-eighteenth-century French original of the *Encyclopédie* was where the term *peste d'Orient* was first used, its English equivalent "Oriental plague" does not seem to appear until slightly later. In the nineteenth century, the term acquired a much wider circulation within the European epidemiological

14 See, for example, Mordach Mackenzie, "Extracts of Several Letters of Mordach Mackenzie, M. D. Concerning the Plague at Constantinople," *Philosophical Transactions (1683–1775)* 47 (1752): 384; Mackenzie, "An Account of the Plague at Constantinople: In a Letter from Mordach Mackenzie, M. D. to Sir James Porter, His Majesty's Envoy Plenipotentiary at Brussels, and F. R. S.," *Philosophical Transactions (1683–1775)* 54 (1764): 69–82; Patrick Russell, *A Treatise of the Plague: Containing an Historical Journal, and Medical Account, of the Plague, at Aleppo, in the Years 1760, 1761, and 1762; Also, Remarks on Quarantines, Lazarettos, and the Administration of Police in Times of Pestilence. To Which Is Added, an Appendix, Containing Cases of the Plague; and an Account of the Weather, during the Pestilential Season* (London: Printed for G. G. J. and J. Robinson, 1791).

15 Louis de Jaucourt, "Peste," in *Encyclopédie, ou dictionnaire raisonné des sciences, des arts et des métiers*, ed. Denis Diderot and Jean le Rond d'Alembert (Paris: Sociétés Typographiques, 1751–72), 12: 452: "la peste nous vient de l'Asie, & depuis deux mille ans toutes les pestes qui ont paru en Europe y ont été transmises par la communication des Sarrasins, des Arabes, des Maures, ou des Turcs avec nous, & toutes les pestes n'ont pas eu chez nous d'autre source."

episteme. This was also an era when medical writers experimented with other similar terms, such as "Asiatic plague" or "true plague," which likewise responded to Europe's new disease experiences and to its newly emerging epidemiological epistemologies. The term "Oriental plague" was used to distinguish plague from other epidemic diseases, such as smallpox, yellow fever, and others. Terminology and nosology, in turn, had implications for policy development, owing to Europe's increased encounters with new and recurring infectious diseases—both at home and abroad. In the nineteenth century, new transportation technologies, such as steamships and railroads, meant that infectious diseases could spread much faster across the globe. Cholera was the ultimate proof of this change.[16] Yet Europe's encounters with disease—whether old or new—were not limited to what reached its shores. It is perhaps no surprise that the coining of the term "Oriental plague" coincided with Napoleon's invasion of Egypt in 1798 and increased French and British involvement in the region.

No matter what its particular taxonomic classification may have been, the Oriental plague pointed toward the physical space of the "Orient." More specifically, the term was used to refer to recurrent outbreaks of plague in the Ottoman Empire. By this time, Europeans could only encounter the disease in the Orient, which meant that their knowledge about it could be drawn from there alone. While reinforcing some ideas that had been circulating since the early modern era, such as because the Orientals were fatalistic, they did not take any precautions to prevent plagues, the disease came to be irrevocably associated with the Oriental space. Soon enough, this spatial association also infiltrated the European epidemiological episteme. The Ottoman experience of plague was studied, interpreted, categorized, and systemized by British and French scientists who worked for imperial projects. Sanitation policies developed by Western European public health officials were also imposed on Oriental bodies. In this backdrop, it is no coincidence that modern epidemiology, in its inception, was closely entwined with the study of the Orient.

The European plague episteme of the early nineteenth century informed policy but not yet historical writing. This would have had to wait for the rise of modern historiography of the Black Death a few decades later. In 1832, German medical historian Justus Friedrich Carl Hecker published his pioneering *Der schwarze Tod im vierzehnten Jahrhundert*, which gave a new life to conceptions of Oriental

---

16 Starting in 1820s and 1830s, cholera pandemics swept across the globe in repeated waves. A term (nearly) contemporary with Oriental plague was "Asiatic Cholera." For a comprehensive archive of texts and images related to cholera, see http://www.nlm.nih.gov.proxy.libraries.rutgers.edu/exhibition/cholera/index.html (accessed January 11, 2017).

plague.[17] Hecker used the term *morgenländische Pest* to refer not only to contemporary outbreaks, but also to past plagues, opening up its use to new possibilities. In other words, Hecker's historical analysis made it possible to imagine pre-nineteenth century plagues in taxonomically similar terms as nineteenth-century Oriental plague. Under such circumstances, the Black Death could be labeled an Oriental plague, though Hecker must have felt that he needed to give the reader a little extra information to distinguish it from other diseases. He noted that the "great pestilence of the fourteenth century ... was an oriental plague, marked by inflammatory boils and tumors of the glands, such as break out in no other febrile disease" and that the "buboes ... are the infallible signs of the oriental plague."[18] In so doing, Hecker irreversibly changed the meaning of the Oriental plague for subsequent medical writers and historians. By the late nineteenth century, the Oriental plague's new temporal scope was entrenched. In an essay written for the Statistical Society of London, British surgeon and medical writer Henry Percy Potter surveyed the great plagues of the Antiquity and the Middle Ages, including the recurrent waves of the Black Death in Europe. He stated: "Epidemics of Oriental plague were noted in 1407, 1427, and 1478, and during the fifteenth century the plague broke out seventeen times in different parts of Europe."[19] Read in this light, the Great Plague of London, Baltic Plagues, the Plague of Marseille were all appearances of Oriental plague.

The extension of Oriental plague's temporal scope (by retrospectively attributing the term to the Black Death and its subsequent outbreaks) was ironic, especially given that plague gradually receded from the Ottoman Empire throughout the nineteenth century. The outbreak in 1812–13 is generally regarded as the last major epidemic in the empire's history.[20] In 1838, the Ottoman administration

---

17 J. F. C. Hecker, *Der schwarze Tod im vierzehnten Jahrhundert* (Berlin: Herbig, 1832).

18 J. F. C. Hecker, *The Epidemics of the Middle Ages*, trans. B. G. Babington (London: Trübner, 1859), 2–3. For further discussion on Hecker's views as "gothic epidemiology," see Faye Marie Getz, "Black Death and the Silver Lining: Meaning, Continuity, and Revolutionary Change in Histories of Medieval Plague," *Journal of the History of Biology* 24, no. 2 (1991): 265–89, for an observation about the orientalist character of this epidemiology, see 276n50.

19 Henry Percy Potter, "The Oriental Plague in Its Social, Economical, Political, and International Relations, Special Reference Being Made to the Labours of John Howard on the Subject," *Journal of the Statistical Society of London* 43, no. 4 (1880): 605–42, 606–13, quote on 608. In his "Historical Sketch," Percy relies on William A. Guy's *Public Health* published a decade earlier. See William A Guy, *Public Health: A Popular Introduction to Sanitary Science* (London: Renshaw, 1870).

20 Panzac, *La peste*, 446–56; Nalan Turna, "İstanbul'un Veba ile İmtihanı: 1811–1812 Veba Salgını Bağlamında Toplum ve Ekonomi," *Studies of the Ottoman Domain* 1, no. 1 (2011):

started to implement maritime and overland quarantines, supplemented by the use of disinfection and sanitary practices.[21] Plague was observed to become less and less frequent in Ottoman cities, even though sporadic outbreaks still occurred in Egypt, Syria, and Iraq.[22] By the end of the century, the plague had become almost a rarity. In 1880, Potter wrote: "The malady known to us as Oriental plague ... has been described under different appellations of pestilential fever, septic or glandular fever, the black death. ... It is of such rare occurrence now-a-days that few modern physicians have had the opportunity of examining or reporting upon a case."[23] Nevertheless, as the actual Oriental plague became a rare occurrence, its meaning continued to become more comprehensive.

The re-conceptualization of Oriental plague's temporality brings to mind questions regarding notions of its spatiality. In late nineteenth-century discussions of Oriental plague, it was commonplace to find the mention of such places as Aleppo, Cairo, Alexandria, Smyrna, and Constantinople. It was true that these were cities where epidemics continued to recur. But also, it was in these places that European observers witnessed, watched, commented on, and opined about the plague. Hence the epidemiological knowledge distilled from these experiences was heavily colored by the Oriental landscape, climate, flora and fauna, as well as its social aspects. As we shall see below in more detail, the spatial anchoring of Oriental plague was heavily contaminated by early modern accounts of Orien-

23–58; Mehmet Ali Beyhan, "1811–1812 İstanbul Veba Salgını, Etkileri ve Alınan Tedbirler," in *1. Uluslararası Türk Tıp Tarihi Kongresi/10. Ulusal Türk Tıp Tarihi Kongresi Bildiri Kitabı (20–24 May 2008)*, ed. Ayşegül Demirhan Erdemir (Konya: Türk Tarih Kurumu, 2008), 2: 1029–36.

21 On Ottoman quarantines, see Bedi Şehsuvaroğlu, "Karantina Tarihi," PhD diss., Istanbul University, 1956; Gülden Sarıyıldız, "Karantina Teşkilatının Kuruluşu ve Faaliyetleri (1838–1876)," MA thesis, Istanbul University, 1986; Sarıyıldız, "Karantina Meclisi'nin Kuruluşu ve Faaliyetleri," *Belleten* 58, no. 222 (1994): 329–76; Sarıyıldız, *Hicaz Karantina Teşkilatı (1865–1914)* (Ankara: Türk Tarih Kurumu, 1996); Robarts, "A Plague on Both Houses?"; Birsen Bulmuş, *Plague, Quarantines, and Geopolitics in the Ottoman Empire* (Edinburgh: Edinburgh University Press, 2012). Also see, Robarts, "Nowhere to Run to, Nowhere to Hide? Society, State, and Epidemic Diseases in the Early Nineteenth-Century Ottoman Balkans," (221–41); Gülden Sarıyıldız and Oya Dağlar Macar, "Cholera, Pilgrimage, and International Politics of Sanitation: The Quarantine Station on the Island of Kamaran," (243–73).

22 Panzac, *La peste*, 456–514.

23 Potter, "Oriental Plague," 605–6. The following note is included on 606: "The author when at Alexandria in 1877, was furnished with opportunities of seeing several individuals who were the victims of large elevated patches on the skin, accompanied with fever which was said to be contagious. The disease only existed in those squalid portions of the town so well known to eastern travellers."

tal travel, which did not fall short in establishing lasting associations between the disease and the Oriental space, even before plague started to subside in Europe.[24] Be that as it may, the landholdings of the Ottoman Empire and its neighbors were typically associated with plague in the nineteenth century, even in the absence of a consensus on the exact limits of the affected zone. For example, Potter wrote in 1880: "When we investigate the geographical range of the Oriental plague, we find that epidemics have chiefly originated in the eastern parts of Europe and western Asia."[25] The following year, August Hirsch, a professor of medicine at the University of Berlin, raised skepticism about this geographical delineation. He wrote: "Until quite recently, everyone considered it settled that Persia was the eastern limit of the area of plague on Asiatic soil, beyond which, during the last five centuries at least, it had never penetrated. But the latest observations in India and China have completely upset that opinion."[26] What Hirsch identifies here was the beginnings of the so-called Third Pandemic in the nineteenth century.[27] Hirsch was part of a medical commission sent by the German government to Central Asia to study a plague epidemic in Astrakhan in 1878–79.[28] During his investigations, he noticed that new centers of epidemic activity emerged in the second half of the nineteenth century, which to him indicated "a new era in the history of the plague."[29]

Under the circumstances, late nineteenth-century definitions of Oriental plague were quite different, both temporally and spatially, from its early conceptions over a century earlier. Yet with the onset of the Third Pandemic (ca. 1855–1956), many long-held precepts about it came under revision. Hirsch was right to think of this time as the beginning of a new era in the history of plague, which triggered discussions about the nosology of the disease (e.g., was it the same

24 For an insightful discussion of how English plague-treatise writers came to attribute plague's origins to foreign landscapes, see Lori Jones, "The Diseased Landscape: Medieval and Early Modern Plaguescapes," *Landscapes* 17, no. 2 (2016): 108–23.

25 Potter, "Oriental Plague," 606.

26 August Hirsch, *Handbook of Geographical and Historical Pathology*, vol. 1, *Acute Infective Diseases*, trans. Charles Creighton (London: The New Sydenham Society, 1883), 508.

27 Hirsch, *Handbook*, 508–11. For a discussion of the Western scholarly opinion regarding the origins of the Black Death on the eve of the Third Pandemic, see George D. Sussman, "Was the Black Death in India and China?," *Bulletin of the History of Medicine* 85, no. 3 (2011): 319–55, especially 324–25. For the origins of the Third Pandemic, see Carol Ann Benedict, *Bubonic Plague in Nineteenth-Century China* (Stanford: Stanford University Press, 1996); for its global spread, see Myron J. Echenberg, *Plague Ports: The Global Urban Impact of Bubonic Plague, 1894–1901* (New York: New York University Press, 2007).

28 Potter, "Oriental Plague," 613.

29 Hirsch, *Handbook*, 511–14.

old "true" plague or something different?),[30] about its spatial extent (e.g., would it penetrate the tropical zone?), or its temporality (e.g., is the current plague related to past plagues?). Geographic, climatic, and ecological differences of the Third Pandemic posed incommensurable challenges that required radical revisions to the epidemiological epistemology. However, more importantly, this was the beginning of the age of modern bacteriology, which culminated in the discovery of the pathogen of plague (*Yersinia pestis*), as well as its hosts and vectors. By the close of the nineteenth century, the Oriental plague of the Third Pandemic had to be reoriented and transplanted to the colonial contexts of South and East Asia.[31]

The Legacy of Oriental Plague in Modern Historiography

Oriental plague and its epidemiological fronts (real or imagined) served a double purpose for the nineteenth-century European mindset. On the one hand, it helped to identify the European difference—a plague-free healthscape, hence a "civilized" society. On the other hand, it facilitated the legitimization of sanitary policies and the imposition of technologies for infectious disease-control. The narrative of epidemiological divisions lent itself remarkably well to modernization projects, not only in Europe but also in the Ottoman Empire itself. While informing public health policy at home, controlling disease allowed governments to assert greater

30 For example, see Adrien Proust, *La défense de l'Europe contre la peste et la Conférence de Venise de 1897* (Paris: Masson, 1897), 104: "mais nous croyons que cette peste offre les mêmes caractères que la peste d'Orient." About two decades before, Potter pointed out that plague's nosological classification was controversial among the European medical establishment. He opined that plague was very similar to typhus. See Potter, "Oriental Plague," 611. In fact, plague's nosology was being debated for quite some time. An example from the turn of the nineteenth century comes from the writings of the Scottish medical writer James Tytler. Following the 1793 yellow fever epidemic in Philadelphia, Tytler compares plague ("Asiatic or True Plague") to yellow fever and concludes that "true plague" is distinguished by its high mortality. See James Tytler, *A Treatise on the Plague and Yellow Fever* (Salem: Printed by Joshua Cushing, for B.B. Macanulty 1799). Even though Tytler's treatise does not use the term "Oriental plague," a very critical review of his book published the next year refers to plague as the "Oriental plague." See "Review of *A Treatise on the Plague and Yellow Fever*, by James Tytler," *Medical Repository* 3, no. 4 (1800): 373–79. In a similar vein, Hecker used the term Oriental plague mostly for taxonomic purposes in the first half of the nineteenth century. See Hecker, *Epidemics*.

31 Despite the different geographic, climatic, historical, social, and cultural conditions that shaped the plague experiences of the Near East and that of East and South Asia, there are interesting overlaps in discussions of plague foci, plague's epidemiological origins, and the directionality of its spread in the writings of European public health officials and scientists. For further discussion, see Varlık, "New Science and Old Sources."

authority over their borders. In the Ottoman example, discussions about public health and quarantine involved anxieties about modernization, border control, and religion.[32]

The legacy of this post-Enlightenment vision has not been limited to cultivating binaries of healthscape and imagining divided histories of disease. Once the narrative of epidemiological fronts was integrated into modern epidemiology and public health policy, it also informed the writing of history. When modern plague historiography emerged in the nineteenth century, it quickly embraced this post-Enlightenment narrative and reproduced it in historical scholarship. As a result, the nineteenth-century epidemiological fronts have gradually become the fronts of academic inquiry in the twentieth. This becomes especially problematic when these epidemiological fronts are applied to pre-nineteenth-century history. Imagined as the source of all plagues that Europe experienced, the Ottoman landscape has come to represent an area that has always been afflicted with disease and its past has often been represented as having a uniformly sickly character.[33] The historiography of medieval and early modern Mediterranean plagues has largely followed the precept of European exceptionalism, while freely drawing from the premise that the Ottoman Empire has been a *timeless* repository of disease.[34] Historians of the Ottoman Empire and later those of Turkish Republic have likewise drawn heavily from this narrative.[35]

---

32 For example, pilgrimage became a growing source of concern starting in the second half of the nineteenth century, owing to increased number of seaborne pilgrims coming from and through British India. See Michael Christopher Low, "Empire and the Hajj: Pilgrims, Plagues, and Pan-Islam under British Surveillance, 1865–1908," *International Journal of Middle East Studies* 40, no. 2 (2008): 269–90; also see note 19 above.

33 A similar case is how, after the Third Pandemic, China came to be imagined as the source of past plague pandemics. This is still a contentious issue among historians. See Paul D. Buell, "Qubilai and the Rats," *Sudhoffs Archiv* Band 96, no. 2 (2012): 127–44; Sussman, "Was the Black Death in India and China?"; Robert Hymes, "Epilogue: A Hypothesis on the East Asian Beginnings of the *Yersinia pestis* Polytomy," *The Medieval Globe* 1 (2014): 285–308.

34 For recent works that have been largely informed by this vision of European exceptionalism, see for example Jane L. Stevens Crawshaw, *Plague Hospitals: Public Health for the City in Early Modern Venice* (Farnham: Ashgate, 2012); Kristy Wilson Bowers, *Plague and Public Health in Early Modern Seville* (Rochester: University of Rochester Press, 2013); Zlata Blažina-Tomić and Vesna Blažina, *Expelling the Plague: The Health Office and the Implementation of Quarantine in Dubrovnik, 1377–1533* (Montreal: McGill-Queen's University Press, 2015).

35 For further discussion, see Varlık, *Plague and Empire in the Early Modern Mediterranean World: The Ottoman Experience, 1347–1600* (Cambridge: Cambridge University Press, 2015), 55–63. Recent scholarship shows a move away from this narrative. See, for example, Kyle

It might be helpful to highlight how this narrative has obscured modern historiography. Privileging the nineteenth-century Eurocentric epidemiologic narratives, this body of scholarship has approached earlier eras from the prism of these narratives and has unquestioningly accepted its projection to late medieval and early modern eras. It has largely failed to problematize the post-Enlightenment European plague episteme (e.g., no discussion of European plague foci (reservoirs), focusing instead on repeated introductions from outside). Instead of recognizing this episteme and its related body of policies as representations that responded to European anxieties of a particular age, modern scholarship has largely accepted it uncritically.[36]

This particular nineteenth-century vision that sought to divide the Mediterranean world into distinct epidemiological regions dominated modern historiography of plague for decades. In fact, explaining the differences in the epidemiological experiences of Europe and the rest of the Mediterranean world has been one of the fundamental problems of the plague historiography since the 1970s. Typically, this body of scholarship has approached the post-Black Death Mediterranean with an assumed epidemiological division, in binary oppositions, such as "Christian" vs. "Muslim" or "Oriental" vs. "Occidental." These invisible divisions of epidemiological experiences came to mark the boundaries of scholarship, hence producing separate histories of plague in Europe and the Middle East/Islamic world.[37] Even for studies that maintained a unified Mediterranean vision, those divisions played a critical role. For example, in his authoritative work on the history of plague in France, Europe, and the Mediterranean, French historian Jean-Noël Biraben offers

T. Evered and Emine Ö. Evered, "Governing Population, Public Health, and Malaria in the Early Turkish Republic," *Journal of Historical Geography* 37, no. 4 (2011): 470–82; Evered and Evered, "State, Peasant, Mosquito: The Biopolitics of Public Health Education and Malaria in Early Republican Turkey," *Political Geography* 31, no. 5 (2012): 311–23; Evered and Evered, "Syphilis and Prostitution in the Socio-Medical Geographies of Turkey's Early Republican Provinces," *Health and Place* 18, no. 3 (2012): 528–35; Emine Ö. Evered and Kyle T. Evered, "Sex and the Capital City: The Political Framing of Syphilis and Prostitution in Early Republican Ankara," *Journal of the History of Medicine and Allied Sciences* 68, no. 2 (2013): 266–99.

36 An exception to this general trend can be found in Hans-Uwe Lammel, "Western European Perception and Representation of Plagues in Eastern Europe, the Ottoman Empire and the Near East, 1650–1800," in *Economic and Biological Interactions in Pre-Industrial Europe from the Thirteenth to Eighteenth Centuries*, ed. Simonetta Cavaciocchi (Florence: Firenze University Press, 2010), 399–421.

37 See for example Michael W. Dols, *The Black Death in the Middle East* (Princeton: Princeton University Press, 1977); Lawrence Conrad, "The Plague in the Early Medieval Near East," PhD diss., Princeton University, 1981.

an epidemiological division between regions he calls *nord-occidental* (north-occidental) and *sud-oriental* (south-oriental).[38] Biraben legitimizes this bipartite view of the Mediterranean in terms of differences in climate, fauna, and, interestingly, attitudes toward disease. However, a close analysis of his division clearly suggests a historically defined construction of the geographical regions, whereby religion is the single most dividing factor. Perhaps even more influential in re-enacting these older stereotypes and "civilizational/religious" differences is the 1976 *Plagues and Peoples* of American historian William McNeill. Failing to see that this narrative of epidemiological binaries was a product of post-Enlightenment European anxieties, McNeill reproduces the same discourse by maintaining that Christian and Muslim responses to plague were fundamentally different. According to him, while the Christian attitude was an active combat with disease, the Muslim response was (or had, by the sixteenth century, become) passive and fatalistic. Interestingly enough, the passage he chooses to illustrate the so-called Turkish fatalism is taken from *The Turkish Letters* of the Habsburg ambassador Ogier Ghiselin de Busbecq, one that involves an interchange with the Ottoman sultan Süleyman (r. 1520–66) regarding right conduct at times of plague. Taking the passage at its face value and failing to identify the exchange of rhetoric there, McNeill reads it as a reflection of a fatalistic stand in the face of disease and does not refrain from generalizing it to Islamic civilization.[39] This position became very influential and left its imprint on succeeding scholarship.[40] Daniel Panzac's 1985 *La peste dans l'empire ottoman* situates the empire as a plague exporter to Europe during the eighteenth and nineteenth centuries, while not fully addressing the roots of the historical divergence in their epidemiological experience.[41]

This trend has surprisingly prevailed until today. Even books published very recently continue to draw from the same repository of epidemiological boundaries.[42] A theme that underlies these studies is a shared agreement about *European*

38 Jean-Noël Biraben, *Les hommes et la peste en France et dans les pays européens et méditerranéens* (Paris: Mouton, 1975), 1: 106.

39 William McNeill, *Plagues and Peoples* (Garden City, NY: Anchor Press, 1976), 198–99.

40 For further discussion, see Varlık, *Plague and Empire*, 72–76.

41 Panzac, *La peste*.

42 For example, historian Sylvia Chiffoleau refers to the Orient as "*terrain privilégié des épidémies*." See Sylvia Chiffoleau, *Genèse de la santé publique internationale: de la peste d'Orient à l'OMS* (Rennes: Presses universitaires de Rennes, 2012), 13. Similarly, a recent book on the natural disasters in the Ottoman Empire works with the premise that the European experience of plague was different than that of the Middle East and seeks to explain why the latter's response was different. See Yaron Ayalon, *Natural Disasters in the Ottoman Empire: Plague, Famine, and Other Misfortunes* (Cambridge: Cambridge University

exceptionalism, as well as an uncritical acceptance of accounts that represented the Oriental landscape as the hotbed of disease and the inability of Oriental governments to deal with it effectively. With a conviction that we can no longer afford to retain this nineteenth-century Eurocentric imagination of divided epidemiological pasts in the Mediterranean world, it might be helpful to consider some methodologies to help us transcend these binding debates. Using the new science of plague, for example, might be one avenue to critically reconsider the narratives that we have inherited.[43] Another possible avenue to explore might be to draw from methodologies recently adopted by environmental historians, which contributed invaluable insights into the reassessment of processes of environmental change.

Environmental Imaginaries and the Revisionist Scholarship

Over the past few decades, historians and anthropologists have become more attentive to environmental imagination in both contemporary and historical sources. In the main, this body of revisionist scholarship has not only contributed to our understanding of the specifics of environmental change in certain regions but has also helped to adjust mainstream thinking in environmental history. Examples of this scholarship have tackled the contentious relationship between nature and human agency in the narratives of environmental change. Disentangling environmental imaginaries from historical and contemporary anthropogenic phenomena makes it possible to rectify the central role of human response in environmental history.

There are excellent examples of this scholarship, especially in the context of the United States and the rest of the Americas, as well as Africa and Europe.[44] In the case of American environmental history, a prolific body of scholarship has reckoned with environmental change in both colonial and pre-colonial eras. This body of works has heavily focused on the frontier environment, forests, agriculture, as well

---

Press, 2015). Also see note 36 above. Recently, the limited geographical scope of the Second Plague Pandemic was reconsidered in Green, ed. *Pandemic Disease in the Medieval World*.

43 For an example of how the "new science" of plague can inform our reading of "old sources," see Varlık, "New Science and Old Sources."

44 For a state-of-the-field of global environmental history over a quarter of a century, see J. R. McNeill, "Observations on the Nature and Culture of Environmental History," *History and Theory* 42, no. 4 (2003): 5–43. For a more recent overview of the field, see J. R. McNeill, "The State of the Field of Environmental History," *Annual Review of Environment and Resources* 35, no. 1 (2010): 345–74, which discusses problems in the field of environmental history including the issue of declensionism.

as hunting and animals.[45] In addition, one of the most contentious subjects of the environmental histories has been the exploitation of nuclear energy resources and management of nuclear waste disposal and its lasting effects in the American West. The ethnographic and ecological research of Valerie Kuletz, for example, takes issue with the imagination of the American West as a wasteland. Kuletz argues that the perception of Euroamerican settlers of desert lands as marginal and as no man's land was endorsed by environmental science and effectively exploited by the U.S. government for nuclear waste disposal, despite the region's rich energy resources and its sacred character for Native American inhabitants. As her work deconstructs the wasteland discourse maintained by military officials, policy makers, and government bureaucrats, the sacred geography of the region becomes visible.[46]

In a similar vein, historical, social anthropological, and ecological research has helped us to understand how some prevailing assumptions about the African environment, long held by scientists and policy makers alike, have been wrong. In the example of Guinea in West Africa, the work of James Fairhead and Melissa Leach offers a corrective to widespread convictions of forest degradation, by showing how the locals indeed carefully and strategically strove to cultivate and maintain forest islands around villages. This analysis not only demonstrates that environmental imaginaries inherited from colonialism are to be reassessed but also allows for a reversal in forest histories by emphasizing enrichment of the environment.[47]

---

45 The field of American environmental history, spearheading the larger field since its rise, has yielded a substantial body of literature, too large to include here. For a recent discussion of the historiography of environmental history in the Americas, see Peter Coates, "Emerging from the Wilderness (or, from Redwoods to Bananas): Recent Environmental History in the United States and the Rest of the Americas," *Environment and History* 10, no. 4 (2004): 407–38. For a recent comprehensive survey, see Carolyn Merchant, *American Environmental History: An Introduction* (New York: Columbia University Press, 2007). For the revisionist literature, see for example, a work that takes issue with representations of Native Americans as ecologists and conservationists: Shepard Krech III, *The Ecological Indian: Myth and History* (New York: Norton, 1999); or a work that challenges the notion of wilderness, William Cronon, "The Trouble with Wilderness; Or, Getting Back to the Wrong Nature," *Environmental History* 1, no. 1 (1996): 7–28. Regional studies have also inspired comparative perspectives. For an example of comparative environmental history of the USA and South Africa, offering a critical evaluation of inherited wisdom about environmental change in both contexts, see William Beinart and Peter Coates, *Environment and History: The Taming of Nature in the USA and South Africa* (London: Routledge, 1995).

46 Valerie Kuletz, *The Tainted Desert: Environmental Ruin in the American West* (New York: Routledge, 1998).

47 James Fairhead and Melissa Leach, *Misreading the African Landscape: Society and Ecology in a Forest-Savanna Mosaic* (Cambridge: Cambridge University Press, 1996). For other works of scholarship that challenge the narrative of environmental degradation, destruction, and

In the field of Middle East studies, environmental history is a recently developing area of scholarship.[48] In open contrast to an older generation of scholarship that largely neglected human agency in the study of Middle Eastern environment, this new scholarship seeks to restore the dialectical relationship between humans and environment. This effort involves adopting different timescales than have previously been used (i.e., years or decades rather than centuries or millennia) as well as exploiting different types of sources (i.e., human-authored historical sources rather than archeological, climatic, or biological data).[49] This fresh approach has already resulted in excellent studies challenging a host of assumptions about the region's history, ranging in topics from climate to agriculture to animals.[50]

One of the threads that the field of environmental history of the Middle East and North Africa (MENA) takes issue with is "environmental imaginaries," which,

---

deforestation in the African landscape, see, for example James C. McCann, "The Plow and the Forest: Narratives of Deforestation in Ethiopia, 1840–1992," *Environmental History* 2, no. 2 (April 1, 1997): 138–59; James C. McCann, *Green Land, Brown Land, Black Land: An Environmental History of Africa, 1800–1990* (Portsmouth, NH: Heinemann, 1999); Paul Richards, *Fighting for the Rain Forest: War, Youth and Resources in Sierra Leone* (Portsmouth, NH: Heinemann, 1996); Melissa Leach and Robin Mearns, *The Lie of the Land: Challenging Received Wisdom on the African Environment* (Oxford; Portsmouth, NH: Heinemann, 1996).

48 For an earlier comprehensive survey of the field, see Jeff Albert, Magnus Bernhardsson, and Roger Kenna, eds., *Transformations of Middle Eastern Natural Environments: Legacies and Lessons* (New Haven: Yale School of Forestry and Environmental Studies, 1998). For more recent surveys, see Diana K. Davis and Edmund Burke III, eds., *Environmental Imaginaries of the Middle East and North Africa* (Athens: Ohio University Press, 2011); Alan Mikhail, ed., *Water on Sand: Environmental Histories of the Middle East and North Africa* (Oxford: Oxford University Press, 2012).

49 For a more detailed discussion of the historiography of Middle East environmental history, see Mikhail, "Introduction: Middle East Environmental History: The Fallow between Two Fields," in *Water on Sand*, 1–25.

50 See, for example, Mikhail, "An Irrigated Empire: The View from Ottoman Fayyum," *International Journal of Middle East Studies* 42, no. 4 (2010): 569–90; Mikhail, *Nature and Empire in Ottoman Egypt: An Environmental History* (Cambridge: Cambridge University Press, 2011); Mikhail, ed., *Water on Sand*; Mikhail, *The Animal in Ottoman Egypt* (Oxford: Oxford University Press, 2013); Sam White, *The Climate of Rebellion in the Early Modern Ottoman Empire* (Cambridge: Cambridge University Press, 2011); Arash Khazeni, *Tribes and Empire on the Margins of Nineteenth-Century Iran* (Seattle: University of Washington Press, 2009); Suraiya Faroqhi, ed., *Animals and People in the Ottoman Empire* (Istanbul: Eren, 2010); Richard W Bulliet, *Cotton, Climate, and Camels in Early Islamic Iran: A Moment in World History* (New York: Columbia University Press, 2009); Richard Bulliet, "The Camel and the Watermill," *International Journal of Middle East Studies* 42, no. 4 (2010): 666–68; Edmund Burke III, "Pastoralism and the Mediterranean Environment," *International Journal of Middle East Studies* 42, no. 4 (2010): 663–65.

historian Diana Davis defines as "the constellation of ideas that groups of humans develop about a given landscape, usually local or regional, that commonly includes assessments about the environment as well as how it came to be in its current state."[51] Studying how the region's landscape has been depicted in historical sources and how those imaginaries served imperialist agendas as well as modernist projects of the nation states in the area, recent studies have compellingly demonstrated the crucial importance of environmental imaginaries. Products of British and French colonial visions of the area, these were later integrated into postcolonial modernization projects. As resilient ways of imagining the environment, these imaginaries informed modernization projects in both colonial and postcolonial eras. One aspect of the larger colonial vision of MENA that served the Anglo-European imperialist project is environmental orientalism.[52]

Conceptualizing epidemics as ecological crises involving both environmental change and human agency, allows us to study them with insights offered by studies that take issue with environmental imaginaries. This, in turn, takes us to an exploration of the methodologies and questions that can be applied to studies of historical epidemiology and the history of public health. More specifically, it is worth considering how we can make use of this tool (i.e., environmental orientalism) in advancing our understanding of the region's epidemiological past. In what follows, we will reconsider representations of the Oriental landscape and its people in the narratives of European travelers with a view to recognizing that the epidemiological orientalism that is embedded in them was a discursive practice used by these authors to process epistemologies of plague within a certain configuration of power.[53]

Epidemiological Orientalism

Kinglake and his contemporaries in the nineteenth century did not build upon an entirely empty terrain in creating narratives of epidemiological fronts. Already, there was a long-standing tradition inherited from the medieval and early mod-

51 Davis, "Introduction: Imperialism, Orientalism, and the Environment in the Middle East," in *Environmental Imaginaries*, 3.

52 Davis and Burke, *Environmental Imaginaries.*

53 For the classic definition of orientalism and its uses, see Edward Said, *Orientalism* (New York: Vintage Book, 1978). Despite its huge influence on many disciplines, orientalism has been severely critiqued over the last three decades. For a recent evaluation of genealogies of orientalism and a call to study historically specific orientalisms, see Edmund Burke III and David Prochaska, eds., *Genealogies of Orientalism: History, Theory, Politics* (Lincoln: University of Nebraska Press, 2008).

ern eras that dictated how to imagine the Oriental landscape and its people. Medieval European imaginaries of the Orient were largely shaped by religious difference, as suggested by medieval pilgrimage accounts that did not fall short of supplying Christendom with stories about a perilous landscape and iniquitous people.[54] In the early modern era, the tradition of Oriental travel and travel writing further expanded and diversified. In the Ottoman case, in particular, the number of European travelers increased considerably after the mid-fifteenth-century Ottoman conquest of Constantinople, and continued to increase throughout the early modern era.[55] In addition, those who authored such works were no longer only pilgrims but increasingly a more diversified group of visitors, including those who traveled for diplomatic, commercial, scholarly, and missionary purposes. Among them were a considerable number of physicians, botanists, pharmacists, and other naturalists.[56]

Being among early sources of information on the Oriental landscape and its people, these sources were exceedingly influential on the European imaginaries of the Orient. Between the writings of travelers, the widespread demand for *Turcica* literature in early-modern Europe, the development of the printing press and the widespread circulation of printed books, it should be possible to account, at least in part, for the spread of these ideas among the European audience. A considerable body of historical scholarship has examined the various aspects of the repre-

54 For medieval European imagination of the Orient, see for example John Victor Tolan, *Saracens: Islam in the Medieval European Imagination* (New York: Columbia University Press, 2002). For medieval pilgrimage accounts, see for example Brett Edward Whalen, ed., *Pilgrimage in the Middle Ages: A Reader* (Toronto: University of Toronto Press, 2011); Colin Morris, "Pilgrimage to Jerusalem in the Late Middle Ages," in *Pilgrimage: The English Experience from Becket to Bunyan*, ed. Colin Morris and Peter Roberts (Cambridge: Cambridge University Press, 2002), 141–63; Nicole Chareyron, *Pilgrims to Jerusalem in the Middle Ages*, trans. Donald Wilson (New York: Columbia University Press, 2005).

55 For a compilation of biographical and bibliographical collection of European travelers to the Ottoman Empire between the fourteenth and seventeenth century, see Stefanos Yerasimos, *Les voyageurs dans l'Empire ottoman, XIVe–XVIe siècles: bibliographie, itinéraires et inventaire des lieux habités* (Ankara: Türk Tarih Kurumu, 1991).

56 Sonja Brentjes, *Travellers from Europe in the Ottoman and Safavid Empires, 16th-17th Centuries: Seeking, Transforming, Discarding Knowledge* (Farnham; Burlington, VT: Ashgate/Variorum, 2010). Also see Gerald M. MacLean, *The Rise of Oriental Travel: English Visitors to the Ottoman Empire, 1580–1720* (New York: Palgrave Macmillan, 2004); Elisabetta Borromeo, *Voyageurs occidentaux dans l'empire ottoman, 1600–1644: inventaire des récits et études sur les itinéraires, les monuments remarqués et les populations rencontrées (Roumélie, Cyclades, Crimée)* (Paris; Istanbul: Maisonneuve & Larose; Institut français d'études anatoliennes, 2007).

sentations of the Orient by travelers and how these contributed to the European imaginaries about it.[57] For example, Amanda Wunder's study of the accounts of educated elite European travelers to the Ottoman Empire in the sixteenth century shows that this body of literature contributed to widening the perceived gap between Europe and the Ottoman Empire by articulating a discourse of difference, especially with respect to their relationship with the classical past and its physical products. Emerging from an analysis of books and printed images was an imagination of difference, whereby the Turks inhabiting lands that once possessed the grandeur of a classical past did not have an appreciation for that past, nor for its physical remains. Wunder argues that these travelers regarded the antiquities of the Ottoman Empire as representations of the classical past, hence the European antiquarian, as the guardian of antiquities, was in charge of protecting these items, and if necessary, was entitled to "rescue" them from the hands of "barbaric" Turks. This narrative made it possible and acceptable to transport vast quantities of manuscripts, coins, and other antiquities to Europe for the appreciation and consumption of elites with the right taste for classical culture. Even though these accounts privileged first-hand observations and impressions of educated European men with a taste for antiquities, they did little to complicate the image of the Turk. In fact, they perhaps contributed to its becoming stereotypical.[58]

The image of the Turk cultivated by sixteenth-century travel accounts found a slightly different context in the eighteenth and nineteenth centuries, when antiquarianism was replaced by Orientalism, as an academic discipline that took the East as subject of study. In the nineteenth century, the Turks were represented along similar lines regarding their affective stand to the historical and cultural legacy of the landscape they inhabited. For example, Ebru Boyar's analysis of representations of Anatolia and its inhabitants in the accounts of late-eighteenth- and nineteenth-century British archeological travelers suggests that these travelers imagined the Anatolian past as an extension of ancient Greece and regarded its archeological legacy as living testimony of that past, in a manner that erased centuries of Turkish presence from that very same landscape. In these accounts,

57 For a recent example, see Bozidar Jezernik, *Imagining "the Turk"* (Newcastle upon Tyne: Cambridge Scholars, 2010); for an example that focuses on visual representations, see James G. Harper, ed., *The Turk and Islam in the Western Eye, 1450–1750: Visual Imagery Before Orientalism* (Farnham: Ashgate, 2011). Also see Daniel J. Vitkus, "Early Modern Orientalism: Representations of Islam in Sixteenth- and Seventeenth-Century Europe," in *Western Views of Islam in Medieval and Early Modern Europe: Perception of Other*, David R. Blanks and Michael Frasetto, eds. (New York: St. Martin's Press, 1999), 207–30.

58 Amanda Wunder, "Western Travelers, Eastern Antiquities, and the Image of the Turk in Early Modern Europe," *Journal of Early Modern History* 7, no. 1–2 (2003): 89–119.

Turks are depicted as lacking any understanding of and appreciation for the landscape's history and archeological heritage, which in turn allows the Europeans to appropriate that past. It only follows that the British, with their deep appreciation of the value of Anatolian archeological remains, would extend claims to protect them, if necessary by moving them to British museums.[59] In fact, the nineteenth century witnessed a big surge of European interest to acquire the antiquities in the Ottoman domains.[60]

These studies are invaluable in sketching the discursive map of the Orient, especially with a view to tracing imaginaries of an infected landscape. Especially after large-scale plague epidemics no longer appeared in Europe, Ottoman cities served as repositories of knowledge about the plague, where the disease could be observed and studied first-hand. In this manner, the Oriental cities were not only the repositories of the disease but of knowledge about it as well. Hence, in the eighteenth and nineteenth centuries, a considerable number of European medical writers went to the Orient, observed the plague, and wrote about it.[61] In this manner, these medical writers joined other travelers who created the discursive map of the Orient as an infected landscape. There is clear evidence that the works of these medical writers informed the European historical scholarship in the nineteenth and twentieth centuries.[62]

The Making of the Epidemiological Other: Reconsidering Epidemiological Imaginaries

There has been a complex relationship between epidemiological fronts and the textual (and visual) representations of divided healthscapes. On the one hand, the particular imagination of the sickly Orient was necessary for imposing and maintaining boundary-making technologies, such as quarantines and *cordons sanitaires*.[63] On the other hand, the same imagination was a product of border-

---

59 Ebru Boyar, "British Archeological Travellers in Nineteenth-Century Anatolia: Anatolia 'Without' Turks," *Eurasian Studies* 1, no. 1 (2002): 97–113.

60 For a recent discussion of the historiography of archeology in the Ottoman Empire, see Zainab Bahrani, Zeynep Çelik, and Edhem Eldem, eds., *Scramble for the Past: A Story of Archaeology in the Ottoman Empire, 1753–1914* (Istanbul: SALT, 2011).

61 For a detailed discussion of the Ottoman "laboratory of plague," see Varlık, "New Science and Old Sources," 201–5.

62 For example, Hirsch was familiar with the writings of first-hand observers of plague in the Ottoman Empire. See Hirsch, *Handbook*, 504–8.

63 Panzac, *Quarantaines et lazarets: l'Europe et la peste d'Orient (XVIIe–XXe siècles)* (Aix-en-Provence: Édisud, 1986). The land border between Hapsburgs and the Ottomans started

control and isolation technologies and the policies that sustained them. In other words, the "epidemiological other" stemmed from the very presence of the division between the healthy and the infected. Throughout the early modern era, plague served as a model disaster to emphasize the difference between "us" and "them" in travel narratives, which, in the nineteenth century, found its way to the public health and epidemiology literature.

The representations of the Oriental healthscape in the writings of European visitors reveal insights about notions of plague's spatiality and temporality. Tracing these accounts not only allows us to trace how plague was anchored in Oriental space and time but also makes it possible to explore how these narratives nurtured the larger plague episteme on the questions of its origin and etiology. To this end, we first turn to early modern European travelogues with respect to epidemiological imaginaries of the Orient.

Historian Diana Davis has argued that European environmental imaginaries represented the Oriental environment "as alien, exotic, fantastic, or 'abnormal,' and frequently as degraded in some way."[64] One of the most prominent examples of the representation of the Ottoman landscape can be found in accounts about urban areas, which are typically represented as lacking the properties of great cities. In the words of Gianfrancesco Morosini, Venetian ambassador to the Porte, "[Constantinople] lacks those amenities that a great city should have, such as beautiful streets, great squares, and handsome palaces. Although Constantinople has many mosques, royal palaces, inns, and public baths, the rest of the city is mazy and filthy."[65] Clearly, the urban environment of the city is represented as "subpar" to a "great city" in some ways.

The urban environment of early modern Ottoman cities lent itself to different types of representations in conjunction with plague. For the most part, travel writers placed an unmistakable emphasis on perceived sources of filth in the urban environment. While some believed that the streets were the source of contagion, others considered graveyards a major challenge to the health of cities. In such rep-

---

out as the military border but later also enforced sanitary border. See G. E. Rothenberg, "The Austrian Sanitary Cordon and the Control of the Bubonic Plague: 1710–1871," *Journal of the History of Medicine and Allied Sciences* 28, no. 1 (1973): 15–23. For further discussion of epidemics, border control, and contagion across the Habsburg and Ottoman Empires, see the articles in Teodora Daniela Sechel, ed., *Medicine Within and Between the Habsburg and Ottoman Empires, 18th–19th Centuries* (Bochum: Dieter Winkler, 2011).

64 Davis, "Introduction," in *Environmental Imaginaries*, 3.

65 Gianfrancesco Morosini, "Turkey is a Republic of Slaves," [Albèri, III, 3: 253–322] in *Pursuit of Power: Venetian Ambassador's Reports on Spain, Turkey, and France in the Age of Phillip II, 1560–1600*, ed. James C. Davis (New York: Harper and Row, 1970), 129.

resentations, the "fault" lay on a physical space that was associated with plague's etiology. In yet other examples of the genre, the "poison" lay instead on social norms, beliefs, and practices. In such cases, it was the Oriental administrative and political structures that came under criticism, being hailed as the cause of the outbreaks of plague. These differences were made more subtly in travel narratives, and often entwined with one another. Whatever form they took, however, such representations sought to establish an association between the Ottoman landscape and plague, and in doing so contributed to the cultivation of an image of the plague as something inherent or indigenous to that very landscape.

Throughout the early modern era, the European travel literature continued to contribute to the plague episteme while carving it into Oriental space. In these accounts, the loci of plague also emerged as *topoi* of the narratives. Among these loci were physical spaces associated with filth, such as streets, graveyards, and the flea market. Early modern European travelers typically described the streets of Ottoman cities as dark, unpaved, and being notoriously filthy. Many travelers noted that the streets were narrow and crooked and often commented on the mud and dirt. Some also commented on the accumulation of garbage and animal carcasses, all depicted as contributing to the heavy stench found in Oriental cities.[66] For example, Michael Heberer von Bretten, a southern German traveler who witnessed a plague outbreak in Istanbul in the early months of 1588, described the streets of the city as filthy and commented on dead rats, horses, and dogs left lying in the alleys, which for him was the cause of the pestilence.[67] The English traveler Fynes Moryson's visit to Istanbul in 1597 led him to comment on the streets as follows: "The streetes of this Citie are narrow ... In many places of the streetes lye carcases, yea sometimes the bodies of dead men, even till they be putrified, and I thinke this uncleanlinesse of the Turks is the chiefe cause that this Citie ... is continually more or lesse infected with the plague."[68] In these accounts, filth, stench, and putrefaction produced by animal carcasses (and human corpses) on the streets were understood as the cause of plague.

---

66 Istanbul was the typical example for these representations. For examples of European travelers' descriptions of Istanbul's streets, see İnalcık, "Istanbul"; Robert Mantran, *Istanbul au siècle de Soliman le Magnifique* (Paris: Hachette, 1994), 105–8; Mehmet Mazak, *Orijinal Belge ve Fotoğraflar Işığında Osmanlı'da Sokak ve Çevre Temizliği* (Istanbul: İSTAÇ, 2001). For a critical discussion of these representations, see Varlık, *Plague and Empire*, 276–79.

67 Johann Michael Heberer, *Aegyptiaca servitus* (Graz: Akademische Druck und Verlagsanstalt, 1967), 303.

68 Fynes Moryson, *An Itinerary: Containing His Ten Yeeres Travell through the Twelve Dominions of Germany, Bohmerland, Sweitzerland, Netherland, Denmarke, Poland, Italy, Turky, France, England, Scotland and Ireland* (Glasgow: J. MacLehose and Sons, 1907), 2: 100–1.

Another perceived source of contamination pointed out by European travelers was Ottoman graveyards.[69] While several travelogues mentioned that graveyards were built outside of cities to keep the city air free form stench and that separate graves were dug for each individual, some other accounts insisted that the graves were not dug deep enough and that they could release harmful odors in the air. The concern about the corpses' contaminating the air was especially distressing to European travelers, since the deceased were buried (unlike in Europe) without a coffin. For example, the early nineteenth-century travelogue of physician John Griffiths of the Royal Medical Society of Edinburgh commented that the "graves are not dug deep."[70] Another near-contemporary testimony comes from the British traveler John Cam Hobhouse who noted that the Muslim graves just outside of Smyrna were dug "only a foot or two in depth, and containing corpses without coffins, were exposed to the burning summer sun." He reasoned that the cypress trees planted in and around burial sites were to offset the stench rising from graves.[71] In this manner, burial practices and graveyards were associated with plagues because they were imagined to contaminate the urban environment.

Another perceived source of filth in early-modern European travel accounts was the flea market in Ottoman cities (Istanbul, in particular), where second-hand clothes trade took place. An early example where plague and the flea market are mentioned together comes from the account of Jérôme Maurand, a French priest who witnessed a plague outbreak in Istanbul in the summer of 1544. In order to emphasize how plague did not bring the lively commercial life of the city to a halt even when it killed about five hundred people everyday, Maurand wrote that the belongings of plague victims were brought to the flea market and sold outside its doors, at reduced prices.[72] Even though there is nothing in this account that asso-

69 For the sixteenth-century European accounts that include discussions of Ottoman burial customs and the state of the graveyards, see for example, Stephan Gerlach, *Türkiye Günlüğü: 1573–1576* (Istanbul: Kitap Yayınevi, 2007); Reinhold Lubenau, *Beschreibung der Reisen des Reinhold Lubenau* (Königsberg: Beyer (Thomas and Oppermann), 1914–15); Salomon Schweigger, *Sultanlar Kentine Yolculuk, 1578–1581* (Istanbul: Kitap Yayınevi, 2004).

70 John Griffiths, *Travels in Europe, Asia Minor and Arabia* (London: T. Cadell and W. Davies, 1805), 146–47.

71 John Cam Hobhouse, *A Journey Through Albania and Other Provinces of Turkey in Europe and Asia, to Constantinople, During the Years 1809–1810* (London: James Cawthorn, 1813), 2: 623.

72 Plague was killing about five hundred people every day. Many residents of the city, especially the Europeans residing in Galata took refuge in the surrounding gardens and vineyards. See Jérôme Maurand, *Itinéraire de Jérome Maurand d'Antibes à Constantinople (1544)* (Paris: E. Leroux, 1901), 204–5, 224–27, 236–37.

ciates the spread of plague to second-hand clothes trade, many later writers commented on the sale of items that formerly belonged to plague victims in the context of discussion of Istanbul's flea market. For example, the Venetian *bailo* Ottaviano Bon (d. 1623) observed that the belongings of plague victims were sold in the flea market, which he criticized severely. Later writers established a more intimate relationship between plague and second-hand clothes trade. Unlike Maurand, they added a causal link to this relationship. In doing so, they not only created a very specific spatial definition to plague's causation and transmission, but also connected it to what they believed was lackadaisical attitudes of the locals. The association between the second-hand clothes trade and the flea market became closely intertwined with narratives of plague, as they became *topoi* repeatedly used by European travelers. By the nineteenth century, the flea market was so tightly interwoven to narratives of plague that the French physician Pouqueville could openly target it as a plague focus.[73]

Examples of European travelogues sometimes emphasized perceived sources of filth in social conventions. They often expressed an aversion to the habits of the locals in their handling the sick and the dead, as well as their burial practices (e.g., washing the body of the deceased). The criticism was most poignant, however, when plague was an issue. Early modern European travelers' accounts abound in descriptions of how the Muslims did not refrain from touching the body or the belongings of plague victims. For example, the Habsburg ambassador Ogier Ghiselin de Busbecq voiced his criticism and contempt for such practices as follows: "They handle the garments and linen in which plague-stricken persons have died, even though they are still wet with the contagion of their sweat; nay, they even wipe their faces with them."[74] Soon after Busbecq, another member of the Habsburg diplomatic mission to the Sublime Porte, the Lutheran preacher Salomon Schweigger, embellished his account with an anecdote. According to it, one day Schweigger witnessed the death of a poor man from plague on a street near the ambassadorial residence. Upon seeing this, people passing by stopped and surrounded the deceased immediately; one took his hat, others his shoes, and in this way, they undressed him down to his underwear. Finally, two men took pity

73 François-Charles-Hugues-Laurent Pouqueville, *Voyage en Morée, à Constantinople, en Albanie et dans plusieurs autres parties de l'Empire othoman pendant les années 1798, 1799, 1800 et 1801* (Paris, 1805), 2: 109–11.

74 Ogier Ghiselin de Busbecq, *The Turkish Letters of Ogier Ghiselin de Busbecq, Imperial Ambassador at Constantinople, 1554–1562: Translated from the Latin of the Elzevir Edition of 1663* (Baton Rouge: Louisiana State University Press, 2005), 189.

and carried the body away to bury.[75] These representations shared an emphasis on undisciplined, undesired, and ultimately transgressive forms of contacts between the healthy and the plague-stricken.

More importantly, these accounts associated the contacts between the healthy and the sick as breeding plague. According to this narrative, because the Ottomans lacked a basic understanding of contagion, they did not take any precautions to protect themselves from plague and this helped to sustain the disease among them. The alleged indifference of Muslims on account of their fatalistic beliefs became a common stock of this genre and a stereotype repeated often across centuries.[76] In this narrative, the locus of plague-causation was not limited to the urban environment alone, but also involved the beliefs and conventions of the society at large. Ultimately, this narrative gave way to one that viewed the urban environment as an index of good governance.

In late nineteenth-century Europe, the health of a society came to be seen as a measure of its civilization. In this vein, even though social conventions and their association with disease remained intact, public health and hygiene were honored as greater public goods. In the words of one medical writer in the late nineteenth century, "The ideal city is one which is not only populated by individuals who zealously observe the laws of personal hygiene, but which is so founded, so arranged, and so managed as to exercise upon all within its gates a healthful influence."[77] Hence, it was understood that "the ideal city" offered the right opportunities for its people to be healthy, were they to follow the right rules of personal hygiene. Moreover, this was supported by a new body of knowledge: the "sanitary science" (i.e., public health). A society governed by knowledge of public health would prevent disease, preserve health, and prolong life.[78]

This new perspective had all the ingredients for the exclusion of Oriental cities from the boundaries of a "civilized" healthscape. The older tropes of the genre of early modern travel literature, such as narrow and crooked streets, burial practices, indifference to plague, and lack of personal hygiene among the Orientals, continued. Moreover, Oriental cities were represented as lacking the form of governance that could sustain a healthy city. By the end of the nineteenth century, old and new representations could be used together freely. In the words of Adrien

75 Schweigger, *Sultanlar Kentine Yolculuk*, 200. This account seems to contradict Schweigger's own description of funerary rites and ceremonies practiced in Istanbul. Cf., for example, 199.

76 For the trope of "Turkish fatalism," see Varlık, *Plague and Empire*, 72–88.

77 J. Hobart Egbert, "Preventable Causes of Ill Health and Disease in Cities," *The Dietetic and Hygienic Gazette* 11, no. 1 (1895): 5–7.

78 Guy, *Public Health*, 6.

Proust, professor of medicine at the University of Paris, the "insalubrious" conditions, such as "the absence of any public health that is felt in all Oriental cities; piles of refuse surrounding the houses and up to the mosques; cemeteries situated in the middle of houses, containing tombs always open and continuously exhaling a cadaverous odor; the narrow and irregular streets," all contributed to the emergence of plague epidemics.[79]

In the late nineteenth century, both old and new anxieties shaped international public health and infectious disease-control policies. The representations of the Orient and the Orientals were intimately entwined with the episteme that informed them. Blaming the Orientals for their beliefs and practices that came to be associated with the transmission of plague prepared the necessary grounds for legitimizing the imposition of international public health and infectious disease-control measures. Nevertheless, new representations that sought to situate the blame in political power made it possible to impose new regulations on governments. It was the International Sanitary Conferences of the nineteenth century that started the process of negotiation between local and international priorities of public health.

Having traced epidemiological imaginaries of the Orient, we now turn our attention to how these imaginaries contributed to the formation of modern epidemiology and its tenets about plague's origins and transmission. In the eighteenth century, when the divergence of epidemiological experience became more visibly pronounced between Europe and the Orient, it was commonly accepted that plague came from there. Yet whether the ultimate geographic origin of the plague lay there or elsewhere was still not settled. For example, English physician Richard Mead's well-known *A Discourse on the Plague* (1720) states that the Ottoman ports were the places where plagues come from even though he believed the real origin of plague to be in Africa (Cairo and Ethiopia, in particular).[80] He writes: "The Plague is a real Poison, which being bred in the Southern Parts of the World, is carried by Commerce into other Countries, particularly into *Turky*, where it maintains itself by a kind of Circulation from Persons to Goods: which is chiefly owing to the Negligence of the People there, who are stupidly careless in

79 Proust, *La défense de l'Europe*, 110-12, quote on 110: "l'absence de toute hygiène publique qui se fait sentir dans toutes les cités orientales; des amas d'immondices entourant les maisons et jusqu'aux mosquées; les cimetières placés au milieu des habitations, contenant des tombeaux toujours ouverts et exhalant continuellement une odeur cadavéreuse; les rues étroites, irrégulières."

80 Richard Mead, *A Discourse on the Plague* ([first edition 1720]; London: Printed for A. Millar, 1744), 21–40. He refers to Cairo and Ethiopia as "the two great Seminaries of the *Plague*," 30 and explains their environmental features that cause plague, 30–34.

this affair."[81] Toward the end of the eighteenth century, however, the idea of Africa as the origin of plague is no longer tenable. For example, James Tytler's *A Treatise on the Plague and Yellow Fever* (1799) discusses the origins of plague without pointing out to a particular direction. Unlike Mead, Tytler does not believe Cairo to be the source of plague and mentions the conflict of opinion about whether Egypt received plagues from Istanbul or vice versa.[82] Even Hecker, writing in the 1830s, did not regard the Anatolian cities and Istanbul as the ultimate geographic origin of plague. Hecker was not fully convinced that all plagues that broke out in Europe were imported from the East. While he acknowledged that Constantinople, being "the capital of commerce, and the medium of connexion between Asia, Europe, and Africa," received the infection from outside, it was (along with port cities of Anatolia) "regarded as the foci of infection; whence it radiated to the most distant seaports and islands."[83]

Nevertheless, the idea that the Ottoman lands harbored plague fit well in the larger plague episteme of the nineteenth century. In the language of the time, it was important to determine the "native habitat of the plague-poison," that is, to identify whether plague was "endemic" to an area or imported from elsewhere. Underlying these discussions, however, was a certain anxiety to distance Europe from its past plagues. In other words, even though it was well known that Europe had suffered from plague for centuries, it was important to show that it was not "native" to it but instead resulted from importation. This effort was facilitated by the ubiquitous presence of plague in the Orient. That there was something inherently wrong with the Oriental landscape, its people, and government that bred the plague made it easy for most European scholars to identify Europe as an exception. In this manner, the nineteenth-century vision of Europe as a healthscape of difference could be projected to the pre-nineteenth-century history. In this line of reasoning, it only followed that a plague focus could have never existed in Europe. A fervent defender of this idea, Hirsch, reasoned: "There is, in my opinion, not a single fact to show that plague ever had an autochthonous origin in Europe in the middle ages or subsequently."[84] Hence the plague, since the Middle Ages, had to

81 Mead, *Discourse*, 78. He designates the Coast of Africa as the origin of Ottoman plagues: "The frequent *Plagues*, which depopulate that Country [*Turkey*], are brought thither from the Coast of *Africa*: inso much that at *Smyrna*, and other Ports of that Coast, they often know the very Ship which brings it. And, in these latter Ages, since our Trade with *Turkey* has been pretty constant, the *Plagues* in these Parts of *Europe* have evidently been brought from thence." 24. There are also references to "Turkish infection." See, for example, 74.

82 Tytler, *Treatise*, 21–24.

83 Hecker, *Epidemics*, 17–19.

84 Hirsch, *Handbook*, 530.

be a result of importation. Hirsch wrote: "Since the seventeenth century, at least, every epidemic on European soil outside Turkey has owed its origin to importation of the morbid poison from the East. ... [T]he diffusion of plague over Europe had *always* to be referred to importation from the East."[85]

Although adamant about Europe's historical position as recipient of the infection from outside, Hirsch was not certain that Europe could never be re-infected again. In his article titled "What Has Europe to Fear in the Future from Oriental Plague?" he raised this distressing question to which he responded, "we are not justified in assuming that we are wholly secure from its recurrence" and vehemently called on European states for better sanitary administration.[86] The possibility that plagues could recur in Europe was a pressing concern shared by many medical authors of the time, especially after a lecture delivered by J. Netten Radcliffe, the President of the Epidemiological Society, at the Society's meeting during its session of 1874–75.[87] Hence it is no surprise to read Potter's warning a few years later: "We dare not say that England is perfectly safe from future infection. Given a tropical summer, a cargo of plague-stricken passengers, and an unhealthy, badly-managed port, the plague may yet be revived."[88] As the case may be, the late nineteenth-century European anxieties about the possibility of plague's recurrence was more pressing than it had been for at last a century and a half (i.e., since the Plague of Marseille). It is no coincidence that this era saw this question in the context of the wider political conjuncture. In the words of Hirsch, this was "a new 'Eastern Question' of a hygienic nature."[89] Yet this "question" would immediately bring to mind associations with Oriental plague and its thorny legacy that became entangled in epidemiological Orientalism.

---

85 Hirsch, *Handbook*, 527, 530. Emphasis mine.

86 Hirsch, "What Has Europe to Fear in the Future from Oriental Plague?," *The Practitioner: A Journal of Therapeutics and Public Health* 19 (1877): 223–40, quote on 239.

87 See for example J. Netten Radcliffe, "On the Prospect of a Reappearance of Plague in this Country and on the Continent of Europe," *Medical Times and Gazette* 1 (Jan 22, 1876): 83–85.

88 Potter, "Oriental Plague," 611–12.

89 Hirsch, "What Has Europe to Fear," 223.

Nükhet Varlık (varlik@andromeda.rutgers.edu) is Associate Professor of History at Rutgers University–Newark. She is a historian of the Ottoman Empire interested in disease, medicine, and public health. Her first book, *Plague and Empire in the Early Modern Mediterranean World: The Ottoman Experience, 1347–1600* (Cambridge University Press, 2015), is the first systematic scholarly study of the Ottoman experience of plague during the Black Death pandemic and the centuries that followed. It received the Middle East Studies Association's Albert Hourani Book Award and the Ottoman and Turkish Studies Association's M. Fuat Köprülü Book Prize. Dr. Varlık has authored several articles and book chapters addressing different aspects of plague epidemics in Ottoman society. She is currently working on a new book, titled *The Ottoman Healing Arts: Healers, Patients, and the State in the Early Modern Era*, which explores the transformations of Ottoman healing traditions in the early modern era. In conjunction with this research, she is also translating and editing a number of sources pertaining to the history of Ottoman medicine. She holds a PhD from the University of Chicago.

PART TWO

DISEASES IN CONTEXT

A MODEL DISASTER: FROM THE GREAT OTTOMAN PANZOOTIC TO THE CATTLE PLAGUES OF EARLY MODERN EUROPE

SAM WHITE
Ohio State University

BY THE LATE sixteenth century, the Ottomans reigned over vast stretches of territory in three continents, covering all or part of thirty present-day countries. Their empire's subjects numbered as many as thirty-five million, and its animals many more. Their capital city and their military, by far the largest in Europe, were supplied from distant provinces with countless ships and caravans of provisions, and herds of sheep and cattle. These were tremendous achievements for an early modern empire—and also tremendous opportunities for some enterprising microbes, especially among the Ottomans' large, vulnerable, and mobile population of livestock.

This chapter examines the history of a devastating but little-known pestilence of Ottoman sheep and cattle in the 1590s, and it makes the case that this contagion set a pattern for major European epizootics (animal epidemics) over the following century and a half. The first part explains how the Ottoman livestock pestilence arose from a conjuncture of three circumstances: rising stock densities and diminishing pasturage; expanding animal supply lines and pressures on supplies during military campaigns; and the recurrence of severe winters typical of the Little Ice Age. These factors aligned to produce a widespread contagion that wiped out as many as nine in ten sheep and cattle over much of the empire, contributing to severe famine, flight, and violence. The second part of the chapter examines how Europe witnessed a similar combination of ecological pressures during the eighteenth century, with similar consequences for its livestock. Changing cattle supply lines and the untimely combination of severe winters and military campaigns triggered Europe-wide panzootics (animal pandemics) of rinderpest in the 1710s and 1740s resulting in losses of millions of cattle. The third and final part of this essay reconsiders some conventional narratives in the history of veterinary medicine in light of these findings. The few scholars who have written on the history of early modern epizootics have tended to champion the early proponents of contagion theories and their efforts to contain invading diseases of livestock, especially in response to the 1710s and 1740s rinderpest outbreaks. Yet contemporary observers, including contagionists, also emphasized local environmental factors in epizootic outbreaks, and their observations should be appreciated as more than mere holdovers from pre-contagionist Galenic medical thought.

The chapter builds on an emerging historiography of epizootics as important human and environmental disasters. This research has begun to investigate social factors—imperial expansion, long-distance trade, and war—as well as environmental conditions, including weather and climate, in the history of animal diseases. It has also highlighted the contribution of animal deaths to economic losses, famines, and disease outbreaks among people. The "Great Famine" of Europe in the 1310s has received particular attention.[1] Similar insights have come from studies of seventeenth-century Korea and Japan,[2] and from eighteenth- and nineteenth-century epizootics in America, Africa, and India.[3]

---

1 William C. Jordan, *The Great Famine: Northern Europe in the Early Fourteenth Century* (Princeton, NJ: Princeton University Press, 1996); Tim Newfield, "A Cattle Panzootic in Early Fourteenth-Century Europe," *Agricultural History Review* 57 (2009): 155–90; idem, "A Great Carolingian Panzootic: The Probable Extent, Diagnosis and Impact of an Early Ninth Century Cattle Pestilence," *Argos: Bulletin van het Veterinair Historisch Genootschap* 46 (2012): 200–10; Philip Slavin, "The Fifth Rider of the Apocalypse: The Great Cattle Plague in England and Wales and Its Economic Consequences, 1319–1350," in *Le interazioni fra economia e ambiente biologico nell'Europa preindustriale secc. XIII–XVIII*, ed. Simonetta Cavaciocchi (Florence: Firenze University Press, 2010), 165–79; idem, "The Great Bovine Pestilence and Its Economic and Environmental Consequences in England and Wales, 1318–51," *The Economic History Review* 65 (2012): 1239–66; idem, "Warfare and Ecological Destruction in Early Fourteenth-Century British Isles," *Environmental History* 19 (2014): 528–50; Bruce M. S. Campbell, "Nature as Historical Protagonist: Environment and Society in Pre-Industrial England," *The Economic History Review* 63 (2010): 281–314; idem, "Physical Shocks, Biological Hazards, and Human Impacts: The Crisis of the Fourteenth Century Revisited," in *Le interazioni fra economia e ambiente biologico nell'Europa preindustriale secc. XIII–XVIII*, ed. Simonetta Cavaciocchi (Florence: Firenze University Press, 2010), 13–32; and idem, *The Great Transition: Climate, Disease and Society in the Late-Medieval World* (Cambridge: Cambridge University Press, 2016).

2 Hiroshi Kishi, "A Historical Study on Outbreaks of Rinderpest during the Yedo Era in Japan," *The Yamaguchi Journal of Veterinary Medicine* 3 (1976): 33–40; Dong Jin Kim, Han Sang Yoo, and Hang Lee, "Effects of the Periodical Spread of Rinderpest on Famine, Epidemic, and Tiger Disasters in the Late 17th Century," *Korean Journal of Medical History* 23 (2014): 1–56.

3 See e.g., Adam R. Hodge, "'In Want of Nourishment for to Keep Them Alive': Climate Fluctuations, Bison Scarcity, and the Smallpox Epidemic of 1780–82 on the Northern Great Plains," *Environmental History* 17 (2012): 365–403; G. Terry Sharrer, "The Great Glanders Epizootic, 1861–1866: A Civil War Legacy," *Agricultural History* 69 (1995): 79–97; Saurabh Mishra, "Cattle, Dearth, and the Colonial State: Famines and Livestock in Colonial India, 1896–1900," *Journal of Social History* 46 (2013): 989–1012; Gwyn Campbell, "Disease, Cattle, and Slaves: The Development of Trade between Natal and Madagascar, 1875–1904," *African Economic History*, 19 (1990): 105–33.

The history of the Great Ottoman Panzootic makes significant contributions to this emerging field of research. It raises the important and often overlooked role of environmental factors in the life of the Ottoman Empire, and it elucidates the ecological pressures that played such a crucial role in the Ottoman crisis of the seventeenth century. At the same time, this study highlights the shared environmental conditions and links between Europe and the Ottoman Empire, revealing facets of their interconnected histories. Finally, as this chapter will consider in the conclusion, a comparative and environmental perspective on the history of preindustrial livestock plagues could point to potential dangers in the current century of intensified animal production, globalization, and climate change.

The Ottoman Panzootic

The Ottoman panzootic of the 1590s, most likely an outbreak of rinderpest, constitutes a previously unappreciated turning point in that empire's long history.[4] By the late 1500s, the Ottoman Empire had enjoyed close to three centuries of nearly unbroken expansion. Beginning as a small band of warriors in western Anatolia, the Ottomans had conquered lands from Hungary to the Hijaz, emerging as one of the great powers of the early modern world. Yet the breadth of Ottoman domains and the growing number of Ottoman subjects posed risks as well as benefits.

As the empire expanded, the imperial administration had to provision growing cities, armies, and navies from ever more distant sources of supply. This logistical project, which I have likened to a sort of "imperial ecology," operated on a far larger scale than anything else in Europe at the time, and encompassed a wide range of goods from wheat to salt to saltpeter.[5] Through regulated sales

4 This account of the Ottoman panzootic builds on previous research in Sam White, *The Climate of Rebellion in the Early Modern Ottoman Empire* (New York: Cambridge University Press, 2011). The disease was never firmly identified, and no archaeologists have yet discovered physical evidence of the pathogen. Rinderpest would be a best guess for the following reasons: (1) it affected sheep and cattle rather than horses; (2) few other animal diseases have produced such high and widespread animal mortality; (3) when it spread to Hungary it was identified as a "cattle plague." For more on diagnosing rinderpest, see Newfield, "Cattle Panzootic." Anthrax remains another possibility. Outbreaks often coincide with major climatic changes—see O. M. Radostits and Stanley H. Done, eds., *Veterinary Medicine: A Textbook of the Diseases of Cattle, Sheep, Pigs, Goats, and Horses*, 10th ed (New York: Elsevier Saunders, 2007), 816—and one Ottoman chronicler noted an outbreak of anthrax among people in Istanbul in 1595—see Gelibolulu Mustafa Âlî, *Gelibolulu Mustafa Âlî ve Künhü'l-ahbâr'ında II. Selim, III. Murat ve III. Mehmet Devirleri*, ed. Faris Çerçi (Kayseri: Erciyes University Press, 2000), 693–94.

5 White, *Climate of Rebellion*, chapter 1. For further studies of Ottoman provisioning,

and forced purchases, or sometimes direct requisitions and *corvée* labor, Ottoman administrators assured that key commodities flowed from regions of surplus to those of deficit. For instance, timber flowed from forests in Anatolia to the treeless Nile Valley, while Egypt sent back rice to the cities of Turkey. Through the mid-sixteenth century, these provisioning systems proved mostly successful at relieving shortages and supplying major cities and military campaigns.

At the same time, as the empire's population expanded, Ottoman officials enacted ambitious measures to promote settlement and agriculture. Through tax incentives, controls on migration, and sometimes forced resettlement, the imperial administration brought subjects out of difficult forested and mountainous lands under imperial control. Through strategically placed settlements, insecure and marginal areas were made safe for agriculture. Nomadic and semi-nomadic pastoralists were taxed and forced into stable transhumance routes, and pastoral regions in Syria and central and eastern Anatolia were increasingly brought under cultivation.

By the last decades of the 1500s, this "imperial ecology" started to fall victim to its own expansion. The population of Istanbul had grown to as many as half a million people, with hundreds of thousands more in the empire's other major cities, largely dependent on bountiful provisions from distant sources. The army, too, had grown to well over a hundred thousand men, with tens of thousands more sailors and auxiliaries. In the empire's incessant wars on distant fronts, major campaigns began to place a growing strain on suppliers and supply routes, some stretching hundreds of miles over land and sea. Meanwhile, the very success of Ottoman settlement policies contributed to a near doubling of the subject population between the late fifteenth and late sixteenth centuries. By the 1580s, agriculture pushed to the limits of cultivable land, above all in the semi-arid zone stretching from central Anatolia through northern Syria and Iraq. More mouths to feed and diminishing returns to agriculture began to cut into surplus for provisioning. Farms already at the margins of subsistence continued to shrink, and landlessness rose alarmingly. While regional conditions varied, extensive Ottoman cadastral surveys and tax records paint a grim picture of falling yields per household in many provinces. The combination of population pressure and the wider "price revolution" of the sixteenth century drove serious inflation, along with rising vagrancy and crime.[6]

---

see e.g., Lütfi Güçer, *Osmanlı İmparatorluğunda Hububat Meselesi ve Hububattan Alınan Vergiler* (Istanbul: Istanbul University Press, 1964) and Gábor Ágoston, *Guns for the Sultan: Technology, Industry, and Military Power in the Ottoman Empire* (Cambridge: Cambridge University Press, 2004).

6 White, *Climate of Rebellion*, chapter 2. For previous studies of inflation, unrest, and

These difficult circumstances left Ottoman lands particularly susceptible to a worsening climate over the late 1500s, associated with a strong phase of the Little Ice Age. Against the background of global cooling that characterized the fourteenth to early nineteenth centuries, the Northern Hemisphere experienced an especially cold climate ca. 1560–1660, marked by pronounced extremes following large tropical volcanic eruptions. This climatic change tended to bring freezing winters and erratic precipitation to Ottoman lands, and these changes are well attested in physical and written records of weather and climate.[7] In Mediterranean regions that depended on a single crop of winter wheat or barley, these conditions spelled agricultural disaster. From the 1560s to 1580s, four serious droughts brought waves of harvest failure and shortages to Ottoman lands, especially in Syria, Anatolia, and the southern Balkans. Each put increasing pressure on overtaxed systems of famine relief and provisioning, especially in times of war; and each drove rising banditry in the provinces, especially Anatolia. Meanwhile, strong El Niños and volcanic eruptions periodically interrupted the East African monsoon, causing the failure of the Nile flood and cutting important provisions from Egypt.[8]

---

population pressure, see especially Mustafa Akdağ, *Türkiye'nin İktisadi ve İçtimai Tarihi* (Ankara: Türk Tarih Kurumu, 1971) and Oktay Özel, "Population Changes in Ottoman Anatolia During the 16th and 17th Centuries: The 'Demographic Crisis' Reconsidered," *International Journal of Middle East Studies* 36 (2004): 183–205.

7 At the time of writing, the state of the art for temperature reconstructions was presented in Moinuddin Ahmed et al., "Continental-Scale Temperature Variability During the Past Two Millennia," *Nature Geoscience* 6 (2013): 339–46, and Martin P. Tingley and Peter Huybers, "Recent Temperature Extremes at High Northern Latitudes Unprecedented in the Past 600 Years," *Nature* 496 (2013): 201–05. For specific evidence of cooling in the Eastern Mediterranean, see Ingo Heinrich et al., "Winter-to-Spring Temperature Dynamics in Turkey Derived from Tree Rings since AD 1125," *Climate Dynamics* 41 (2013): 1685–1701, and D. Kaniewski et al., "The Medieval Climate Anomaly and the Little Ice Age in Coastal Syria Inferred from Pollen-Derived Palaeoclimatic Patterns," *Global and Planetary Change* 78 (2011): 178–87.

8 White, *Climate of Rebellion*, chapters 3 and 5, and references therein. For an overview of Mediterranean climate in the Little Ice Age, see Jürg Luterbacher et al., "Mediterranean Climate Variability over the Last Centuries: A Review," in *The Mediterranean Climate: An Overview of the Main Characteristics and Issues*, ed. P. Lionello, P. Malanotte-Rizzoli, and R. Boscolo (Amsterdam: Elsevier, 2006), 27–148, and Jürg Luterbacher et al., "A Review of 2000 Years of Paleoclimatic Evidence in the Mediterranean," in *The Climate of the Mediterranean Region*, ed. P. Lionello (London: Elsevier, 2012), 87–185. Particularly useful have been tree-ring studies reconstructing Eastern Mediterranean precipitation—see e.g., Ramzi Touchan et al., "Reconstructions of Spring/Summer Precipitation for the Eastern Mediterranean from Tree-Ring Widths and Its Connection to Large-Scale Atmospheric Circulation," *Climate*

Yet the worst breakdowns in the Ottoman imperial ecology came not in the grain supply, but the supply of livestock. It is hard to overstate the importance of animals to the preindustrial Ottoman economy.[9] They provided essential labor, food, and clothing. Livestock represented the most valuable possessions of a typical peasant household, and its only recourse when harvests failed. Moreover, live animals and animal products constituted one of the largest elements in Ottoman imperial provisioning. Huge drives brought hundreds of thousands of sheep each year from the Danube region, with deliveries of tens or hundreds of thousands more coming from east and central Anatolia. By the late 1500s, well over a million animals were driven to Istanbul each year (around 70,000 sheep for the imperial kitchens alone) and perhaps another million to other cities, along with significant deliveries of lard, tallow, and clarified butter. Armies on campaign demanded enormous deliveries of animals on the hoof to provide transportation and protein to the soldiers. Yet by the 1580s, live animal and animal product deliveries faced rampant price inflation and chronic disruptions, putting civilian and military supplies at risk.[10]

Often these breakdowns in supply stemmed from systemic weaknesses in the Ottoman livestock provisioning system. Unlike timber and grain, the empire did not directly administer deliveries of livestock. Instead, the imperial government tried to impose an artificial price gradient between cheaper areas of supply and more expensive areas of demand. It then ordered wealthy individuals, called *celeps*, to buy up sheep in the one and sell to the other at fixed prices. Yet as inflation picked up in the late sixteenth century, the imperial government failed to adjust its fixed prices accordingly, which encouraged widespread smuggling

---

Dynamics 25 (2005): 75–98. For the influence of ENSO and volcanic eruptions on the African monsoon and Nile flood see Peter Whetton, Ian Rutherford, and Robert Allan, "Historical ENSO Teleconnections in the Eastern Hemisphere," *Climatic Change* 28 (1994): 221–53, and Luke Oman et al., "High-Latitude Eruptions Cast Shadow over the African Monsoon and the Flow of the Nile," *Geophysical Research Letters* 33 (2006): L18711.

9 See Alan Mikhail, "Unleashing the Beast: Animals, Energy, and the Economy of Labor in Ottoman Egypt," *American Historical Review* 118 (2013): 317–48.

10 For studies of the Ottoman sheep provisioning system, see: Anthony Greenwood, "Istanbul's Meat Provisioning: A Study of the Celep-Keşan System," PhD diss., University of Chicago, 1988; idem, "Meat Provisioning and Ottoman Economic Administration," in *Abdullah Kuran İçin Yazılar*, ed. Çiğdem Kafesçioğlu and Lucienne Thys-Şenocak (Istanbul: Yapı Kredi Yayınları, 1999), 191–210; Bistra A. Cvetkova, "Le service des celeps et le ravitaillement en bétail dans l'Empire ottoman (XVe–XVIIIe s.)," *Études Historiques* 3 (1966): 145–72; and Suraiya Faroqhi, *Towns and Townsmen of Ottoman Anatolia* (New York: Cambridge University Press, 1984), chapter 9. Late sixteenth-century famines and breakdowns in supply are discussed in White, *Climate of Rebellion*, chapter 3.

and evasion. Unable to purchase enough animals or forced to buy at inflated black market rates, many *celeps* simply went bankrupt or absconded. Anxious to preserve the supply of protein for the cities and army, successive sultans resorted to heavier and more urgent demands from more distant provinces, including east and central Anatolia.

Nevertheless, the underlying reasons for the shortages were environmental. The cattle and especially sheep of Ottoman lands proved particularly vulnerable to the empire's intensifying ecological pressures and the extreme seasons characteristic of the Little Ice Age. Paradoxically, rising population pressure had led Ottoman peasants to depend more, not less, on pastoralism and to raise even more animals per person, especially in semi-arid regions. In those areas, simple farming technologies, limited capital, and poor water supplies hindered the intensification of agriculture. Peasants extended land use into ever more marginal zones and tried to diversify to reduce risk: both strategies that encouraged more pastoralism. Animals, besides, were a more secure and portable form of wealth, easier to transport and sell in growing urban markets. Where grain harvests were precarious, they could be seen as sort of insurance policy against the vagaries of man and weather. Consequently, ever more animals must have been feeding on inferior pasturage. At the same time, the expansion of village settlement restricted the migration of pastoral nomadic tribes, forcing their flocks onto more limited grazing land.[11] As a result, the livestock to supply imperial cities and armies had to make ever longer treks with less adequate nourishment along the way. Meanwhile, the onset of the Little Ice Age left them exposed to harsher weather along the journey.

Through the 1570s and 1580s, we find occasional evidence of serious mortality among Ottoman flocks and herds. For instance, one report to Istanbul mentions how oxen in parts of northern Anatolia and Gallipoli fell sick and died, delaying deliveries of timber;[12] another describes how armies on the march to Persia lost their animals to exposure and sickness.[13] The impact of such losses proved more serious and enduring than that from crop failures. When one harvest fell short, farmers could always plant their seed-corn again and hope for the best next spring. But when flocks and herds were decimated, peasants lost their breeding stock as well, reducing numbers for years to come.

---

11 White, *Climate of Rebellion*, chapter 2.

12 T.C. Başbakanlık Osmanlı Arşivi, Mühimme Defterleri 10/217, 16/570, 35/74, and 35/462. (Hereafter abbreviated "MD" and cited by *defter* and entry number only.) The *Mühimme Defterleri* are notebooks of copied imperial orders, usually prefaced by summaries of petitions from the provinces.

13 See e.g., MD 32/468.

Matters came to a head in the 1590s, a decade that brought one of the worst droughts in the empire's long history and one of its most costly wars. As attested by contemporaries, and confirmed in tree-ring and lake varve studies, from 1591 to 1596 much of the Eastern Mediterranean suffered a continuous shortage of rain.[14] Year after year, harvest failures stretched Ottoman provisioning systems to the breaking point while many regions, especially in the semi-arid zone, faced unprecedented famine. At the same time, Ottoman armies on the Habsburg frontier drained precious resources from the countryside for a protracted and ultimately unsuccessful war launched in 1593. Unscrupulous officials and soldiers departing for the front fleeced an already starving peasantry. Desperation drove flight and banditry, especially in central Anatolia, where a series of harsh Little Ice Age winters aggravated the mortality from famine and violence.[15]

However, as contemporary sources make clear, it was the Ottoman sheep and cattle who suffered most. Already short of good pasture, the animals now faced years of drought that dried up their fodder and pasturage, as well as freezing winters that weakened their immune systems. Imperial orders began to note disruptions in provisioning as animals died in the cold and snow.[16] Once the empire mobilized for the Habsburg war, the army demanded ever more sheep for food, horses for cavalry, and oxen for pulling carts. As the conflict disrupted Balkan supplies, the imperial administration turned increasingly to animals from central and eastern Anatolia. These weakened animals, traveling hundreds of miles across the empire, proved an effective vehicle for a deadly panzootic.

The great Ottoman sheep and cattle pestilence may have begun as early as 1591. The most detailed description comes from the chronicler Mustafa Ali (d. 1600), who was serving as an official in east-central Anatolia at the time:

> ...One by one the cattle and sheep and other breeds died. Their corpses became one with the black earth. Indeed, in the capital Constantinople in the years 1001 and 1002 (1592–4) clarified butter stopped coming. When they inquired for the reason of this shortage and famine, they found proof that in those provinces there was an animal plague (*kırgun*) and no oxen or cows remained. Afterwards, it apparently came from these parts spreading into Persia, and in the fourth year it appeared from Iraq. It reached first Diyarbakır (southeast Anatolia), then Zülkadriyye and the land of Rum (east-central Anatolia). In Muharrem 1004 (September

14 Neil Roberts et al., "Palaeolimnological Evidence for an East–West Climate See-Saw in the Mediterranean Since AD 900," *Global and Planetary Change* 84–85 (2012): 23–34.

15 See White, *Climate of Rebellion*, chapter 6.

16 See e.g., MD 73/789.

> 1595), this poor man—that is, the writer of this history—was appointed to the two offices of secretary (*defterdar*) to the treasury of Rum and general (*mirliva*) of Amasya... Among the towns and cities I visited...it so happened there were neighborhoods where not a single cow remained, and villages where the inhabitants were relieved that one or two cows were left from four or five hundred.[17]

Other sources largely confirm Ali's description. Imperial orders from the period made frequent reference to "wasting" (*telef*) and "perishing" (*zayi*) sheep.[18] As early as October 1593, in a demand for fats from Caffa, in the Crimea, it was noted that "in this blessed year, an animal sickness has appeared and most have died."[19] Yet around one year later the governor of Caffa wrote back to Istanbul that "In these parts a murrain had appeared among the sheep, and some who had four or five hundred had only ten or twenty left." A second wave of sickness soon followed, and "the remaining sheep and cattle perished. In the province of Crimea, not one sack of clarified butter remains to be gathered."[20]

Around 1596, there may have been a lull in the panzootic as the rapid spread of the pathogen exhausted the supply of fresh hosts to infect. Then it appears to have broken out in Anatolia again a year later, spreading with renewed vigor, a pattern sometimes observed in rinderpest.[21] In June of 1598 the Venetian ambassador wrote a dispatch that mentioned "the shortage of everything but principally of meat, since the animals that are usually brought here in other times for the use of the city in this season come from Anatolia, which has been almost emptied of every sort of animal by a mortality that came through the year before."[22] From Anatolia it spread rapidly through the Balkans, where the contemporary English chronicler Richard Knolles noted "the wonderful Mortality of their Cattel"[23] among the Ottoman army. As the contagion crossed the Danube, Hungarian sources described it as the worst cattle plague in generations, wiping out nineteen in twenty animals or more in some parts of the country.[24]

---

17 Âlî, *Künhü'l-ahbâr*, 675–77.

18 See e.g., MD 72/335, 72/905, and 74/181.

19 MD 71/214.

20 MD 72/6.

21 See Clive A. Spinage, *Cattle Plague: A History* (New York: Kluwer, 2003), 22.

22 *Archivio di Stato di Venezia, Dispacci - Costantinopoli* filza 47, dated 13 June 1598.

23 Richard Knolles, *The Turkish History from the Original of that Nation ...* (London: 1687), 779.

24 My sincere thanks to Prof. Lajos Rácz for sharing and translating the relevant passages from the following sources: István Kaprinai, *Collectione Miscell. B. Excerpta nonnulla e ms. Diario Zavoczkiano* (Manuscript, Tom. LXXIX, Library of Budapest University); Gáspár

Coming at such a critical moment, the panzootic pushed the empire into crisis. The livestock provisioning system broke down almost entirely. Imperial orders complained repeatedly of severe shortages of meat, butter, and lard in the capital and army. Sultans Murad III (r. 1574–95) then Mehmed III (r. 1595–1603) took ever more arbitrary measures to preserve supplies. These included banning private shipowners from oiling their ships, in order to save fat, and even forbidding sheep consumption across the Balkans to keep animals flowing to the capital.[25] Meanwhile, the death of animals contributed as much as the drought and military requisitions to the growing famine in Anatolia and parts of Syria and the Balkans. The loss of cattle in particular took away vital meat, milk, and labor. As Mustafa Ali descibed:

> With the cattle plague not only was there a shortage of cheese and yoghurt, but of the basic sustenance—barley and wheat. As the cattle died, they went without. Now in these circumstances in the province of Rum I saw that some peasants (*reaya*) were hitched up and made to plow in place of oxen, and some of them even planted wheat and barley seeds and tilled the land with a hoe.[26]

The panzootic also played a central role in the outbreak of a destructive rural uprising known as the Celali Rebellion. Like any major historical event, the Celali Rebellion had a number of underlying causes, some already taken up by Ottomanists and others still to be discovered.[27] Nevertheless, Ottoman and Venetian sources make it clear that the immediate factors behind the uprising were famine, desperation, and resistance to heavy wartime taxes and requisitions.[28] Contemporary accounts even suggest that the trigger for revolt was a crisis over Ottoman sheep.

Upon his accession in 1595, the new sultan Mehmed III decided to consolidate his authority by leading his army in person against the Habsburgs. This campaign would lead to an important though inconclusive victory at the Battle of Mezőkeresztes (Haçova) in 1596. Yet its most significant effects took place at home the previous autumn, as officials scrambled to secure the vast provisions

---

Hain, ed., *Lőcsei krónikája (Chronicle of Lőcse)* (Lőcse, 1910–13); and Szilágyi Sándor, ed., *Szamosközi, István történeti maradványai (Chronicle of István Szamosközi)* (Budapest, 1889).

25 MD 71/150, MD72/340, and MD 73/460.

26 Âlî, *Künhü'l-ahbâr*, 677.

27 See Oktay Özel, "The Reign of Violence: The *celâlis* c. 1550–1700," in *The Ottoman World*, ed. Christine Woodhead (New York: Routledge, 2012), 184–202.

28 White, *Climate of Rebellion*, chapter 6.

necessary for the royal campaign. The imperial government in Istanbul must have been aware of conditions in countryside. Nevertheless, with the ongoing Habsburg war and extreme cold cutting off supplies from the Danube, the imperial government may have had no choice but to turn to already murrain- and famine-stricken provinces of Anatolia for further requisitions of sheep. The remaining flocks were forced onto a long and dangerous trek across the peninsula, sometimes all the way to the army in Hungary, leaving the sultan to issue vain exhortations not to let the animals sicken or perish.[29] Frustrated with the poor results, it seems Mehmed III took to blaming central Anatolian officials for siphoning off supply.

The tipping point came with an extraordinary order for 200,000 sheep in late 1595 from the poor south-central Anatolian province of Karaman.[30] This demand would have been onerous even in normal times. In the middle of an unprecedented famine and dearth of livestock it fanned the flames of rebellion. The chronicler Selaniki Mustafa Efendi (d. [1600]) recorded how the order sparked a local uprising in the name of a pretender to the pre-Ottoman Karamanid dynasty.[31] Over the following year, as the disorder in the province reached a new pitch, a larger rebellion gathered in the town of Larende. And it was from this uprising, as the chronicler ʿAbdülkâdir Efendi (d. [1644]) and the Venetian ambassador recorded, that the first major Celali leader, Karayazıcı (the "Black Scribe"), built his rebel army, joining common bandits, discontented locals, unruly tribes, and provincial mercenary bands.[32]

For more than a decade, a succession of rebel armies defied imperial troops and laid waste to the countryside in Anatolia and Syria. Peasants fled their villages in a movement known as the "Great Flight," and perhaps millions died of starvation and disease in the ongoing famine and extreme Little Ice Age cold.[33] By the

---

29 Cf. Madeleine Ferrières, *Sacred Cow, Mad Cow: A History of Food Fears*, trans. Jody Gladding (New York: Columbia University Press, 2006), 175, citing similar proclamations by Louis XVI when faced with provisioning difficulties during the rinderpest outbreaks of the 1700s.

30 On population pressure in Karaman, see Osman Gümüşçü, *Tarihî Coğrafya Açısından Bir Araştırma: XVI. Yüzyıl Larende (Karaman) Kazasında Yerleşme ve Nüfus* (Ankara: Türk Tarih Kurumu, 2001). The order for sheep is in MD 73/964.

31 Selânikî Mustafa Efendi, *Tarih-i Selânikî*, ed. Mehmet İpşirli (Ankara: Türk Tarih Kurumu, 1999), 581.

32 *Tarih-i Selânikî*, 751; *Topçular Kâtibi ʿAbdülkâdir Efendi Tarihi*, ed. Ziya Yılmazer (Ankara: Türk Tarih Kurumu, 2003), 321; *Archivio di Stato di Venezia, Dispacci – Costantinopoli* filza 49, dated 7 Aug. 1599.

33 For narratives of the rebellion, see especially Mustafa Akdağ, *Celâlî İsyanları* (Ankara: Ankara University Press, 1964); William Griswold, *The Great Anatolian Rebellion, 1591–1611*

time the rebels were finally defeated in 1608, parts of the empire had been almost emptied of inhabitants. Nor did the end of the rebellion put an end to Ottoman troubles. The vacuum of abandoned land drew a widespread invasion of nomadic and semi-nomadic tribes in the following decade; and the ongoing stream of rural-to-urban migrants fleeing famine and unrest contributed to endemic and epidemic disease and an ongoing demographic drain. Recent work in Ottoman sources has revealed that considerable regions of Anatolia, the southern Balkans, and the Levant lost over half their settlements and population by the 1630s, and that Ottoman numbers overall did not fully recover until the nineteenth century.[34] And so, a combination of ecological pressures and the Little Ice Age created a livestock plague that triggered the most costly rebellion in Ottoman history.

From the Ottoman Panzootic to Europe's Cattle Plagues

Beyond its significance for Ottoman history, the panzootic of the 1590s also sheds new light on Europe's great "cattle plagues" of the 1700s. These outbreaks, usually identified as rinderpest, circulated through Europe during much of the century, reaching two peaks during the 1710s and 1740s. Europe had faced rinderpest since antiquity, but the eighteenth-century outbreaks were the most widespread and fatal since the Great Famine of the 1310s.[35] These panzootics did not come from Ottoman lands, as is sometimes supposed. Yet in important ways the rinderpest outbreaks of the eighteenth century emerged from the same combination of social and environmental pressures experienced in the Ottoman Empire during the 1590s: long-distance livestock deliveries, warfare, and severe winters.

Eighteenth- and nineteenth-century observers of the panzootics could often only guess at the source of the infection, and most simply assumed it came from somewhere in the East. Typical of nineteenth-century historians, W. Dieckerhoff stated, "Its source was, as always, the Orient."[36] Italian observers, including some

(Berlin: Klaus Schwarz Verlag, 1983); and White, *Climate of Rebellion*, chapter 7.

34 See e.g., Özel, "Demographic Crisis"; Leila Erder, "Population Rise and Fall in Anatolia 1550–1620," *Middle East Studies* 15 (1979): 322–45; idem, "Osmanlı Anadolu'sunda Terkedilmiş/Kayıp Köyler Sorunu (17–19. Yüzyıllar)," in *Ötekilerin Peşinde: Ahmet Yaşar Ocak'a Armağan*, ed. Mehmet Öz and Fatih Yeşil (Istanbul: Timaş, 2015), 557–91; and White, *Climate of Rebellion*, chapters 9 to 11.

35 For European sources on ancient and medieval animal plagues, including rinderpest, see George Fleming, *Animal Plagues: Their History, Nature, and Prevention* (London: Champman and Hall, 1871).

36 W. Dieckerhoff, *Geschichte der Rinderpest und ihrer Literatur* (Berlin: T. C. F. Enslin, 1890), 32.

major figures in the history of veterinary medicine, ascribed the outbreaks to contagion from Hungarian animals, suggesting origins in Ottoman lands. These influential sources have led some modern authors to continue writing of "Hungarian cattle plague," obscuring the real sources of the epizootics.[37]

It is possible that the association of rinderpest with Ottoman lands and Hungary dates back to the Ottoman panzootic recounted in the previous section. Passing from Ottoman into Habsburg lands during the 1590s, that outbreak spread into Germany in 1598–99, and thence into parts of Western Europe. In northern Italy and France officials responded with some of the first concerted efforts in European history to control an epizootic through restriction on sales and the culling of infected animals.[38] However, this panzootic was probably the last of its kind to originate in Ottoman territory and spread to Western Europe through Hungary. Over the following centuries, Ottoman lands continued to witness periodic murrains.[39] Yet there was nothing on the scale of the 1590s epizootic until the great Anatolian famine of the 1870s, when parts of Turkey again lost around 90 percent of their sheep and cattle during a major drought and freezing winters.[40] However, that epizootic never spread into Europe. Hungarian sources reveal no further epizootics of a similar magnitude until the 1810s, in the wake of the Tambora eruption and the fatal "year without a summer."[41] Even during the European cattle

37 See e.g., Ferrières, *Mad Cow*, chapter 9, and Karl Appuhn, "Ecologies of Beef: Eighteenth-Century Epizootics and the Environmental History of Early Modern Europe," *Environmental History* 15 (2010): 268–87.

38 Spinage, *Cattle Plague*, 98, which draws on original sources reproduced in Fleming, *Animal Plagues*, 138. See also Dieckerhoff, *Geschichte der Rinderpest*, 32–33; and Johann Kanold, *Historische Relation von der Pestilenz des Hornviehes welche anno 1711 und 1712 in Schlesien* [etc.] (Breslau: Ben Esaia Fellgiebels, 1713), 71. On disease control efforts, see Jean Blancou, *History of the Surveillance and Control of Transmissible Animal Diseases* (Paris: Office International des Épizooties, 2003), 171–73.

39 See e.g., Thomas Roe, *The Negotiations of Sir Thomas Roe, in His Embassy in the Ottoman Porte, from the Year 1621 to 1628 Inclusive* (London, 1740), 420: "The same day (July 14, 1625) proclamation was made in the cyttye, that no butcher should kyll mutton; a murraine, or plague, whither in uncerteyne, having take that sort of cattle so violently, that dye in multitudes, with soares, in the fields; and wee know not what to eate, not where safely to provide yt."

40 The event is described in *The Famine in Asia Minor: Its History Compiled from the Pages of the Levant Herald* [1875] (Istanbul: Isis Press, 1989) and Mehmet Erler, *Osmanlı Devleti'nde Kuraklık ve Kıtlık Olayları (1800–1880)* (Istanbul: Libra Yayınevi, 2010). Recent reconstructions of Anatolian drought in Roberts et al., "Palaeolimnological Evidence."

41 Again I thank Prof. Rácz for sharing data he has collected on the subject. For a thorough study of the "year without a summer" and its impacts, see John D. Post, *The Last Great Sub-*

panzootics of the 1710s and 1740s, Hungary was not particularly affected, and probably served as only a minor corridor for the disease.[42]

There are further reasons why Western European observers may have inaccurately attributed eighteenth-century outbreaks to Ottoman lands, or Hungary in particular. First, as the historian of rinderpest Clive Spinage has noted, "It is convenient to explain away the origin of a disease as coming from the most remote and almost unknown places."[43] Both contemporary observers and later historians had little fear of contradiction or criticism if they blamed Ottoman lands for the epizootics. Moreover, by the eighteenth century the idea of "Oriental plague" was already something of a trope among Western and Central European observers, one that could distort their understanding of plagues and their origins. Rather than an endemic problem, many were tempted to see disease as a sort of foreign invader, especially from Muslim lands.[44] At the time of the panzootics, several European states were already constructing *cordons sanitaires* to isolate the Ottoman Empire and its microbes.[45] Finally, Hungary was (and to an extent, still is) known for its grassy Central Plain and its characteristic herds of tough gray cattle, reminiscent of the Eurasian steppe. These herds had been major suppliers of beef for late medieval Europeans; and it was not unreasonable to imagine these wild-looking, free-ranging cattle could be the carriers of distant diseases.[46]

---

sistence Crisis in the Western World (Baltimore: The Johns Hopkins University Press, 1977).

42 Kanold, *Historische Relation*, 36, makes it clear that the 1710 rinderpest only spread *through* Hungary, not from it. There are some accounts of animal disease in 1708–10, but only of a general sort, evidently related to the weather and to locust swarms—see Johanne Baptista and Antonio Loick, *Historia Pestis quae ab Anno 1708 ad 1713 Transylvaniam, Hungariam, Austriam, Pragam & Ratisbonam, Aliasque Conterminas Provincias Depopulabatur [etc.]* (Styria: Joseph Grünewald, 1715). See also Dénes Karasszon, *A Concise History of Veterinary Medicine* (Budapest: Akadémiai Kiadó, 1988), 300.

43 Spinage, *Cattle Plague*, 55.

44 See Hans-Uwe Lammel, "Western European Perception and Representation of Plagues in Eastern Europe, the Ottoman Empire and the Near East, 1650–1800," in *Le interazioni fra economia e ambiente biologico nell'Europa preindustriale secc. XIII–XVIII*, ed. Simonetta Cavaciocchi (Florence: Firenze University Press, 2010), 399–421, and Aaron D. Shakow, "Marks of Contagion: The Plague, The Bourse, the Word and the Law in the Early-Modern Mediterranean, 1720–1762," PhD diss., Harvard University, 2009. On "Oriental plague," also see Nükhet Varlık "'Oriental Plague' or Epidemiological Orientalism? Revisiting the Plague Episteme of the Early Modern Mediterranean," (57–87).

45 See Daniel Panzac, *Quarantaines et lazarets: l'Europe et la peste d'Orient (XVIIe–XXe siècles)* (Aix-en-Provence: Édisud, 1986), 59, 62, 82, 88.

46 For an overview of Hungary's environmental history, including the rise of its cattle herding, see Lajos Rácz, "The Price of Survival: Transformations in Environmental Conditions

To understand where and how the great rinderpest panzootics actually originated we need first to reconsider two important factors: the long-distance livestock trade and the biological consequences of large-scale husbandry on the margins of Europe. Karl Appuhn has taken an important step in this direction with his recent work on beef supplies and cattle plagues in eighteenth-century Venice. Appuhn argues that Western European livestock imports were a way of displacing ecological pressures from an emerging economic and demographic core onto Europe's periphery. He suggests that the rinderpest outbreaks of the 1710s and 1740s formed part of early modern Europe's intensifying environmental interactions with the wider world.[47]

Nevertheless, Appuhn's study focuses exclusively on Venice in the eighteenth century and therefore overlooks broader long-term shifts in the cattle trade. The wide ecological footprint of eighteenth-century European consumers was nothing new and not the exclusive cause of the panzootics. As Richard Hoffmann has shown, European city-dwellers had been "ecological omnivores" since the later middle ages, drawing considerably on imported resources, including livestock.[48] Historians have carried out considerable research on the development of the preindustrial European cattle trade, a major enterprise which rivaled the grain trade in volume and value. This research demonstrates that early eighteenth-century imports were certainly on the rise, but only in comparison to the depressed and crisis-ridden 1600s. They had already reached similar levels in the 1500s.[49]

Between the sixteenth and eighteenth centuries the major sources of supply for Central and Western Europe had shifted farther north and east. Hungarian herds had dominated Western European markets between the 1300s and mid-1500s particularly those of Italian cities.[50] Hungarian cattle exports had soared from the late fifteenth to mid-sixteenth century, reaching a peak of around

---

and Subsistence Systems in Hungary in the Age of Ottoman Occupation," *Hungarian Studies* 24 (2010): 21–39, and idem, *The Steppe to Europe: An Environmental History of Hungary in the Traditional Age* (Cambridge: White Horse Press, 2013).

47 Appuhn, "Ecologies of Beef."

48 Richard Hoffman, "Frontier Food for Late Medieval Consumers: Culture, Economy, Ecology," *Environment and History* 7 (2001): 131–67. Hoffmann notes that the characteristic gray steppe cattle breed was probably a creation of the cattle trade itself.

49 See especially Ian Blanchard, "The Continental European Cattle Trades, 1400–1600," *Economic History Review* 39 (1986): 427–60.

50 Blanchard, "Continental European Cattle Trades," 429–31, and Othmar Pickl, "Der Viehhandel von Ungarn nach Oberitalien vom 14. bis zum 17. Jahrhundert," in *Internationaler Ochsenhandel (1350–1750)*, ed. Ekkehard Westermann (Stuttgart: Klett-Cotta, 1979), 39–81, at 39.

100,000–200,000 animals a year before 1570, with perhaps 20,000 going to Venice alone.[51] Denmark, the next largest supplier, had also boomed since the later fifteenth century, peaking at over 50,000 cattle around 1610.[52] However, Hungarian exports to Europe had started falling off sharply in the 1580s, victim to Ottoman requisitions and Ottoman-Habsburg border wars. They had declined to only 50,000–60,000 per year during the early seventeenth to early eighteenth centuries, which could explain why Hungarian cattle ceased to be a major source of European epizootics.[53] Danish deliveries also declined sharply in the early seventeenth century, a victim to Dutch tariffs.

In place of Hungary and Denmark, Poland grew into Europe's largest cattle supplier by the 1700s. Its exports had risen from perhaps 40,000 a year in the 1500s to around 80,000 by the time of the rinderpest panzootics in the early eighteenth century.[54] And within Poland itself the major supply regions were shifting farther east. The kingdom then known as Poland spread well beyond the boundaries of the modern state, and its animals often came from remote regions of its wide borderlands. During the fifteenth century, most so-called Polish cattle had originated in the independent principality of Moldavia (present-day Moldova and parts of Romania). In the sixteenth century, as those lands fell under Ottoman control, imperial officials began to re-route those cattle to Istanbul, so European cattle merchants had to seek out more distant supplies.[55] Fortuitously, the Union of Lublin in 1569 expanded the borders of the Poland-Lithuanian Commonwealth deep

---

51 For various estimates see, Blanchard, "Continental European Cattle Trades," 434; Rácz, "Price of Survival," 38; István N. Kiss, "Die Bedeutung der ungarischen Viehzucht für Ungarn und Mitteleuropa vom 16. bis zum 18. Jahrhundert," in *Internationaler Ochsenhandel (1350–1750)*, ed. Ekkehard Westermann (Stuttgart: Klett-Cotta, 1979), 83–124, at 108–09; and Pickl, "Viehhandel von Ungarn," 49.

52 Blanchard, "Continental European Cattle Trades," 431–33; Wilhelmina Maria Gijsbers, "Kapitale Ossen: De Internationale Handel in Slachtvee in Noordwest-Europa (1300–1750)," PhD diss., University of Amsterdam, 1999, 474; and Erling Ladewig Petersen and Ekkehard Westermann, "Production and Trade in Oxen 1450–1750: Denmark," in *Internationaler Ochsenhandel (1350–1750)*, ed. Ekkehard Westermann (Stuttgart: Klett-Cotta, 1979), 137–70, at 145. For general aspects of the trade, see also Wilhelmina Maria Gijsbers and Peter A. Koolmees, "Food on Foot: Long-Distance Trade in Slaughter Oxen Between Denmark and the Netherlands (14th-18th Century)," *Historia Medicinae Veterinariae* 26 (2001): 115–27.

53 Rácz, "Price of Survival," 38; and Kiss, "Bedeutung der ungarischen Viehzucht," 108–09.

54 Jan Baszanowski, "Ochsenzuchtgebiete und Ochsenausfuhr aus Polen vom 16. bis 18. Jahrhundert," in *Internationaler Ochsenhandel (1350–1750)*, ed. Ekkehard Westermann (Stuttgart: Klett-Cotta, 1979), 125–36, at 133.

55 Blanchard, "Continental European Cattle Trades," 440.

into the Russian and Ukrainian steppe; and cattle from these easternmost reaches soon came to dominate Polish exports.[56]

In short, by the eighteenth century new herds from deep inside Eurasia had replaced closer Hungarian and Danish supplies to Central and Western European markets, and those markets were just recovering to peak levels of demand. At the time of the great panzootics of the early 1700s, animals were not just coming from Europe's periphery to its center. They were making long treks from distant grazing grounds with harder winter conditions.

Facing severe weather and long drives to market, the cattle would have been more exposed to infection, with more compromised immune systems, and therefore more likely to spread rinderpest to herds in Central and Western Europe. As recent research has demonstrated, both climatic shifts and changes in long-distance migration exacerbate vulnerabilities to disease, even in migratory and cold-adapted species. Recent research on the ecoimmunology of sheep, for instance, has demonstrated a natural limit to the animal's ability to withstand infections in cold weather, because otherwise the immune response would seriously impair reproductive capacity.[57] Studies of early modern Italian and Spanish transhumance offer anecdotal evidence that sheep herds regularly suffered disease outbreaks following the worst cold spells and droughts of the Little Ice Age.[58] While we have no specific studies of the effects of climate and migration on rinderpest, there is circumstantial evidence suggesting that long-distance winter travel in the steppe would have put European herds at risk. In his discussion of the disease, Clive Spinage points to the dangers of stress, malnutrition, and the crowding of animals in stalls and around waterholes. He cites older studies arguing that the cattle plague could incubate very slowly among Russian and Podolian steppe cattle trekking west. According to some observers, the animals "could leave the steppes apparently healthy, and after three months from arrival at their destina-

56 Blanchard, "Continental European Cattle Trades," 441, 446–8; and Baszanowski, "Ochsenzuchtgebiete," 125.

57 Lynn B. Martin and Courtney A. C. Coon, "Infection Protection and Natural Selection," *Science* 330 (2010): 602–03. See also Sonia Altizer, Rebecca Bartel, and Barbara A. Han, "Animal Migration and Infectious Disease Risk," *Science* 331 (2011): 296–302.

58 John Marino, *Pastoral Economics in the Kingdom of Naples* (Baltimore: Johns Hopkins University Press, 1988), 56–57; Alfonso Rodríguez Grajera and Mireille Mousnier, "Les Maladies et l'état sanitaire des animaux dans la couronne de Castille à l'époque moderne," in *Les animaux malades en Europe occidentale (VIe–XIXe siècle)* (Toulouse: Presses Universitaires du Mirail, 2005), 153–78; and Francis Brumont, "Les Moutons de la grange de Quintanajuar en vieille-Castille (1623–1834)," in ibid., 117–24.

tion, the disease might appear, induced by the long marches and privation."[59] In twentieth-century Africa, outbreaks often emerged from contact between the cattle of settled populations and the migrating herds of nomads.[60] We may never be certain of the source of the eighteenth-century panzootics, but some of our closest witnesses implicate Polish imports in the outbreak of 1709,[61] and according to Spinage, the disease was still circulating among Polish cattle at the time of the 1740 wave of pestilence.[62]

The timing of the two waves of rinderpest also implicates weather and warfare in the spread of infection. Overall the early eighteenth century may have been the mildest period of the Little Ice Age, but 1709 and 1740 were the two of the coldest European winters in the past millennium. Moreover, both were years of major European military campaigns, separated by the unusually long European peace between the War of the Spanish Succession (1701–14) and the War of the Austrian Succession (1740–48). Climate and conflict again proved the triggers for major outbreaks of livestock disease.

The winter of 1708–9 was widely regarded at the time as the worst in memory. It stands out in some climate reconstructions as Europe's coldest winter in at least the past five hundred years.[63] In January a strong polar air mass brought unprecedented cold that persisted a month or more. Londoners held another frost fair on the Thames. Parts of France suffered famine and high mortality, as the weather turned so cold that wine burst its casks and sea water froze in the Bay of Marseilles.[64]

The winter was even more destructive in Northeastern Europe, then at the climax of the Great Northern War (1700–21). Following his stunning victories over Denmark and Poland, Charles XII of Sweden had turned his army eastward to Lithuania and marched into Russia in summer 1708. Czar Peter the Great answered with scorched-earthed tactics, leaving the Swedish forces starving and exposed during the first frozen months of 1709. Having lost around a third of its men from

---

59 Spinage, *Cattle Plague*, 7, 19.

60 Rodostits and Done, *Veterinary Medicine*, 1238.

61 Spinage, *Cattle Plague*, 102–06; Kanold, *Historische Relation*, 8, 18, 34.

62 *Cattle Plague*, 116.

63 Jürg Luterbacher et al., "European Seasonal and Annual Temperature Variability, Trends, and Extremes Since 1500," *Science* 303 (2004): 1499–503.

64 For an in-depth study of the winter, see W. Gregory Monahan, *Year of Sorrows: The Great Famine of 1709 in Lyon* (Columbus: Ohio State University Press, 1993). For a contemporary description, see e.g., William Derham, "The History of the Great Frost in the Last Winter, 1708 and 1708/9," *Philosophical Transactions of the Royal Society* 26 (1708–1709): 477.

cold and disease, Charles's army fell to Russian forces at the critical Battle of Poltava the following summer.[65] The winter changed not only the outcome of the war but also the political map of Eastern Europe. Yet the combined effect of cold and conflict had still wider repercussions for the human and animal populations of the region. Armies in the Northern War had to stay on the move and live off the land in order to survive, creating another vehicle for contagions. Armies wasted provisions and drove up the price of food and fodder, leaving local populations hungry and vulnerable to infection. It is probably no coincidence that the Great Northern War also brought the last great bubonic plague epidemic in the Baltic region, reaching its peak in 1709–13.[66] The outbreak of the cattle panzootic formed part of a wider environmental disaster that also affected humans and other animals. While human quarantine measures helped contain the human plague, however, the cattle pestilence spread into the rest of Europe with the growing Continental meat trade.

The most detailed eye-witness account of the panzootic, that of Johann Kanold in Breslau (now Wrocław), took particular note of environmental factors leading up to the outbreak. He described the severe winter of 1709 and locust invasions in Poland and other infected lands during 1710.[67] Likewise, Kanold noted a variety of other contagious diseases among animals, including a disease of horses, which he blamed on the bad weather and poor fodder.[68] Since rinderpest does not infect equids, Kanold's description suggests that the environment was already conducive to animal infections.

The situation in 1740 proved remarkably similar to that of 1709. The winter of 1739–40 was almost as harsh as that of 1709, with the cold persisting even later into the season. In some parts of Europe, unusual extremes of temperature and precipitation continued over the following two years, leading to some of the

65 On the conduct of the Great Northern War, see Robert Frost, *The Northern Wars* (New York: Longman, 2000), chapters 9 and 10. For Eastern European temperature reconstructions, see e.g., Ulf Büntgen et al., "Filling the Eastern European Gap in Millennium-Long Temperature Reconstructions," *Proceedings of the National Academy of Sciences* 110 (2013): 1773–78; Ye. P. Borisenkov, "Documentary Evidence from the U.S.S.R.," in *Climate Since A.D. 1500*, ed. R. S. Bradley and P. D. Jones (London: Routledge, 1995), 171–83; and Vladimir Klimenko and Olga Solomina, "Climatic Variations in the East European Plain During the Last Millennium: State of the Art," in *The Polish Climate in the European Context: An Historical Overview*, ed. Rajmund Przybylak et al. (Berlin: Springer, 2010), 71–101.

66 See Karl-Erik Frandsen, *The Last Plague in the Baltic Region 1709–1713* (Copenhagen: Museum Tusculanum Press, 2010).

67 Kanold, *Historische Relation*, 18 and 45–50.

68 Ibid., 55 and chapter 5 *passim*.

highest food prices and mortality rates of the century.[69] At the same time, the War of the Austrian Succession raised demands for provisions; and moving armies, including the Prussian invasion of Silesia in 1740, may have helped spread the disease around the Continent.

Examples across Europe demonstrate that extreme cold, poor pasture, and harvest failures had fatally weakened livestock in advance of the panzootic. As one contemporary tract on the cattle plague observed, "It hath generally been observed that pestilential and contagious Distempers are check'd, at least, if not wholly put a stop to, by the coming in of cold Weather; whereas, on the contrary, the Violence of this Disease has been increased: for it has been observed to have been much more fatal during the Frosts which we have lately had, than at any other Time, since its Appearance."[70] In Germany, livestock mortality accelerated during the severe cold of late 1739, and reached an "alarming rate" after the complete failure of fodder crops in 1740. By that point, some peasants supposedly fed animals the very thatch from their roofs.[71] Even the more advanced agricultural economy of England endured a great loss of sheep as snow and ice covered the ground, and long winters and prolonged stall feeding aggravated shortages of fodder.[72] Yet by far the worst impacts were felt in more marginal environments. Ireland faced the second-worst famine in its history. The country lost "a vast number of sheep" for want of fodder and suffered an epizootic of horses as well.[73] Meanwhile the Highlands of Scotland faced "critical" shortages of cattle.[74] Scandinavia was worse affected still. So many cattle were lost for lack of fodder, or consequently died of disease, that not enough land could be plowed for the following two years, contributing to widespread starvation, especially in Norway.[75]

---

69 For a detailed study of these years, see John Post, *Food Shortage, Climatic Variability, and Epidemic Disease in Preindustrial Europe* (Ithaca: Cornell University Press, 1985). For further analysis of the climatic anomaly, see P. D. Jones and K. R. Briffa, "Unusual Climate in Northwest Europe During the Period 1730 to 1745 Based on Instrumental and Documentary Data," *Climatic Change* 79 (2006): 361–79.

70 John Barker, *An Account of the Present Epidemical Distemper Amongst the Black Cattle* (London: A. Millar, 1745), 13.

71 Post, *Food Shortage*, 105; and Spinage, *Cattle Plague*, 116.

72 Post, *Food Shortage*, 62, 82.

73 S. Engler et al., "The Irish Famine of 1740–1741: Famine Vulnerability and 'Climate Migration'," *Climate of the Past* 9 (2013): 1161–79; Post, *Food Shortage*, 64, 97.

74 Ibid., 95.

75 Ibid., 108–13. Norway had suffered a similar disaster in the 1690s-1710s as well: see Jean Grove and A. Battagel, "Tax Records from Western Norway as an Index of the Little Ice Age Environmental and Economic Deterioration," *Climatic Change* 3 (1983): 265–82.

Developments in the Netherlands and Denmark point to further environmental factors in the spread of the panzootic. In Holland and neighboring provinces, a series of severe winters, floods, poor harvests, and then infectious diseases produced a severe mortality among cattle in advance of the principal panzootic.[76] Consequently, the Netherlands had to reopen its borders to Danish cattle imports in the late 1730s. Denmark, however, was in the midst of what historian Thorstein Kjaegaard has described as an ecological crisis.[77] Centuries of deforestation had left sand dunes drifting into arable and pasture, and the land suffered rampant overstocking and overgrazing. Fuel ran so short that farmers had to burn fodder, leaving their livestock weakened and vulnerable. Consequently, the 1740 rinderpest struck Jutland worst of all and persisted there for decades.[78] The Netherlands' brief opening to Danish cattle exposed its herds to one of the most severe outbreaks of the whole panzootic, with perhaps 80 percent of Dutch cattle infected by 1745 and herd losses as high as 70 percent.[79]

Thus in eighteenth-century Europe, as in the sixteenth-century Ottoman Empire, the high mortality of livestock was the consequence not only of a pathogen but also a particular historical and environmental conjuncture. Expanding supply lines and growing demand for livestock laid the groundwork for the spread of infection, while adverse climate and military campaigns sparked the worst outbreaks.

Revising the History of the Panzootics and the Rise of Modern Veterinary Medicine

Europe's early modern rinderpest outbreaks traditionally mark a turning point in the story of veterinary medicine. Standard accounts of the period have tended to focus on a series of medical writers beginning with Girolamo Fracastoro (ca.1478–1553) and continuing through Bernardino Ramazzini (1633–1714), Giovanni Maria Lancisi (1654–1720), and Carlo Franceso Cogrossi (1682–1769),

76 Gijsbers, "Kapitale Ossen," 93, and Post, *Food Shortage*, 103.

77 Thorkild Kjaegaard, *The Danish Revolution, 1500–1800: An Ecohistorical Interpretation*, trans. David Hohnen (New York: Cambridge University Press, 1994).

78 See Robert Dossie, *Memoirs of Agriculture and Other Oeconomical Arts* (London: J. Nourse, 1771), 2: 375.

79 Gijsbers, "Kapitale Ossen"; J. A. Faber, "Cattle-Plague in the Netherlands During the Eighteenth Century," *Medelingen van de Lanbouwhogeschool te Wageningen* 62 (1962): 1–7; and Peter A. Koolmees, "Epizootic Diseases in the Netherlands, 1713–2002," in *Healing the Herds: Disease, Livestock Economies, and the Globalization of Veterinary Medicine*, ed. Karen Brown and Daniel Gilfoyle (Athens, OH: Ohio University Press, 2010), 19–41.

and how they advanced a more modern understanding of human and animal disease contagion in place of classical Galenic theories of humoral imbalances and environmental causation.[80] A number of studies have also emphasized the important role of the panzootics in the founding of veterinary colleges and the development of human and animal public health, as European states began to take aggressive measures to cull infected herds and guard against contagion from infected skins and meat.[81] The story has usually been one of cumulative advances in knowledge and more effective disease prevention, particularly the rise of germ theory and its application to public health.

Putting epizootics into a comparative and environmental perspective calls into question parts of this conventional narrative. While Renaissance theories of contagion eventually contributed to a modern understanding of epidemiology, they were neither as revolutionary as often supposed nor such a self-evident advance over the prevailing Galenic understanding of disease. As Vivian Nutton has argued, Fracastoro's contemporaries already understood disease as "the result of a multiplicity of causes, which afforded a variety of levels of explanation and action." Environmental approaches to disease did not preclude the presence of some particular disease-causing agent. Harmful air, bad weather, miasma, even astronomical conjunctions or the wrath of God could be understood as predisposing condi-

80 See e.g., Karasszon, *Concise History of Veterinary Medicine*, 291–327; Lise Wilkinson, *Animals and Disease: An Introduction to the History of Comparative Medicine* (New York: Cambridge University Press, 1992), chapters 3–5; Robert H. Dunlop and David J. Williams, *Veterinary Medicine: An Illustrated History* (St. Louis: Mosby, 1996), 277–81; and Joanna Swabe, *Animals, Disease and Human Society* (London: Routledge, 1999), 85–117. Swabe also discusses the historiography of veterinary medicine. More recently, Louise Hill Curth, *The Care of Brute Beasts: A Social and Cultural Study of Veterinary Medicine in Early Modern England* (Leiden: Brill, 2010) has argued that the impact of the epizootic and the new veterinary institutions of the eighteenth century may have been less revolutionary for medical theories and public health than previously supposed.

81 See e.g., Reinhold Dorwart, "Cattle Disease (Rinderpest?): Prevention and Cure in Brandenburg, 1665–1732," *Agricultural History* 33 (1959): 79–85; J. Broad, "Cattle Plague in Eighteenth-Century England," *Agricultural History Review* 31 (1983): 104–15; Carsten Stühring, "Managing Epizootic Diseases in 18th-Century Bavaria," in *Le interazioni fra economia e ambiente biologico nell'Europa preindustriale secc. XIII–XVIII*, ed. Simonetta Cavaciocchi (Florence: Firenze University Press, 2010), 473–80; Dominik Hünniger, "Policing Epizootics: Legislation and Administration During Outbreaks of Cattle Plague in Eighteenth-Century Northern Germany as Continuous Crisis Management," in *Healing the Herds: Disease, Livestock Economies, and the Globalization of Veterinary Medicine*, ed. Karen Brown and Daniel Gilfoyle (Athens, OH: Ohio University Press, 2010), 92–107; and Dorothee Brantz, "'Risky Business': Disease, Disaster and the Unintended Consequences of Epizootics in Eighteenth- and Nineteenth-Century France and Germany," *Environment and History* 17 (2011): 35–51.

tions for transmission of some unknown seed of infection—something Fracastoro himself and many of his successors never denied.[82]

Nutton's point is even more pertinent to the history of livestock disease and veterinary medicine. Notions of contagion among animals were likely even older and more widely accepted than contagion among humans. Nutton quotes a third-century Christian preacher who recommended the segregation of sinful virgins "like infected sheep or diseased cattle"[83]; and by Fracastoro's time it was typical for writers on animal disease to assume some form of animal-to-animal transmission.[84] Moreover, those seventeenth- and eighteenth-century writers usually cited as pioneers in the science of animal epidemiology and public health sometimes proposed theories of multiple causation as well. Starting in the 1690s, Ramazzini made detailed observations of severe and variable weather in relation to insect invasions and animal plagues in northern Italy.[85] In his treatise on the cattle plague of the 1710s, he attributed the disease to "foul air, or rotten food, or ... a contagious seed" and made reference to "contagious miasma" as well.[86] Cogrossi, too, could not help noting unusual weather leading up to the 1709 panzootic.[87] However, historians of veterinary medicine have tended to focus on these writers' more simplified pronouncements about epizootic contagion, perhaps to emphasize their role as forerunners of the bacteriological revolution. For instance, Lancisi and Cogrossi both stated that a "single Hungarian ox" like a "Trojan horse" had brought the entire panzootic to Europe—a verdict that became influential among eighteenth- and nineteenth-century proponents of contagion theories and more aggressive public health measurements.[88]

---

82 Vivian Nutton, "The Reception of Fracastoro's Theory of Contagion: The Seed that Fell among Thorns?," *Osiris* 6 (1990): 196–234, quote on 230. I have elsewhere argued that Ottoman understandings of disease were broadly similar: Sam White, "Rethinking Disease in Ottoman History," *International Journal of Middle East Studies* 42 (2010): 549–67.

83 Nutton, "Reception of Fracastoro's Theory," 229.

84 See e.g., Leonard Mascall, *The First Booke of Cattell* (London: John Harison, 1610), 66–67.

85 Translated and quoted at length in Fleming, *Animal Plagues*, 158–72 *passim*.

86 Bernardino Ramazzini, *De Contagiosa Epidemia Quae in Patavino Agro, & Tota Fere Veneta Ditione in Boves Irrepsit Dissertatio* (Padua: Gio. Batt. Conzatti, 1712), 14, 21: "Omnibus epidemiis, si a sporadicis affectibus differe debent, id peculiare inest, quod communem causam habeant, sive ab Aeris vitio, sive a corruptis alimentis, aut aliduo contagioso fomite prognata fuerit, qui ab uno corpore in aliud transmigret."

87 Carlo Francesco Cogrossi, *Nuova Idea del Male Contagioso de' Buoi* [1714] (Rome: Società Italiana di Microbiologia, 1953), 28–30.

88 Giovanni Maria Lancisi, *Dissertatio Historica de Bovilla Peste, Quae ex Campaniae Finibus Anno 1713 Latio Importata* [etc.] (Rome: G.M. Salvoni, 1715), 1; Cogrossi, *Nuova Idea*, 21–22.

In light of the findings in this chapter, it seems appropriate to re-evaluate early modern theories of multiple causation in animal disease. That is not to say that Galenic medicine had an unrecognized scientific foundation, but that most early modern observers were being perfectly reasonable in associating epizootics with factors such as weather, rather than dismissing environmental causation altogether and adopting a precursor of germ theory. It did not necessarily make sense to emphasize the action of still unknown pathogens in these outbreaks when social and environmental factors were evidently so important in their timing. An exclusive focus on microbial contagion was (and perhaps still is) a dangerously simplified way to understand the origins of epizootics. This recognition calls for a re-evaluation of some common-sense observations of contemporaries, who are otherwise forgotten or dismissed as mere holdouts against germ theory.[89] In this regard, Robert Dossie's 1771 discussion of the cattle plague left an unusually insightful account of how changes in the long-distance cattle trade and the timing of military campaigns interacted with extreme winters to create one of the worst European disasters of the century:

> Where the infection does not before subsist, it never comes, but after some general cause has weakened the habit of the beasts in general: such as very severe cold;—long continued want of a sufficient quantity of wholesome food;—repeated alternations of heat and cold in the weather;—moist air, replete with putrid vapours;—a long continuance of easterly winds;—or, what is more frequent, a combination of two or more of these causes together.—Thus we find this contagion invading every part of Europe after the year 1711, when the season had been so inclement the year before, as to destroy a great part of the sheep in England; and again in 1741, as mentioned above, after a very intense frost, which lasted from December to April; and, by rigour of cold, and scarcity of fodder, had reduced the cattle in general to a debilitated state: which was still aggravated by the almost constant easterly winds that blew the summer and autumn following. It results, therefore, from these circumstances, that though infection conveyed from some beast diseased with it, is the efficient cause of the murrain in cattle, yet there is a predisponent cause, or particular state of the subject, absolutely necessary to its acting or taking effect ... It appears also, that this weak state of the beast may arise from general causes, either of an epidemic nature, affecting whole regions, such as inclemency of season or scarcity of wholesome food.[90]

See also Wilkinson, *Animals and Disease*, 38–39.

89 Cf. Spinage, *Cattle Plague*, 52–53.

90 Dossie, *Memoirs*, vol. 2, 375–78.

Conclusion

Since the seminal publication of William McNeill's *Plagues and Peoples* in 1976, historians have come to appreciate both the important role of disease in human history and also the role of social and environmental factors in the history of diseases. Animal infections now deserve the same reconsideration. At times, the health of livestock has also played an important part in the fate of empires; and many of the same historical factors that have shaped human plagues have governed their animal equivalents, including commerce, war, climate, population growth, and resource pressures. As this chapter has argued, animals have also been surprisingly mobile, cosmopolitan actors in history, and the study of past animal diseases could also benefit from a more comparative and environmental approach.

In 2011, the Food and Agriculture Organization of the United Nations officially declared that rinderpest had been eradicated, closing the history of the sheep and cattle plagues described in this chapter. Nevertheless, during the past decade diseases such as avian influenza and swine flu have come to remind us that microbes may adapt faster than medical technologies to the new conditions of globalization. Once more, a focus on contagion and containment alone may not be enough to control these infections, as global trade and travel accelerate, as large-scale intensive livestock operations expand into developing countries with weaker public health systems, and as the overuse of antibiotics in animal feeding operations threatens to render them less effective. Environmental factors will likely continue to play a central role in epizootic outbreaks. New systems of confinement, especially stressed animals in enormous and densely crowded production facilities, will provide breeding grounds for new diseases. With the onset of global warming, climate change may once again add to the dangers of infection, exposing animals to new environmental conditions and new disease vectors.[91] Preindustrial livestock disease may seem a dark and remote chapter of world history, and in some ways it surely is. Nevertheless, the history of Little Ice Age epizootics could yet prove troublingly relevant for the future.

---

91 See e.g., Smita Sirohi and Axel Michaelowa, "Sufferer and Cause: Indian Livestock and Climate Change," *Climatic Change* 85 (2007): 285–98; Roland Zell, "Global Climate Change and the Emergence/Re-emergence of Infectious Diseases," *International Journal of Medical Microbiology* 293 Suppl 37 (2004): 16–26; Kenneth L. Gage et al., "Climate and Vectorborne Diseases," *American Journal of Preventive Medicine* 35 (2008): 436–50; Irene Hoffmann, "Climate Change and the Characterization, Breeding and Conservation of Animal Genetic Resources," *Animal Genetics* 41 Suppl 1 (2010): 32–46; and Sally J. Cutler, Anthony R. Fooks, and Wim H. M. van der Poel, "Public Health Threat of New, Reemerging, and Neglected Zoonoses in the Industrialized World," *Emerging Infectious Diseases* 16 (2010): 1–7; Brian D. Perry, Delia Grace, and Keith Sones, "Current Drivers and Future Directions of Global Livestock Disease Dynamics," *Proceedings of the National Academy of Sciences* 110 (2013): 20871–77.

Sam White (white.2426@osu.edu) is associate professor of environmental history at the Ohio State University and author of *The Climate of Rebellion in the Early Modern Ottoman Empire* (Cambridge University Press, 2011), which examines environmental pressures in the empire's crisis and transformation during the sixteenth and seventeenth centuries. It received the Middle East Studies Association Albert Hourani award and the Turkish Studies Association M. Fuat Köprülü book prize. Prof. White has authored various articles and chapters on climate, disease, and animals in history, and a second monograph (forthcoming) on the influence of climate in early European exploration and colonization of North America. He is the lead editor of the *Palgrave Handbook of Climate History* and co-founder and co-director of the Climate History Network (climatehistory.net).

VETERINARY MEDICINE IN NINETEENTH-CENTURY EGYPT

ALAN MIKHAIL
Yale University

THE HUMAN-ANIMAL RELATIONSHIP is an essential aspect of understanding the past and present of all societies.[1] This chapter offers an account and analysis of one small slice of this relationship—a history of veterinary medicine in nineteenth-century Egypt. The human application of medical knowledge and technology to the lives of other animals has been a constant in the history of interspecies relations in Egypt.[2] Indeed, some of the earliest sources from Egypt evince the beginnings of this long history of veterinary knowledge.[3] The story of veterinary medicine in Egypt is obviously therefore an enormous and complicated one with many twists and turns.[4] In focusing on just one recent piece of this history, I

---

1 On this topic in Ottoman Egypt, see Alan Mikhail, *The Animal in Ottoman Egypt* (Oxford: Oxford University Press, 2014), from which portions of this chapter are adapted.

2 Generally on the history of veterinary medicine, see Joanna Swabe, *Animals, Disease, and Human Society: Human-Animal Relations and the Rise of Veterinary Medicine* (London: Routledge, 1999); Karen Brown and Daniel Gilfoyle, eds., *Healing the Herds: Disease, Livestock Economies, and the Globalization of Veterinary Medicine* (Athens: Ohio University Press, 2010); Susan D. Jones, *Valuing Animals: Veterinarians and Their Patients in Modern America* (Baltimore: Johns Hopkins University Press, 2002); Housni Alkhateeb Shehada, *Mamluks and Animals: Veterinary Medicine in Medieval Islam* (Leiden: Brill, 2013).

3 A. R. Williams, "Animal Mummies," *National Geographic* (November 2009): http://ngm.nationalgeographic.com/2009/11/animal-mummies/williams-text/1 (accessed July 6, 2014). More generally on animals in ancient Egypt, see Patrick F. Houlihan, "Animals in Egyptian Art and Hieroglyphs," in *A History of the Animal World in the Ancient Near East*, ed. Billie Jean Collins (Leiden: Brill, 2002), 97–143; Emily Teeter, "Animals in Egyptian Literature," in *A History of the Animal World in the Ancient Near East*, ed. Billie Jean Collins (Leiden: Brill, 2002), 251–70; idem, "Animals in Egyptian Religion," in *A History of the Animal World in the Ancient Near East*, ed. Billie Jean Collins (Leiden: Brill, 2002), 335–60; Douglas Brewer, "Hunting, Animal Husbandry and Diet in Ancient Egypt," in *A History of the Animal World in the Ancient Near East*, ed. Billie Jean Collins (Leiden: Brill, 2002), 427–56; Dorothea Arnold, "An Egyptian Bestiary," *Metropolitan Museum of Art Bulletin* 52 (1995): 1 and 7–64.

4 For an extremely important study of Mamluk veterinary medicine, see Shehada, *Mamluks and Animals*. Generally on Arab and Islamic zoology, see Herbert Eisenstein, *Einführung in die arabische Zoographie: Das tierkundliche Wissen in der arabisch-islamischen Literatur* (Berlin: Dietrich Reimer, 1990); Manfred Ullmann, *Die Natur- und Geheimwissenschaften im Islam* (Leiden: Brill, 1972), 5–61.

will show that the nineteenth century was a period of marked change in the kinds and techniques of veterinary medicine used in Egypt. There were two reasons for this change in the nineteenth century.

First, veterinary knowledge was centralized in an institution—the Egyptian School of Veterinary Medicine. The school sought to regulate, regularize, and monopolize how veterinary medicine was used in Egypt. Instead of the animal body being approached through experience, localized knowledge, and home remedies as had previously been the case, in the nineteenth century animals came to be seen as disease carriers that had to be understood primarily through epidemiology and zoology, knowledge held, deployed, and controlled by the school of veterinary medicine. Second, as never before in Egypt, the history of animal diseases in the nineteenth century was a global one. That is, to understand why and how Egypt's animals became sick, we must understand Egypt's place in a global economy and network of connections. The influence of these global ties on Egypt's animals is an essential aspect of its nineteenth-century history, one indeed unprecedented in the millennia of human-animal interactions in Egypt.

The Egyptian School of Veterinary Medicine

The school of veterinary medicine was founded in 1827 to address one of the oldest issues affecting the human-animal relationship—disease—through several new techniques. The first was the employment of French expertise to help with the founding and operation of the new animal institution—an outgrowth of both the French expedition to Egypt between 1798 and 1801 and the many educational delegations that took Egyptian students to France in the nineteenth century.[5] Second was the school's clear objective to instrumentalize and maintain healthy animals for warfare. The third was the new notion that medical understandings of the animal body were the best means to forge a more productive and sustainable society.[6]

---

5 For useful insights from the literature on colonial veterinary medicine, see Diana K. Davis, "Prescribing Progress: French Veterinary Medicine in the Service of Empire," *Veterinary Heritage* 29 (2006): 1–7; idem, "Brutes, Beasts, and Empire: Veterinary Medicine and Environmental Policy in French North Africa and British India," *Journal of Historical Geography* 34 (2008): 242–67; Brown and Gilfoyle, *Healing the Herds*; Shaun Milton, "Western Veterinary Medicine in Colonial Africa: A Survey, 1902–1963," *Argos* 18 (1998): 313–22; Richard Waller, "'Clean' and 'Dirty': Cattle Disease and Control Policy in Colonial Kenya, 1900–40," *Journal of African History* 45 (2004): 45–80. On the Egyptian student delegations, see Alain Silvera, "The First Egyptian Student Mission to France under Muḥammad Ali," *Middle Eastern Studies* 16 (1980): 1–22.

6 Although I do not focus on it here, the animal body itself was of course also variously understood as having its own inherent medicinal properties. For a discussion of the historic

Disease in all its forms—human, animal, social—was a problem that had to be removed from Egypt in the nineteenth century, and the school of veterinary medicine was a major part of the effort to do that.

The Egyptian School of Veterinary Medicine was not the first opportunity for French scientists to study Egyptian animals. Indeed, Napoleon's expedition to Egypt at the turn of the nineteenth century led to gigantic leaps forward in French and wider European zoology, anatomy, and botany.[7] The person most immediately responsible for the zoological work that came out of the expedition was Étienne Geoffroy Saint-Hilaire.[8] He spent much of his time in Egypt examining fish, ostriches, and crocodiles, and collecting mummified animal bodies and other zoological specimens to take back with him to Paris.[9] His major contribution to nineteenth-century zoology and anatomy was his idea of the "unity of type," which for the first time put forth the notion that homologous structures existed across organisms, a concept that angered many of his contemporaries but would later prove to be a major influence on Charles Darwin.[10] Identifying homologous anatomical features shared by seemingly unrelated species quickly led to recognizing the roles of evolutionary relationships and environmental factors in natural selec-

---

uses of various animals' body parts as *materia medica* in Yemen, see Hanne Schönig, "Reflections on the Use of Animal Drugs in Yemen," *Quaderni di Studi Arabi* 20/21 (2002–03): 157–84.

7 On Arab and Islamic zoology, see Eisenstein, *Einführung in die arabische Zoographie*; Ullmann, *Die Natur- und Geheimwissenschaften*, 5–61.

8 For accounts of Geoffroy Saint-Hilaire's life and work, see Isidore Geoffroy Saint-Hilaire, *Vie, travaux et doctrine scientifique d'Étienne Geoffroy Saint-Hilaire* (Paris: P. Bertrand, 1847); Théophile Cahn, *La vie et l'oeuvre d'Étienne Geoffroy Saint-Hilaire* (Paris: Presses universitaires de France, 1962); Hervé Le Guyader, *Étienne Geoffroy Saint-Hilaire, 1772–1844: A Visionary Naturalist*, trans. Marjorie Grene (Chicago: University of Chicago Press, 2004); Michael A. Osborne, "Zoos in the Family: The Geoffroy Saint-Hilaire Clan and the Three Zoos of Paris," in *New Worlds, New Animals: From Menagerie to Zoological Park in the Nineteenth Century*, ed. R. J. Hoage and William A. Deiss (Baltimore: Johns Hopkins University Press, 1996), 33–42.

9 For accounts of Geoffroy Saint-Hilaire's time in Egypt, see Geoffroy Saint-Hilaire, *Vie, travaux et doctrine scientifique*, 74–123; Nina Burleigh, *Mirage: Napoleon's Scientists and the Unveiling of Egypt* (New York: HarperCollins, 2007), 195–207. For some of his writings about Egypt, see Étienne Geoffroy Saint-Hilaire, "Miscellaneous Notes in Egypt (1798–1801 and 1830s)," Étienne Geoffroy Saint Hilaire Collection, Mss.B.G287p, American Philosophical Society, Philadelphia.

10 Toby A. Appel, *The Cuvier-Geoffroy Debate: French Biology in the Decades before Darwin* (New York: Oxford University Press, 1987).

tion. Darwin understood the importance of Geoffroy Saint-Hilaire's contributions to nineteenth-century science and to his own work.[11] He wrote:

> This is the most interesting department of natural history, and may be said to be its very soul. What can be more curious than that the hand of a man, formed for grasping, that of a mole for digging, the leg of the horse, the paddle of the porpoise, and the wing of the bat, should all be constructed on the same pattern, and should include the same bones, in the same relative positions? Geoffroy St. Hilaire has insisted strongly on the high importance of relative connexion in homologous organs: the parts may change to almost any extent in form and size, and yet they always remain connected together in the same order.[12]

Zoology was quickly becoming the primary means through which humans were engaging with and understanding animals.[13] More importantly, the human experience of animals in Egypt heavily shaped European and other globalizing scientific understandings of the animal world.

Epizootics increasingly came to be understood and dealt with through veterinary medicine and zoological conceptions of animals' bodies. In point of fact, the immediate impetus for the founding of the Egyptian School of Veterinary Medicine was an epizootic among livestock working in rice fields in Rosetta in 1827. Ever the believer in European expertise, Mehmet ʿAli, Egypt's Ottoman governor general in the first half of the nineteenth century, hired two French veterinarians to deal with this crisis in 1827.[14] Pierre Nicolas Hamont and his associate Pretot were both distinguished graduates of the renowned French National Veterinary School of Alfort.[15] In dealing with the Rosetta epizootic, Hamont identified a com-

---

11 One biographer goes so far as to liken Geoffroy Saint-Hilaire's time in Egypt to Darwin's voyage on the *Beagle*. Le Guyader, *Étienne Geoffroy Saint-Hilaire*, 21–22.

12 Charles Darwin, *On the Origin of Species by Means of Natural Selection, or the Preservation of Favoured Races in the Struggle for Life* (London: John Murray, 1859), 434.

13 For a collection of studies of early modern, mostly European, zoology, see Karl A. E. Enenkel and Paul J. Smith, eds., *Early Modern Zoology: The Construction of Animals in Science, Literature and the Visual Arts*, 2 vols. (Leiden: Brill, 2007).

14 Aḥmad ʿIzzat ʿAbd al-Karīm, *Tārīkh al-Taʿlīm fī ʿAṣr Muḥammad ʿAlī* (Cairo: Maktabat al-Nahḍa al-Miṣriyya, 1938), 309.

15 Antoine Barthélemy Clot-Bey, *Aperçu general sur l'Égypte*, 2 vols. (Bruxelles: Meline, Cans, 1840), 2: 440. Of the two, Hamont would play the more important role in the history of veterinary medicine in Egypt since Pretot quickly fell ill upon his arrival in Egypt and soon returned to France where he died less than a year after first coming to Egypt. ʿAbd al-Karīm, *Tārīkh al-Taʿlīm*, 309. James Heyworth-Dunne writes that Pretot died in Smyrna. James Heyworth-Dunne, *An Introduction to the History of Education in Modern Egypt*

bination of mostly climatic factors as the main cause of the animals' diseases—high rates of humidity, exposure to extreme winter rainfall, inadequate amounts of food, and too much work.[16] He and Pretot quickly set out to ameliorate these conditions by constructing better stables and by preventing animals from drinking from the Nile. Pleased with these results, Mehmet ʿAli quickly took advantage of the veterinarians' expertise. He sent them ten students from the military academy to Rosetta to be trained in techniques useful in the prevention of animal diseases. Unlike almost all of the major educational institutions founded in Egypt in the first third of the nineteenth century, the school of veterinary medicine did not initially operate in Cairo.[17] A short time after the first ten students were sent to the coastal city of Rosetta in 1827, a few more were dispatched by Mehmet ʿAli to train with Hamont, and the school started to improve and extend its facilities, adding stables and drinking troughs for horses, dorms for students, kitchens, more doctors, and an administrative structure. Soon, however, the school began to face many problems. Hamont bitterly complained that the students lacked concentration and seriousness and that the translators employed by the school did not have the veterinary expertise needed to adequately express in Arabic the concepts Hamont related in French.[18] Moreover, Hamont grumbled that the chief translator was lazy and would often speak badly of him to the governor of Rosetta.

(London: Luzac, 1939), 133. For Hamont's general comments on Egypt's animals, see P. N. Hamont, *L'Egypt sous Méhémet-Ali*, 2 vols. (Paris: Léautey et Lecointe, 1843), 1: 523–61. Hamont also knew Étienne Geoffroy Saint-Hilaire and consulted him on various veterinary matters in Egypt. See, for example, Pierre Nicolas Hamont, "Observations communiqué par M. P.N. Hamont, medecin vétérinaire d'Alfot professeur de medecine veterinaire en Egypte au Service se S.A. Mehamet Ali Pacha (27 April 1829)," Étienne Geoffroy Saint Hilaire Collection, Mss.B.G287p, American Philosophical Society, Philadelphia.

16 ʿAbd al-Karīm, *Tārīkh al-Taʿlīm*, 310. On these points, ʿAbd al-Karīm cites Hamont, *L'Egypt sous Méhémet-Ali*, 2: 122–24.

17 Generally, on the history of the school of veterinary medicine, see Clot-Bey, *Aperçu general*, 2: 437–48.

18 Interestingly, the only book on science or technology to be published in both Turkish and Arabic by Mehmet ʿAli's new Būlāq Press (founded in 1822) was a textbook of veterinary medicine. Richard N. Verdery, "The Publications of the Būlāq Press under Muḥammad ʿAlī of Egypt," *Journal of the American Oriental Society* 91 (1971), 131. For a complete list of the books available from the Būlāq Press in 1845, including nine on veterinary medicine, two of which were the Arabic and Turkish versions of the text just mentioned (*Ṭibb Bayṭarī Qānūnnāmesi*), see the following press catalog: *Mısır'da Bir Kütüphaneye ait Fihrist*, Süleymaniye Kütüphanesi (Istanbul), Hüsrev Paşa 828. On the general history of the Būlāq Press and its publications, see Abū al-Futūḥ Raḍwān, *Tārīkh Maṭbaʿat Būlāq wa Lamḥa fī Tārīkh al-Ṭibāʿa fī Buldān al-Sharq al-Awsaṭ* (Cairo: al-Maṭbaʿa al-Amīriyya,

Discussions about moving the school to Abu Zaʿabel near Cairo began in 1829, but the move did not actually occur until two years later.[19] In addition to being near the capital and having better facilities, the new location was closer to the school of medicine. Since both schools taught their students anatomy and surgery, Mehmet ʿAli's government thought the institutions could usefully combine resources to share facilities and teaching responsibilities. Hamont strongly resisted merging the schools of human and animal medicine under one administration and pedagogical structure and sent a letter to Ibrahim Pasha making his case that a country as dependent on agriculture as Egypt had to maintain an independent and autonomous school of veterinary medicine. He added that each cavalry division should employ at least two of the school's graduates to oversee the well-being of its horses.[20]

These reasons aside, Hamont's primary opposition to combining the two schools came from his professional competition with his fellow countryman Antoine Barthélemy Clot-Bey, whom Mehmet ʿAli had also recently hired to establish a school of human medicine in Egypt.[21] One of Clot-Bey's assistants, a doctor named Bouzari who headed up the Medical Council in the 1830s, repeatedly told Hamont that it would be nearly impossible to establish a regime of human medicine in Egypt as long as he continued to demand a separate veterinary school.[22] Nevertheless, Hamont proved largely successful in maintaining his independent school in Abu Zaʿabel in these early years. A separate veterinary facility was built, complete with classrooms, lecture halls, surgical theaters, chemical labs, a pharmacy, and a recovery unit large enough for 140 horses. Student dormitories and housing for professors were also constructed. Between fifty and one hundred students were enrolled in the school in any given year in the early 1830s.[23]

1953); J. Heyworth-Dunne, "Printing and Translations under Muḥammad ʿAlī of Egypt: The Foundation of Modern Arabic," *Journal of the Royal Asiatic Society* 72 (1940): 325–49.

19 ʿAbd al-Karīm, *Tārīkh al-Taʿlīm*, 313; Heyworth-Dunne, *History of Education in Modern Egypt*, 133.

20 ʿAbd al-Karīm, *Tārīkh al-Taʿlīm*, 313.

21 For his part, Clot-Bey was also very interested in Egypt's animals. Clot-Bey, *Aperçu general*, 1: 203–40.

22 ʿAbd al-Karīm, *Tārīkh al-Taʿlīm*, 313.

23 There is some discrepancy here. Amira el-Azhary Sonbol puts the enrollment at one hundred, while ʿAbd al-Laṭīf Muḥammad al-Ṣabbāgh claims only fifty students were enrolled. Amira el-Azhary Sonbol, *The Creation of a Medical Profession in Egypt, 1800–1922* (Syracuse, NY: Syracuse University Press, 1991), 43; ʿAbd al-Laṭīf Muḥammad al-Ṣabbāgh, "al-Ṭibb al-Bayṭarī fī Miṣr (1828–1849): Dirāsa Wathāʾiqiyya," *Miṣr al-Ḥadītha* 8 (2009), 24.

In the early 1830s, Hamont also began overseeing the health of Egyptian cavalry horses in the stables of Shubra. Much of his effort went toward ensuring a sizable animal fighting force for various missions of the Egyptian army in this period. In addition to training the army's horses, the cavalry school consistently had an enrollment of two hundred to five hundred soldiers studying the various military uses of horses.[24] Not coincidently, the major push for veterinary medicine in Egypt came at the end of the 1820s and through the 1830s, when Mehmet ʿAli invaded Greater Syria and parts of Anatolia with the aim of marching to Istanbul to bring down the entire Ottoman Empire.[25]

When Hamont first arrived to the stables in Shubra, he found the cavalry horses inadequately fed and exercised.[26] Many were sick, and these sick horses were allowed to mix freely with the healthy animals.[27] Hamont's first task was therefore to institute a new system of feeding and exercising the horses. This effort yielded immediate results, greatly improving the animals' overall health.

Despite these early successes, pressure to combine the veterinary school with the school of medicine remained strong. When the school of medicine's main hospital was transferred to Qasr al-ʿAini in 1837, Clot-Bey pushed hard to fold the veterinary school into the new facility. The animal institution was nevertheless able to remain essentially independent, thanks mostly to its indispensable military function. In 1837, the year the school was moved to Shubra, it reached its highest enrollment—122 students.[28]

A compromise was eventually reached between the school of veterinary medicine and the medical school whereby veterinary students would complete their first year of preparatory training at the school of medicine before undertaking more specialized training with animals at Shubra.[29] In 1846, the system was slightly modified to allow students to spend all four years at the veterinary school,

24 Heyworth-Dunne, *History of Education in Modern Egypt*, 136.

25 About this military confrontation, see Khaled Fahmy, *All the Pasha's Men: Mehmed Ali, His Army and the Making of Modern Egypt* (Cambridge: Cambridge University Press, 1997); Muhammad H. Kutluoğlu, *The Egyptian Question (1831–1841): The Expansionist Policy of Mehmed Ali Paşa in Syria and Asia Minor and the Reaction of the Sublime Porte* (Istanbul: Eren, 1998).

26 Hamont, *L'Egypt sous Méhémet-Ali*, 1: 523–39 and 562–73.

27 Hamont's rival Clot-Bey also made special note of the very poor state of Egypt's horses. Clot-Bey, *Aperçu general*, 2: 439–40.

28 ʿAbd al-Karīm, *Tārīkh al-Taʿlīm*, 319. In 1836, the Agriculture School was also transferred to Shubra. Hamont would come to oversee both institutions. Heyworth-Dunne, *History of Education in Modern Egypt*, 134 and 152.

29 Clot-Bey, *Aperçu general*, 2: 445–48.

with a professor of medicine brought in during the students' first year to teach them physics, chemistry, and botany.[30] In addition to these general subjects, students studied muscular and skeletal structures and general anatomy in year one; surgery, pathology, specialized anatomy, and physiology in year two; and internal medicine, surgery, general and endemic disease pathologies, physiology, and general medicine in the third and fourth years.[31] French was studied in all years. The academic year was nine months long, split into three three-month segments.[32] The first of these was spent in book study and classroom lecture; the last two consisted of various practica.

Upon graduation, new veterinarians were dispersed throughout Egypt to oversee animal health in all the country's provinces. Given the delta's higher concentration of agricultural land, the majority were sent there, though many were dispatched to Fayyum and the south as well. They maintained connections with Cairo once in the field, mostly to secure medicines, equipment, and other necessities that were doled out by the capital's central veterinary administration.[33] One of the first major reform efforts pushed by these veterinarians was to prevent animal labor during the hottest periods of the summer for fear of increasing pulse rates and certain inflammatory diseases.[34] Mehmet ʿAli's new veterinarians recommended that animals not be used during the afternoon, that they be housed in shaded quarters, that they be given copious amounts of drinking water, and that the ground underneath them be regularly watered to keep it cool. This burgeoning veterinary establishment also recommended how long and at what times of day each animal in the countryside was to work and rest. Livestock used to push waterwheels and threshers (*al-nawārij*) were only to perform these tasks for one and a half hours each day. Buffalo cows were not to labor in the afternoons, and camel labor was recommended only at the harvest and then only at sunset. Furthermore, Mehmet ʿAli's government directed that trees be planted near waterwheels and other areas where livestock worked so as to provide them with adequate shade.

These efforts to reform the agricultural utilization of animals show that the relationship between Egyptian farmers and beasts of burden was becoming

30 al-Ṣabbāgh, "al-Ṭibb al-Bayṭarī," 30–31.

31 Ibid., 31.

32 ʿAbd al-Munʿim Ibrāhīm al-Jumayʿī, ed., *Wathāʾiq al-Taʿlīm al-ʿĀlī fī Miṣr khilāl al-Qarn al-Tāsiʿ ʿAshar* (Cairo: Dār al-Kutub wa al-Wathāʾiq al-Qawmiyya, 2004), 290.

33 al-Ṣabbāgh, "al-Ṭibb al-Bayṭarī," 43. Given the distances involved and the organizational time needed, veterinarians in the countryside were instructed to stock up on medicines to make sure they did not run out.

34 Ibid., 39–40.

increasingly subsumed under the scientific gaze of the medical bureaucracy that purported to understand this relationship better than peasants who had been using animals their entire lives. The interspecies relationship was to be managed and controlled to ensure the most effective uses of animal productivity and to defend human and animal populations from disease. Veterinarians' recommendations were ultimately meant to fundamentally reconfigure various aspects of the countryside. It was no longer the intense intimacy between humans and animals that was the primary motor force of the human-animal relationship—and hence of the social world built around it—but rather a logic of order, separation, cleanliness, and disease prevention driven by "objective science."

Needless to say, Egypt's new veterinarians worked hard to prevent the incidence and spread of certain animal diseases. Especially in the northern delta, where the majority of Egypt's rice was cultivated, large populations of flies and mosquitoes were sustained in the wide pools of standing water that covered rice fields. In 1847, the veterinarian assigned to Kafr al-Shaykh made provisions for large swaths of canvas to cover camels in the city in an effort to protect them from insects and heat.[35] The following year the veterinary council outlawed the importation of southern (*ṣaʿīdī*) buffalo cows to Sharqiyya and elsewhere in the delta. Most animals brought from the south died quickly in their new homes of angina and liver failure resulting from—it was determined—elevated temperatures and increased humidity in the north and exposure to insects living in the standing water of rice fields and in heavily weeded areas.[36] Temperature fluctuations caused further problems.[37] The cooling of fall and the attendant increase in humidity and precipitation resulted in a spike in the incidence of typhoid, dropsy, fevers, tapeworms, respiratory diseases, and skin infections.[38] Fall, therefore, brought with it various regulations and rules the veterinary establishment believed would curb the severity of these outbreaks. Maximum effort was to be undertaken to ensure that animals were well-fed and especially that they consumed enough salts.[39] They were not to drink from the Nile after the flood or to

35 Ibid., 40.

36 Ibid.

37 Another example of extreme temperatures leading to problems for animal populations is the following case from the late nineteenth century about very cold weather preventing the transport of dogs, chickens, and pigeons to the imperial palace in Istanbul: Başbakanlık Osmanlı Arşivi (Prime Ministry's Ottoman Archive, Istanbul; hereafter BOA), Yıldız Perakende Evrakı Mabeyn Başkitabeti 38.67 (2 Cemaziyelahir 1312/1 Dec. 1894).

38 al-Ṣabbāgh, "al-Ṭibb al-Bayṭarī," 40–41.

39 Egyptian veterinarians were generally very concerned with what animals ate, and there

wade in canals. They were only to consume filtered well water, and their coats were to be washed and cleaned twice a day.

For those animals who nevertheless succumbed there were also new rules about the disposal of their bodies.[40] Whereas previously peasants might have left the bodies of their dead animals on roads or in fields, or thrown them into sewage ditches or canals, early nineteenth-century veterinarians outlawed these practices, which they deemed to be unclean, unfit, uncivilized, and unhelpful in the prevention of disease. Veterinarians performed autopsies on dead animals in the countryside to determine their cause of death and would then quickly bury the carcasses after their investigations. Furthermore, living animals found to be stricken with contagion were immediately slaughtered and their bodies burned in the hopes of preventing an epizootic. The slaughter site would then be doused with lime or ammonia.[41] In cases in which an animal was clearly sick and on the brink of death, it was often buried alive (*waʾada*) so that no human would be exposed to the sick body or diseased blood while killing the creature. If it was feared that a contagion might have already spread in a certain location, veterinarians were given the necessary resources to establish a quarantine in the suspected area and were required to send daily reports to Cairo about the situation.[42]

Other efforts to manage and harness the fertility, fecundity, and reproductive capacities of animals exemplify how the school of veterinary medicine contributed to the bureaucratic control of the biological lives of animals and their commodification in the service of a growing capitalist economy. Every Friday, veterinary students undertook controlled breeding operations aimed at increasing the number of desirable animals in Egypt.[43] There were always enough suitable females, but securing an adequate number of healthy and fit males as mates proved a consistent problem, due mostly to their slaughter for meat and, less so, to their use in the countryside. Thus in 1839, Mehmet ʿAli issued several decrees outlawing the slaughter of bulls

thus developed a whole section of the veterinary establishment charged with overseeing dietary health. Ibid., 41.

40 Ibid.

41 Ammonia in the form of sal ammoniac was made in Giza through the crystallization of gas produced by the slow burning of a mixture of animal dung and straw. Mary Kerr, "Savary's Letters on Egypt. 1786," Notes on Visits to Various Country Houses and Towns in Great Britain, 1789–1826, Rare Books and Manuscripts, Yale Center for British Art, Yale University (New Haven), 10.

42 For a comparison with human quarantines in this period, see Alan Mikhail, *Nature and Empire in Ottoman Egypt: An Environmental History* (Cambridge: Cambridge University Press, 2011), 230–41.

43 al-Ṣabbāgh, "al-Ṭibb al-Bayṭarī," 44.

and also limiting the duration and amount of labor they were allowed to perform on rural estates. Cows too were not to be killed before they reached a productive age. Anyone caught breaking these rules would be severely punished.

Mehmet ʿAli furthermore sent some of his own veterinarians and hired others to secure premium animals from outside of Egypt to mate with domestic females and thereby "improve" Egypt's gene pool.[44] In the late 1820s and throughout the 1830s, oxen were regularly imported from Marseille and mules and donkeys from Italy. In the early 1830s, Mehmet ʿAli sought new kinds of sheep because the wool of most Egyptian sheep varieties was not suitable for commercial manufacturing. He serendipitously acquired sheep in 1834 when the King of Sardinia, in recognition of the appointment of a new Egyptian consul to the island, sent Mehmet ʿAli a gift of 150 Spanish merinos—prized, of course, for their fine soft wool.[45] The king also sent along twelve shepherds to show their Egyptian counterparts how best to care for the animals. As part of the effort to maintain this flock and to improve local sheep stocks, the Egyptian veterinarians put in charge of the merinos demanded that Bedouin shepherds provide them with local (*baladī*) sheep of two or three years of age that, if found suitable after an examination, would be bred with the imported animals.[46] To keep his supply going, Mehmet ʿAli also regularly sent some of his officials to Sardinia and Spain to secure more male merinos. As a sign of his gratitude, Mehmet ʿAli also sent the King of Sardinia an elephant.[47]

With the veterinary school, Mehmet ʿAli's government instituted a very deliberate biopolitical program to control the bodies, muscular output, pathologies, and reproductive capacities of various animal species in Egypt. This was the state's first major attempt to systematically manage the biological lives of animals—nonhuman

44 Such breeding efforts would continue throughout the nineteenth century. For example, in 1891, British viceroy of Egypt Lord Cromer sent a letter from Cairo on behalf of the Egyptian Khedive to one of his fellow colonial officers in the Arabian Peninsula stating that "the Egyptian Government wish to buy a good donkey stallion for breeding purposes—one of the large Hedjaz breed." The National Archives of the United Kingdom (Kew; hereafter TNA), Foreign Office (hereafter FO) 633/5 (22 Apr. 1891). For a useful analysis of colonial breeding attempts aimed as species "improvement," see Greg Bankoff, "A Question of Breeding: Zootechny and Colonial Attitudes toward the Tropical Environment in the Late Nineteenth-Century Philippines," *Journal of Asian Studies* 60 (2001): 413–37.

45 al-Ṣabbāgh, "al-Ṭibb al-Bayṭarī," 44.

46 For a discussion of other Ottoman attempts to undertake merino breeding in the nineteenth century, see M. Erdem Kabadayı, "The Introduction of Merino Sheep Breeding in the Ottoman Empire: Successes and Failures," in *Animals and People in the Ottoman Empire*, ed. Suraiya Faroqhi (Istanbul: Eren, 2010), 153–69.

47 al-Ṣabbāgh, "al-Ṭibb al-Bayṭarī," 44.

or otherwise—and interspecies interactions. These efforts resulted in a growing separation between the worlds of human and animal as objective science, experimentation, veterinarians, surgical tools, capitalist desires for production, and market-driven reproductive demands became the most important factors determining how humans viewed, used, and related to animals. The intimacy an individual farmer had developed with his own ox or cow, with whom he had lived and worked for years, was no longer the dominant mode of interaction between human and animal. While this dynamic did not entirely disappear from Egypt, it was no longer how the vast majority of Egyptians engaged with animals. Lingering remnants of this older human-animal relationship were no match for the powerful march toward a very different anthrozoological world in the nineteenth century, a world embodied by the emergence of new institutions like the Egyptian School of Veterinary Medicine.

The school came to an end nearly as quickly as it began. Twenty-two years after its founding in 1827, an order by Mehmet ʿAli's grandson and successor ʿAbbas on March 24, 1849, closed it down. Many structural problems with the school's training and the implementation of its mission contributed to its closing.[48] Declining enrollments clearly evidenced some of the school's troubles.[49] Too few veterinarians were being produced to meet the large demand for their services. By the middle of the 1840s, each of the school's graduates was responsible for an average of twenty villages. The distances between these villages were often very great, and it proved impossible for one person to oversee so many animals in so many different places. It also became impossible to effect any unity of action among the country's veterinarians. Some implemented orders immediately, some only when it was in their personal interests, and some never. Moreover, the small number of suitable veterinary facilities in the countryside also meant that animals could often not be transported quickly enough to receive the treatment they needed. And as they did with their sick familial relations, many peasants hid their sick animals from authorities for fear of losing them forever if taken to a government clinic.[50]

All of this contributed to a general sense among some government officials and the populace at large that the veterinary school did not serve an identifiable and useful purpose. It was ultimately unclear whether the school's gradu-

48 Ibid., 31–32 and 45–47.

49 From the time of its transfer to Shubra in 1837 to its closing twelve years later, the school's enrollment steadily dropped: from 122 in 1837 to 79 in 1839, to 64 in 1841, to 50 in 1842, to 11 in 1843. ʿAbd al-Karīm, *Tārīkh al-Taʿlīm*, 319.

50 On Egyptians' efforts to hide sick relatives from medical officials, see LaVerne Kuhnke, *Lives at Risk: Public Health in Nineteenth-Century Egypt* (Berkeley: University of California Press, 1990), 91; Mikhail, *Nature and Empire*, 230–36.

ates improved the lives, productivity, quality, or usability of Egypt's animals or increased their number. By the middle of the 1840s, it was determined to be much more cost effective and efficacious to send a few Egyptian students to Paris for veterinary training than to maintain a fledging domestic school.[51] For ʿAbbas, the ineffectiveness and futility of the school were made patently obvious when several of his favorite horses fell sick in 1849. He brought a few veterinarians from the school to try to save his animals, but they could not. Their failure, he wrote, was "as clear as the sun," and he ordered the school to be shut down immediately.[52]

Everywhere Epizootics

Although the over twenty-year experiment of the school of veterinary medicine was judged a failure, near-constant epizootics made clear that the original justification for the school remained. As Egypt became ever more deeply enmeshed in the global animal economy, the regularity and severity of its disease outbreaks increased dramatically. Unlike epizootics in the early modern period or earlier, those in the middle of the nineteenth century did not result from solely domestic environmental phenomena like drought or famine; rather, these diseases very often came to Egypt through the various trading links that connected Egypt to the world.[53] This intertwined history of epizootics and animal movement was not always simply the story of animals bringing diseases to Egypt. A year before the closing of the veterinary school, for example, so many animals were dying in Egypt that Ottoman authorities successfully moved *healthy* cows and oxen from Teke and Hamid in Anatolia to replace the Egyptian livestock.[54] Still, in most cases the movement of animals across the seas caused rather than solved the problem of widespread epizootic death.

Throughout the 1850s, 1860s, and 1870s, there were numerous outbreaks of various epizootics triggered by animals brought to Egypt through its increasingly

51 ʿAbd al-Karīm, *Tārīkh al-Taʿlīm*, 320–22.

52 *Ẓāhir ẓuhūr al-shams*.

53 For a discussion of early modern epizootics and the environmental factors that contributed to them, both in the Ottoman Empire and outside of it, see Sam White "A Model Disaster: From the Great Ottoman Panzootic to the Cattle Plagues of Early Modern Europe," (91–116).

54 BOA, Sadaret Mektubî Kalemi 160.94 (29 Zilhicce 1264/26 Nov. 1848). For another example of the export of animals from Teke and Hamid to Egypt, see BOA, İradeler Mısır 11.295 (21 Zilkade 1260/2 Dec. 1844). For later examples of the importation of animals from Anatolia and Greater Syria to Egypt during epizootics, see BOA, Yıldız Esas ve Sadrazam Kâmil Paşa 129.96 (18 Rebiülevvel 1317/27 July 1899); BOA, Meclis-i Vükelâ Mazbataları 93.3 (11 Rebiülevvel 1315/10 Aug. 1897).

global economic connections.[55] In the late 1860s, an outbreak of typhus and rinderpest in Ismailia, Port Said, and other cities in the canal zone caused the Egyptian government to momentarily regret its decision to close the school of veterinary medicine. The French Compagnie Universelle, which managed the canal's construction and later operation, had its own professional veterinarian—itself a sign of the frequency and severity of epizootics in Egypt—who wrote to the Egyptian government about an outbreak of animal disease in late 1865 and early 1866. In a letter dated February 15, 1866, this veterinarian reported on the autopsies he had performed on a dozen cows.[56] He had continually observed these animals from their first signs of disease until their quick deaths twenty-four to thirty-six hours later. Their autopsies revealed hemorrhaged intestines, traces of emphysema, weakened muscles, ulcerations of the rectum, large amounts of phlegm, and lacerations of the esophagus. The epizootics of the late 1860s and early 1870s were indeed very deadly, with numerous reports of extremely high mortality rates. For example, of 347 infected animals in two villages in 1871, 223 of them died.[57] Other villages also frequently reported animal deaths numbering in the hundreds.

In the face of these serious epizootics in the canal zone, Khedive Ismail entertained the possibility of restarting government-sponsored veterinary instruction in Egypt. In October 1865 he therefore hired yet another French veterinarian to train a group of soldiers in the military academy.[58] These new attempts to raise a fresh crop of Egyptian veterinarians did not get very far however. They were hampered by a shortage of equipment and books and, as before, a lack of qualified translators.[59] In the face of the Egyptian government's failures to stop disease, the French Canal Company's veterinarian suggested two possible strategies to break the cycle of epizootics ravaging Egypt in the late 1860s.

The first was to keep animals isolated from one another as much as possible. Animal owners were instructed to prevent their animals from mixing as best they could.[60]

55 BOA, Sadaret Mühimme Kalemi Evrakı 270.86 (6 Safer 1280/23 July 1863); TNA, FO 83/349 (1856–66); TNA, FO 143/10 (1873–78); TNA, FO 143/11 (1880–82).

56 Dār al-Wathā'iq al-Qawmiyya (National Archives of Egypt, Cairo; hereafter DWQ), ʿAṣr Ismāʿīl - Documents concernant Le régime de Khédive Ismail (hereafter ʿAI), Agriculture, 12/2 (15 Feb. 1866).

57 DWQ, ʿAI, Agriculture, 12/2 (22 May 1871).

58 al-Ṣabbāgh, "al-Ṭibb al-Bayṭarī," 47.

59 Khedive Ismail tried to overcome these problems by rehiring some of the best of the veterinary school's former staff, including a teacher named ʿAbd al-Hadi Effendi Ismail who had taught at the school in the 1830s and 1840s.

60 DWQ, ʿAI, Agriculture, 12/2 (22 May 1871).

At Gabari near Alexandria, for example, cows were separated by variety and kept in different barns in an old cotton mill.[61] In addition to these rudimentary quarantine efforts, various simple bovine vaccines, such as coal tar, were also used.[62] Coal tar was not available in large quantities in the canal zone and therefore had to be sent from Cairo, which added cost and complexity to the operation.[63] Other medicinal solutions to cattle plagues included ensuring that livestock stables were kept clean and that animals were adequately fed. The Canal Company's veterinarian also wrote that he had had some success in reducing the incidence of various epizootics by washing animals' mouths daily with vinegar, salt, and crushed garlic. He also cleaned their eyes with phenol diluted in water and made them consume twenty-five grams of phenol dissolved in a large bucket of water daily. He also regularly performed enemas on animals using coal tar and phenol. As all of this suggests, the strategy was to keep all of the animals' orifices as clean as possible.

Of greatest concern was explaining the etiology of the epizootics of the 1860s and 1870s. Determining how and whence infections came to Egypt was part of a nineteenth-century competition among nations to measure and compare the relative epidemiological and civilizational health and disease of each against the others. Health became a marker of civilization. The globalization of disease etiology was also of course a consequence of the rapidly increasing trade and movement of animals in this period. It was thought, for instance, that the typhus and cattle plague that came to Egypt in the 1860s originated in the Russian steppe.[64] As a result, Ottoman authorities temporarily outlawed the importation of animals from Odessa to Egypt in 1863.[65] To make up for some of the animals lost in Egypt in this year, geldings (*bargir*) and mares (*kısrak*) were imported from unspecified areas of Rumelia.[66] There was such high demand and short supply in 1863 that even when a universal ban was imposed on exporting livestock from Adana due to a

61 DWQ, ʿAI, Agriculture, 12/2 (7 Dec. 1871).

62 DWQ, ʿAI, Agriculture, 12/2 (15 Feb. 1866).

63 DWQ, ʿAI, Agriculture, 12/2 (23 Dec. 1871).

64 DWQ, ʿAI, Agriculture, 12/2 (17 Feb. 1866). The Russian steppe was often thought to be the origin of many human diseases as well. See, for example, the following case from the nineteenth century about the quarantine of Tatar *ḥajj* pilgrims in Alexandria: Topkapı Sarayı Müzesi Arşivi (Istanbul), Evrak 5026/242 (n.d.).

65 BOA, Sadaret Mühimme Kalemi Evrakı 283.60 (22 Cemaziyelevvel 1280/4 Nov. 1863); BOA, Sadaret Mühimme Kalemi Evrakı 282.63 (22 Cemaziyelevvel 1280/4 Nov. 1863). For contemporaneous British concerns about the spread of cattle plague from Odessa, see TNA, FO 83/349 (14 Mar. 1866).

66 BOA, Sadaret Mühimme Kalemi Evrakı 270.86 (21 Muharrem 1280/8 July 1863).

disease outbreak there, an official exception was made, despite the risks, to send to Egypt those animals deemed healthy enough for travel.[67]

Cattle plague moving from the Russian steppe to the Ottoman Empire was thought to (and most likely did) spread from the Danube basin through Hungary to Trieste, Istanbul, and beyond.[68] Many of these cities, and even ports further afield in England and France, took measures in the 1860s and 1870s to prevent the spread of epizootics from the steppe and the Ottoman Empire.[69] British officials in Egypt and elsewhere were particularly worried about the global spread of diseases like rinderpest and wrote a great deal about various diseases' origins, symptoms, and pathways.[70] They too placed most epizootics' origins in the Russian steppe.[71] Cattle imported to Egypt from the Danube basin usually traveled from Trieste to Alexandria, and from there would be distributed to various locations throughout Egypt. Those on their way to Cairo would first be transported to Tanta in the central delta. Those destined for the canal zone would go east to Damietta and then on to Port Said. Other animals were sent to various smaller towns all across the delta—al-Manṣūra, Kafr al-Shaykh, and Damanhūr, for example.

Alongside concerns about the importation of cattle plague from Europe, there was also a great deal of attention devoted to the threat of animal diseases coming from Egypt's southern Red Sea ports.[72] Arabian horses—renowned for their strength, size, speed, and beauty[73]—were often brought to Egypt through Red Sea

67 BOA, Sadaret Mühimme Kalemi Evrakı 296.37 (29 Ramazan 1279/20 Mar. 1863).

68 Even animals in cities at some distance from major ports were affected by epizootics in this period. For a case about the spread of cattle plague in landlocked Kayseri in 1849, see BOA, Sadaret Mektubî Kalemi Deavî Yazışmaları 13.60 (21 Safer 1265/16 Jan. 1849).

69 DWQ, ʿAI, Agriculture, 12/2 (15 Feb. 1866).

70 TNA, FO 83/349 (1856–66); TNA, FO 83/350 (1869); TNA, FO 83/351 (1870); TNA, FO 83/352 (1870); TNA, FO 83/353 (1870).

71 See, for example, the following letter dated May 30, 1856, written by a British official named J. A. Blackwell stationed in the Hanseatic port of Lübeck on the Baltic Sea: TNA, FO 83/349 (1856–66).

72 On the history of one of these ports—Qusayr—see Daniel Crecelius, "The Importance of Qusayr in the Late Eighteenth Century," *Journal of the American Research Center in Egypt* 24 (1987): 53–60.

73 On the history of Arabian horse breeding, see Margaret E. Derry, *Bred for Perfection: Shorthorn Cattle, Collies, and Arabian Horses since 1800* (Baltimore: Johns Hopkins University Press, 2003), 103–55; Charles Gladitz, *Horse Breeding in the Medieval World* (Dublin: Four Courts Press, 1997). On Egyptian Arabians in particular, see Philippe Paraskevas, *Breeding the Arabian Horse*, vol. 1 of *The Egyptian Alternative* (Exeter: Obelisque Publications, 2010); idem, *In Search of the Identity of the Egyptian Arabian Bloodlines*, vol. 2 of *The Egyptian Alternative* (Exeter: Obelisque Publications, 2012); Nasr Marei, *The Arabian Horse of Egypt*

shipping channels both for domestic purposes and to be transported to other parts of the Mediterranean world.[74] Many cattle were also often imported from the Hijaz to Egypt. During the epizootic scares of the late 1860s and 1870s, horses and cattle imported from Jidda and other Red Sea ports became subject to intense quarantine regimes and other restrictions on their movement.[75] Before being allowed to dock, Red Sea ship captains were required to provide proper bills of health and other paperwork for the animals onboard their vessels.[76] From their offices in Jidda, British officials regularly dispatched reports about the state of cattle plague in this period.[77] Throughout the 1870s, there were numerous quarantines placed on cattle and horses arriving from the Arabian Peninsula to Egypt and parts of the Sudan.[78] In the spring of 1880, horses arriving in Egypt from the Hijaz were placed in quarantine for twenty-one days.[79] All of these applications of disease prevention regimes on animals, of course, came alongside those regularly imposed on humans arriving in Egypt from the Hijaz and other points south and east.[80]

The foreign importation of disease was not the only reason animals coming to Egypt from across the Mediterranean and Red Seas fell sick and died once in country. Healthy arrivals regularly fell ill on their journeys from Alexandria or Suez after drinking from the Nile or its tributaries. On one such occasion in 1866, waterborne diseases hit a convoy of cattle being transported from Alexandria through Damietta to Port Said so severely that corpses began piling up in the river near Damietta to the point that dogs were able to cross from one bank

(Cairo: American University in Cairo Press, 2010).

74 For an example of the quarantine of animals sent from Egypt, see the following case about quarantine in the Anatolian port of Mersin: BOA, Cevdet Sıhhiye 611 (24 Şaʿban 1259/19 Sept. 1843). See also the following case from the end of the nineteenth century about preventing the movement of animals, leather, and wool from Egypt during an epizootic: BOA, Sadaret Mühimme Kalemi Evrakı 578.19 (19 Safer 1317/29 June 1899).

75 For a later attempt by the Ottoman imperial administration to prevent the spread of epizootics by outlawing the importation of animals to Egypt from Anatolia and Greater Syria, see BOA, Dahiliye Mektubi Kalemi 2306.116 (15 Şevval 1317/16 Feb. 1900).

76 TNA, FO 143/10 (1873–78).

77 See, for instance, TNA, FO 141/70 (19 Nov. 1869).

78 TNA, FO 143/10 (1873–78); TNA, FO 143/11 (1880–82).

79 TNA, FO 143/11 (1880–82).

80 For some of the many examples of efforts to quarantine humans in this period, see TNA, FO 141/131 (1879); TNA, FO 633/3 (1880–83). For a general discussion of quarantine in nineteenth-century Egypt, see Kuhnke, *Lives at Risk*, 89–110 and 154–57. For a discussion of quarantine in the Red Sea, see Gülden Sarıyıldız and Oya Dağlar Macar, "Cholera, Pilgrimage, and International Politics of Sanitation: The Quarantine Station on the Island of Kamaran," (243–73).

of the Nile's tributary to the other (a distance measured at the time to be nearly two thousand feet) by walking on the animals' carcasses.[81] In an ironic—if rather revolting—twist of fate, many of these dead animals did eventually make it to their final destination, as a number of their corpses were found washed up on empty beaches around Port Said. Given the sources, it is impossible to determine the exact etiology of intense epizootics like this one or the many others that hit Egypt and elsewhere in the 1860s. One thing the sources do make clear, however, is that Egyptians understood epizootics to be a result of the regular movement of animals across the Mediterranean and Red Seas.

Conclusion

While Egyptians had of course been dealing with animal diseases for millennia, two developments in the history of epizootics in the nineteenth century set this period apart from all that came before it. First, more than at any other time in Egypt's recorded history, the health of its animals was deeply impacted by global commerce, exchange, and transport. Etiological and epizoological forces outside of Egypt could now kill its domestic animals. The second innovation was how the proposed institutional means for dealing with these animal diseases—chief among them veterinary medicine and quarantine—changed the human-animal relationship.[82] In a world in which animals were increasingly treated as potential disease vectors and commodities to be exchanged on capitalist world markets, new technologies of disease management, as this chapter has shown, became some of the primary means through which humans and animals interacted. This medicalization of interspecies relations was a central aspect of the new human-animal relationship developing in nineteenth-century Egypt—a relationship now based on the increasing separation of large numbers of animals from humans.

Alan Mikhail (alan.mikhail@yale.edu) is Professor of History at Yale University. He is the author of *Under Osman's Tree: The Ottoman Empire, Egypt and Environmental History*, *The Animal in Ottoman Egypt*, and *Nature and Empire in Ottoman Egypt: An Environmental History*; and the editor of *Water on Sand: Environmental Histories of the Middle East and North Africa*.

81 DWQ, ʿAI, Agriculture, 12/2 (15 Feb. 1866).

82 For examples of early modern quarantine efforts aimed at human plague, see Daniel Panzac, *Quarantaines et lazarets: l'Europe et la peste d'Orient (XVIIe–XXe siècles)* (Aix-en-Provence: Édisud, 1986); Charles Carrière, Marcel Courdurié, and Ferréol Rebuffat, *Marseille ville morte: la peste de 1720* (Marseille: M. Garçon, 1968).

SMALLPOX IN THE HAREM: COMMUNICABLE DISEASES AND THE OTTOMAN FEAR OF DYNASTIC EXTINCTION DURING THE EARLY SULTANATE OF AHMED I (R. 1603–17)

GÜNHAN BÖREKÇİ*
İstanbul Şehir University

DURING THE FIRST half of the seventeenth century, the Ottoman dynasty repeatedly faced serious threats of extinction in ways hitherto unseen since the beginning of their monarchical rule in the early 1300s. While the primary factor behind this problem was the coming to the throne of a series of underage and/or childless sultans between 1603 and 1648, it was the incessant military rebellions in the capital city of Istanbul directly targeting the Ottoman ruler that often deepened the political/dynastic crisis prevailing in the same period. Meanwhile frequent outbreaks of epidemic diseases in the densely populated capital—most importantly those of plague—only worsened the precarious situation of the royal family, particularly since all of its male members were by then residing in the Topkapı Palace and thus exposed to the fatal threats of such biological calamities. Hence, under these circumstances, the Ottoman royal family tried to secure not only the well-being of their reigning young sultan and, if any, his male siblings and children, but also the critical problem of dynastic continuity with the introduction of new patrilineal principles of succession, namely that of seniority.[1]

Scholars of early modern Ottoman history typically emphasize that the Ottoman male line came close to extinction only during the last years of Sultan Murad IV's reign (1623–40) and the early years of Sultan İbrahim's (1640–48).[2] Toward

* I am most grateful to our editor Nükhet Varlık for her much valuable comments on earlier drafts, and to Maurizio Alfioldi for providing the transcriptions of the Venetian ambassadorial dispatches utilized in this study. The following discussion is partly based on my PhD dissertation: Günhan Börekçi, "Factions and Favorites at the Courts of Ahmed I (r. 1603-1617) and His Immediate Predecessors," PhD diss., Ohio State University, 2010. The initial research for this article was carried out under the generous fellowships by the American Research Institute in Turkey (ARIT) and the Research Center for Anatolian Civilizations (RCAC) of the Koç University back in 2007 and 2008, respectively.

1 On the introduction of the principle of seniority in Ottoman succession tradition, see *Diyanet Vakfı İslâm Ansiklopedisi* [hereafter *DİA*], s.v. "Cülûs," by Abdülkadir Özcan and s.v. "Osmanlılar," by Feridun Emecen.

2 For instance, see Caroline Finkel, *Osman's Dream: The Story of the Ottoman Empire, 1300–1922* (London: John Murray, 2005), 202. Also see *Encyclopaedia of Islam,* second

the end of his reign, Murad IV ordered the execution of all of his living brothers except Prince İbrahim, who succeeded to the throne in 1640 as the childless sole male member of the dynasty. It was two years before Sultan İbrahim managed to father a child, and during this period, the House of Osman came perilously close to stepping over what I have elsewhere called the "threshold of extinction."[3] The birth of Prince Mehmed (the future Mehmed IV, r. 1648–87) in early January 1642 finally lifted the pall of uncertainty that surrounded the Ottoman throne in the early 1640s.[4] However, most scholars often overlook the fact that the threat of dynastic end actually emerged decades earlier, immediately after the enthronement of Ahmed I (r. 1603–17) and under the exigencies of communicable diseases.

By primarily utilizing the unpublished reports of the contemporary Venetian ambassadors resident in Istanbul, this essay aims to shed new light on the early seventeenth-century Ottoman dynastic crisis by demonstrating how communicable diseases and unexpected health problems of the reigning sultans critically intertwined with the problems that the Ottomans faced in their efforts to secure their fragile male line when ongoing wars and military uprisings were undermining the political and financial stability of the Ottoman imperial establishment. My discussion will largely focus on the early reign of Ahmed I who, upon the sudden death of his father Mehmed III (r. 1595–1603), became the first Ottoman sultan to assume the throne childless, at a time when there was no other adult male in the dynastic family. I will establish that, with Ahmed's enthronement, the Ottoman dynasty experienced their first serious fear of genealogical extinction when the thirteen-year-old new sultan and the only other male member of the dynasty, his four-year-old brother Mustafa (the future Mustafa I, r. 1617–18; 1622–23), survived a near-fatal bout of smallpox in February-March 1604.[5]

---

edition [hereafter *EI2*], s.v. "Murād IV," by Alexander H. de Groot; and *İslam Ansiklopedisi* [hereafter *İA*], s.v. "İbrâhim," by M. Tayyib Gökbilgin.

3 Günhan Börekçi, "İnkırâzın Eşiğinde Bir Hanedan: III. Mehmed, I. Ahmed, I. Mustafa ve 17. Yüzyıl Osmanlı Siyasî Krizi," *Dîvân: Disiplinlerarası Çalışmalar Dergisi* 26 (2009): 45–96.

4 As Derin Terzioğlu, "Sufi and Dissident in the Ottoman Empire: Niyazî-i Mısrî (1618–1694)," PhD diss., Harvard University, 1999, 346–54, aptly notes, "the uncertainty about the future of the Ottoman throne [under Sultan İbrahim] gave rise to speculations about a possible transfer of the throne to the Girays [i.e., the Crimean khan family descended from the line of Chingiz Khan]."

5 In conventional Ottoman historiography, the date of Mustafa I's birth is typically given as ca. 1592. However, new studies based on hitherto overlooked evidence show that he was most likely born at the turn of the seventeenth century. Thus, he was around four years old at the time of Ahmed I's enthronement. For futher details regarding Mustafa I's age, see below.

A Fragile Dynasty

To begin with, the roots of the dynastic problems that marked Ahmed I's early reign can be located in the sultanate of his father Mehmed III, who ascended the throne in 1595 upon the death of his father Murad III (r. 1574–95) and reigned for only eight years. Mehmed III's short sultanate was a period of crisis in the true sense of the term in that it passed with multi-front wars, social disturbances, military revolts, financial difficulties, and intense factionalism within the court and the royal family. Sultan Mehmed inherited from his late father an empire that had been engaged for two years in a war against the Habsburgs in Hungary. In the ensuing years, the Ottoman-Habsburg Long War of 1593–1606 intensified, and not a single year passed without a military confrontation between the two imperial rivals.

In the meantime, a new and much more serious problem beleaguered Mehmed III as numerous towns and villages in the Anatolian countryside fell under the ever-escalating attacks of the rebellious Celâli armies, which were composed mostly of mercenary soldiers, generally known as *sekbans*. These irregular soldiers were recruited from the peasant population on a regular basis to meet the growing need for arms-bearing infantry in Ottoman military forces, then discharged after serving in a campaign or two. Yet instead of returning to their villages, most of these soldiers became bandits or joined the uprisings already in progress in Anatolia. Around the turn of the seventeenth century, the Celâli problem acquired a much more complex character since a number of Ottoman district governors and officials, as well as an increasing number of rank-and-file soldiers in the sultan's military forces, now had similar recourse to either rebellious or unlawful activities.[6]

These multi-front and prolonged military engagements and the deepening social turmoil created no small amount of financial and political problems for Mehmed III and his court in Istanbul. By 1600, the coffers of the state were almost empty and the campaign-weary soldiers turned their discontent into open rebellion, often triggered by the payment of their three-monthly salaries with debased currency. In 1600, 1601, and 1603, the palace cavalry (*sipahis*) and their support-

6 For the Celâli rebellions during this period, see Mustafa Akdağ, *Celâlî İsyanları, 1550–1603* (Ankara: Ankara Üniversitesi Basımevi, 1963); idem, *Türk Halkının Dirlik ve Düzenlik Kavgası* (Ankara: Bilgi, 1975); William Griswold, *The Great Anatolian Rebellion, 1591–1611* (Berlin: Klaus Schwarz, 1983); and Suraiya Faroqhi, "Seeking Wisdom in China: An Attempt to Make Sense of the Celâli Rebellions," in *Zafar-nama: Memorial Volume to Felix Tauer*, eds. Rudolf Vesely and Eduard Gombar (Prague: Enigma, 1996), 101–24. For a detailed discussion of the Celâlis, see Oktay Özel, "The Reign of Violence: The *celâlis*, c. 1550–1700," in *The Ottoman World*, ed. Christine Woodhead (London: Routledge, 2012), 184–202.

ers rose up against their sultan and his court three times, in the last two cases threatening Mehmed III with deposition.[7] Furthermore, seven months before his death in December 1603, Sultan Mehmed ordered the execution of his eldest son, Prince Mahmud, on the suspicion that he was plotting to seize the throne.[8] This act not only paved the way for Prince Ahmed to succeed his father at a young age, but also suddenly put the continuation of the male line of the Ottoman dynasty in jeopardy in a time of challenging wars and rebellions.

Unlike his grandfather, Selim II (r. 1566–74), and his father, Murad III, both of whom were succeeded by their first-born sons, Mehmed III had a tragic experience with his sons. In 1597, his eldest son, Prince Selim, suddenly died at the age of thirteen, most likely of illness.[9] With Selim's death, the issue of dynastic continuity would become a major concern for Mehmed as he was likely left with only two young sons, ten-year-old Mahmud and seven-year-old Ahmed, at a time when, according to one rumor, he had grown very fat and had health problems that curtailed his reproductive powers.[10] Luckily, bad news about Mehmed III's health soon proved wrong and he fathered another son, Mustafa, born in Istanbul around 1601–1602.[11]

7 For a detailed discussion of these rebellions, see my "Factions and Favorites," 48–63.

8 On Prince Mahmud's execution, see İsmail Hakkı Uzunçarşılı, "Üçüncü Mehmed'in Oğlu Şehzade Mahmud'un Ölümü," *Belleten* 94 (1960), 263–67; Börekçi, "İnkırâzın Eşiğinde Bir Hanedan," 74–86.

9 According to Katip Çelebi, *Fezleke*, in Zeynep Aycibin, ed., "Kâtip Çelebi, *Fezleke*: Tahlil ve Metin," PhD diss., Mimar Sinan University, 2007, 452, Prince Selim died on April 20, 1597. The report of the Venetian *bailo* Girolamo Cappello, dated 1600, points to a suspicion regarding Safiye Sultan's possible role in accelerating the death of Prince Selim. According to Cappello, Selim was considered by many to be a good replacement for Mehmed III because of his vigor and because he was expected to diminish the power of Safiye Sultan. Maria Pedani-Fabris, ed., *Relazioni di ambasciatori veneti al senato*, 14: *Costantinopoli, Relazioni inedite (1512–1789)* (Padua: Bottega d'Erasmo, 1996), 399–400. Also mentioned by Baki Tezcan, "Searching for Osman: A Reassessment of the Deposition of the Ottoman Sultan Osman II (1618–1622)," PhD diss., Princeton University, 2001, 329n23.

10 *Calendar of State Papers and Manuscripts Relating to English Affairs in the Archives and Collections of Venice and in Other Libraries of Northern Italy*, Volume IX: 1592–1603, Searchable Text Edition, ed. Allen B. Hinds (Ontario: TannerRitchie Publishing and The University of St. Andrews, 2007), 269 (henceforth, *Calendar of State Papers – Venetian*). It is certain that Mehmed III had grown very fat during these years. His contemporary images testify to this point. Compare, for instance, Pietro Bertelli, *Vite Degl'imperatori de Turchi* ([NP], ca. 1596), 54; Talīkīzāde, *Şehnāme-i Sultān-ı Selātīn-i Cihān* or *Eğri Fethi Ta'rīhi*, Topkapı Sarayı Müzesi Kütüphanesi (TSMK), ms. H. 1609, 68b–69a; and Ganīzāde Mehmed, *Dīvān-ı Nādirī*, TSMK, ms. H. 889, 7a, 8b.

11 According to the conventional Ottoman historiography, Mustafa I was born ca. 1592. See *İA*, s.v. "Mustafâ I," by M. Münir Aktepe; *EI2*, s.v. "Mustafâ I," by John H. Kramers; *DİA*,

In 1602, however, the sultan lost another son, Cihangir, about whom we know only that he was born in Istanbul and died at a very young age.[12]

Thus, barely a year before his death, Sultan Mehmed had only three sons left: Mahmud, Ahmed, and Mustafa, none of whom had been sent to govern a province or even circumcised. In the past, an Ottoman prince was to be appointed governor of a province at around the age of fifteen so as to acquire training for the sultanate and the business of rule while establishing his own court and household, which would form the nucleus of his government when he acceded to the throne.[13] Such a provincial appointment was typically arranged soon after the prince was circumcised at a festival organized by the royal family and celebrated by the public in the capital. In this regard, Mehmed's eldest son Prince Mahmud was probably anxiously awaiting his provincial assignment. However, according to Agostino Nani, the Venetian *bailo* resident in Istanbul between 1600 and 1603, this had to wait for the war in Hungary and the rebellions in Anatolia to come to an end.[14]

An anecdote later related by Ahmed I to one of his favorite viziers, Hafız Ahmed Pasha, is revealing in this regard. According to the chronicler Peçevi, who heard the story from Ahmed Pasha, Ahmed had occasionally witnessed his elder brother impatiently asking their father to send him to Anatolia with an army so that he could personally eliminate the Celâli rebels and bring relief to the sultan, whom

s.v. "Mustafâ I," by Feridun Emecen. Among modern scholars, only Baki Tezcan has observed that a much later birthdate is given in published contemporary Ottoman and non-Ottoman narrative sources. Karaçelebizade Abdülaziz, *Ravzatü'l-ebrār* (Bulaq: Al-Matbaʿa al-Amīriyya, H. 1248/1832), 494 [hereafter Karaçelebizade], mentions that he was born in H. 1011 (1602/1603), while the Venetian *bailo* Ottaviano Bon, in his report dated 1609, gives his age as ten: Pedani-Fabris, ed., *Relazioni di ambasciatori veneti*, 514; also cited by Tezcan, "Searching for Osman," 330n30. Whereas Tezcan (90–92) has cast serious doubt on Mustafa's accepted age and is inclined to accept a later birthdate (ca. 1600), Leslie Peirce, *The Imperial Harem: Women and Sovereignty in the Ottoman Empire* (Oxford: Oxford University Press, 1993), 99, mentions Mustafa's age as nine at the time of Ahmed I's enthronement but provides no reference. The later birthdate is upheld by the unpublished observations of the Venetian *bailo* Francesco Contarini; see Börekçi, "İnkırâzın Eşiğinde Bir Hanedan," 73–74 and 77–78.

12 *EI2*, s.v. "Mehemmed III," by Susan Skilliter.

13 Peirce, *Imperial Harem*, 46; Metin Kunt, "Sultan, Dynasty and State in the Ottoman Empire: Political Institutions in the Sixteenth Century," *The Medieval History Journal* 6, no. 2 (2003): 217–30; and idem, "A Prince Goes Forth (Perchance to Return)," in *Identity and Identity Formation in the Ottoman World: A Volume of Essays in Honor of Norman Itzkowitz*, eds. Baki Tezcan and Karl K. Barbir (Madison: University of Wisconsin Press, 2007), 63–71.

14 Luigi Firpo, ed., *Relazioni di ambasciatori veneti al senato, tratte dalle migliori edizioni disponibili e ordinate cronologicamente,* 13: *Costantinopoli (1590–1793)* (Torino: Bottega d'Erasmo, 1984), 399.

he observed growing seriously demoralized by their ever-escalating attacks. Ironically, however, Mahmud's importuning led Mehmed III to suspect that he actually sought to usurp the throne.[15]

On June 7, 1603, while the repercussions of the above-mentioned *sipahi* rebellion were still unfolding in the capital, Mehmed III ordered Prince Mahmud's execution. According to the contemporary sources, this decision was triggered when the prince's mother, Halime Sultan, asked a Sufi sheikh to tell her son's fortune.[16] The sheikh's letter of reply predicted that Mahmud would succeed to the throne within six months, after unpleasant things happened to his father. However, the letter was intercepted by the chief eunuch of the imperial harem, Abdürrezzak Agha, who then gave it to Mehmed III and his mother Safiye Sultan instead of delivering it to the prince's mother.[17]

For a sultan who had faced three military revolts and been threatened with deposition twice in the past three years, such a letter would no doubt have raised suspicions of treason, particularly at a time when his son was so eager to leave the court for the battlefield and was said to have begun "to grieve and murmur to see how his father was altogether led by the old Sultana his grandmother and the state went to ruin."[18] "Grown so fat and physically unfit that his doctors warned him

---

15 İbrahim Peçevî, Ta'rīh-*i Peçevī*, Beyazıt Devlet Kütüphanesi, ms. Veliyüddin Efendi 2353, 183a: "Her bār ki celālīlerün ʿısyānı ve tuğyānı vüzerā tarafından pādişāh-ı mağfūrun semʿ-i şerīflerine vārid ve vāsıl oldukda, ol gün gāyetde muteʾellim olurdı ve ekl-i taʿāmdan kalurdı. Şehzāde-i mūmā-ileyh bu hāllerini gördükde, 'Hey Hünkārum! Niçün zahmet çekersin? Bana bir mikdār ʿasker taʿyīn idüb gönder. Bu cümle muʿānidīni kalʿ [u] kamʿ idüb bi'z-zarūrī serfürū itdürin' dirdi. Hattā saʿādetlü pādişāh, 'Nice idersin?' didükde, 'Kimin tīğ ile ve kimin medār[-ı kelām] ile iderüm,' dirdi ... Her zemān [böyle] söyledükçe menʿ iderdüm, zīrā saʿādetlü pādişāh bī-huzūr olduğın müşāhede iderdüm."

16 Prince Mahmud and Mustafa I were, in fact, full brothers, sons of a mother whose name has thus far remained unknown in Ottoman historiography. An overlooked dynastic genealogy preserved in a nineteenth-century manuscript reveals that her name was Halime: Milli Kütüphane, ms. 06 Hk 11/3, 5a: "*Vālide-i Sultān Mustafā Hān-ı evvel, Halīme Sultān, Ayasofya'da oğlınun türbesinde medfūndur.*" For further information on Mahmud's mother, see Börekçi, "İnkırâzın Eşiğinde Bir Hanedan," 75–79.

17 Nezihi Aykut, ed., *Hasan Bey-zâde Târîhi*, 3 vols. (Ankara: Türk Tarih Kurumu, 2004), 3: 765 [hereafter Hasan Beyzade]. One of Contarini's dispatches reveals the timing of these events. Archivio di Stato di Venezia (ASVe), Senato, Dispacci Costantinopoli (SDC), filza 57, 209v-210r (dated May 13, 1603): "Volendo la madre del Principe per curiosità sapere da certo astrologo qualche particolare che potesse occorrere al figliolo, mentre che un Negro eunuco portava il pronostico, per darglielo, le fu tolto di mano da un altro, et dato al Gran Signore, il quale si alterò grandemente, perché in esso si conteneva che il Principe doveva subentra presto al commando di questo Imperio."

18 *The Report of Lello*, 14 [I have modernized the spelling].

against campaigning," Leslie Peirce observes, "the sultan was particularly threatened by this augury because of Mahmud's popularity with the Janissaries."[19] Moreover Francesco Contarini, the Venetian *bailo* resident in Istanbul, heard rumors about a conspiracy to poison Mehmed III in order to "bring the Prince [Mahmud] to the command of the empire."[20] In the end, after a brief period of imprisonment, interrogation and even torture to make him confess, Prince Mahmud was strangled for plotting to seize the throne.

Only seven months after this tragic event, on the night of December 20, 1603, Mehmed III suddenly passed away in his bedchambers at the Topkapı Palace. He was only thirty-seven years old and had no apparent health problems, apart from obesity. Shortly after his death, the doctors had second thoughts as to why the sultan had suddenly died. According to Contarini, some doctors believed he died from the plague, but for most, the cause was a stroke.[21] In any case, as Baki Tezcan insightfully notes, Mehmed III's death was among the most critical demographic accidents to hit the House of Osman in the latter part of the sixteenth century. While he was most probably the first Ottoman sultan to die at such a young age, his son's reign was the first to begin during the monarch's minority and continued uninterruptedly into his adult years.[22]

A Childless Sultan and the First Fear of Dynastic Extinction

The following morning, an impromptu official ceremony was held at the palace to announce the enthronement of Ahmed I.[23] This was truly an unusual event in many respects and it marks a critical point of transformation in the early modern

19 Peirce, *Imperial Harem*, 231.

20 ASVe, SDC, filza 57, 314r (dated June 14, 1603).

21 ASVe, SDC, filza 58, 254r (dated January 3, 1604): "sono li medici discordi tra di loro di opinione secondo il solito circa la infirmità che ha condotto a morte il Re, alcuni hanno affirmato che sia stato di Peste, rispetto alle petecchie che dopo si sono vedute; raccontano che che ... habbia maneggiato cierte robbe che le furono donate. Altri dicono altri mali, ma la maggior parte acconsente che sia stata di apoplessia." Also see a brief excerpt from this dispatch in *Calendar of State Papers - Venetian*, 10: 127.

22 Tezcan, "Searching for Osman," 92.

23 I should note that Ahmed I's enthronement definitely took place on Sunday, December 21, 1603 (H. 17 Receb 1012), not on the next day, as the established historiography still holds. For example, see *İA*, s.v. "Ahmed I," by Cavid Baysun; *EI2*, s.v. "Ahmad I," by Robert Mantran; and *DİA*, s.v. "Ahmed I," by Mücteba İlgürel. The above-mentioned Venetian *bailo*, Francesco Contarini, wrote a detailed dispatch about the event on the same day: ASVe, SDC, filza 58, 231r-v (dated December 21, 1603).

Ottoman dynastic and imperial establishment. To begin with, for the first time in Ottoman history, the issue of dynastic succession was resolved within the confines of the palace harem, immediately after the death of a sultan, yet before any high-ranking government official, such as the grand vizier, or any non-government opinion leader, such as the mufti, had been informed of, or consulted with, on the matter. In other words, a faction in the inner palace established a *fait accompli* by arranging the succession of Prince Ahmed.

In fact, Ahmed I had to take the throne at all costs since the only other surviving male member of the dynasty, his brother Prince Mustafa, was around four years old and thus too young to be considered a viable alternative. Hence, Ahmed I's enthronement stemmed from the need to retain the Ottoman traditional pattern of father-to-son sequential succession while sustaining hope that the Ottoman dynasty could survive. However, being the first sultan to assume the throne childless at a time when there was no other adult male in the dynastic family, Ahmed had to quickly prove his biological ability to father a child and, most critically, had to have at least one healthy son in order to secure the unbroken 300-year-old male line of dynastic succession.[24] The Ottomans had never faced such a problem of continuity owing to an under-aged sultan ascending the throne. The closest example was that of Mehmed II (r. 1444–46; 1451–81), who was similarly twelve years old and childless in 1444, when his father Murad II (r. 1421–44; 1446–51) abdicated in his favor. Though Mehmed II had no known living or mature brothers during his short first reign, his father was alive and in his early forties, still capable of fathering a child. Thus, Mehmed's childlessness did not create a potential dynastic crisis as in Ahmed's case.

This extraordinary situation helps to explain why Ahmed I did not apply the Ottoman custom of fratricide (*kardeş katli*), which allowed a new sultan to order the execution of all his living brothers.[25] Unlike his grandfather Murad III and his father Mehmed III, who had been free to engage in fratricide immediately upon their enthronements since they each had several sons, Ahmed had to keep his

---

24 For details, see Anthony D. Alderson, *The Structure of the Ottoman Dynasty* (Oxford: Oxford University Press, 1956), tables I–XXVII.

25 On the Ottoman custom of fratricide, see, e.g., Halil İnalcık, "Osmanlılarda Saltanat Veraset Usulü ve Türk Hakimiyet Telâkkisiyle İlgisi," *Ankara Üniversitesi Siyasal Bilgiler Fakültesi Dergisi* 14 (1959): 69–94; Joseph Fletcher, "Turco-Mongolian Monarchic Tradition in the Ottoman Empire," *Harvard Ukranian Studies* 3–4 (1979–80): 236–51; and Mehmet Akman, *Osmanlı Devletinde Kardeş Katli* (Istanbul: Eren Yayıncılık, 1997). This custom was legally justified by a law (*kānūn*) attributed to Mehmed II. For the text of the law and a discussion of its authenticity, see Abdülkadir Özcan, ed., *Kânûnnâme-i Âl-i Osman: Tahlil ve Karşılaştırmalı Metin* (Istanbul: Kitabevi, 2003).

brother alive so as not to risk the extinction of the dynasty.[26] In addition, given the extraordinary political circumstances, Mustafa was apparently not considered a potential threat to Ahmed's sovereign power, and the young sultan was accordingly advised not to take any action against him. The unpublished observations of Contarini are very telling in this respect:

> He has not otherwise had to *have his only brother put to death*, because the Sultan has said that *he wishes to keep and cherish him like a son*, but one must suppose that, for that purpose, he might have been persuaded by those who advise him. *Since he does not yet have any children, they have considered it opportune for the continuation of the House of Osman not to rest solely in him* in the face of such danger [i.e., of accidental death], *especially since his brother is about four years old*, so that little is to be feared from him, but it is best to wait some length of time for this eventuality, *until the Sultan can secure his posterity*.[27]

By the time of Ahmed's enthronement, then, the reproduction of the dynasty rested solely on the health and virility of a pubescent sultan who was not circumcised yet. Though this reality is not yet recognized by the established historiography, the House of Osman had never before faced such a serious risk of genealogical extinction. Contemporary evidence suggests that Ahmed I was in poor health at the time of his enthronement and may have been unwell for some time. For instance, Contarini reported that Ahmed was "thirteen years old, of white complexion and displayed a weak constitution, as was also understood to be true."[28]

Furthermore, the fear of dynastic extinction reached a climax when Ahmed and his small brother both contracted smallpox three months later, in early March 1604. In conventional historiography, Ahmed's suffering from smallpox is rela-

26 Also noted in the same context by Baki Tezcan, *The Second Ottoman Empire: Political and Social Transformation in the Early Modern World* (Cambridge: Cambridge University Press, 2010), 60–61. Murad III had five and Mehmed III nineteen brothers killed at their successions. Ahmed I, on the other hand, would never apply the custom, a decision which would eventually change the patterns of Ottoman dynastic succession.

27 ASVe, SDC, filza 58, 255v (dated January 3, 1604): "Non è stato altrimenti fatto morir l'unico fratello perché il Gran Signore ha detto che vuol tenerlo come figliolo, et lo accarezza, ma si deve supponere che a ciò sia stato persuaso da chi lo consiglia poiché non havendo ancora figlioli haveranno giudicato conveniente di non tenire in lui solo con tanto pericolo la continuatione della casa Otthomana, massimamente che il fratello è in età di circa quattro anni, onde non si può di lui dubitar tanto, ma ben aspettare questa effettuazione, per qualche spatio di tempo, poiché in tanto il Gran Signore potria assicurare la sua posterità."

28 ASVe, SDC, filza 58, 231r-231v (dated December 21, 1603): "È di età di anni tredeci, di color bianco, et mostra debole complessione, come anco si intende che sia veramente."

tively well-known, but his brother's case not. The Venetian *bailo*'s brief account leaves no doubt that Prince Mustafa contracted the same disease at the same time, if not before. Fortunately, both brothers recovered, but it later became publicly known that Ahmed's condition had been so grave that some observed certain indications that "pointed to him dying or at least to his being dangerously ill."[29] The prospect was so horrifying that, according to the contemporary chronicler Hasan Beyzade, the members of the government and the court altogether "lost their minds and were near death from fear and anxiety." The death of the childless sultan would have easily thrown the whole imperial system into chaos since the only possible successor was his four-year-old brother; moreover, the Habsburgs could have mobilized a larger force and pushed for a full invasion at a time when the Ottomans were preoccupied with the resilient Celâli armies in Anatolia.[30]

Naturally enough, speculations about Ahmed I's health started to circulate throughout the capital, since the sultan had not been seen in public for a while. Based on the testimony of contemporary writers, we can infer that Ahmed had been sick and out of sight for at least a month.[31] Hence, as soon as the young sultan felt better, he had to make a public appearance in order to stop the rumors. Once again, Contarini provides us with a detailed account:

> On account of so much discussion and continuous whispers ... concerning the health and life of the Sultan, who truly had been in some danger, it was necessary for his Majesty to allow himself to be seen in the audience chamber. He planned this in advance; on that occasion, inside the palace were seen and heard several times signs of joy, with fires and the playing of castanets and trumpets. His first departure from the palace had been to the Mosque of Hagia Sophia, and on the following day [he went] through Constantinople to visit some mosques where some of their saints were buried, and there was seen on his face some signs of the pox.[32]

29 ASVe, SDC, filza 59, 68r (dated March 27, 1604): "Si è susurato non poco li giorni passati intorno la persona del Gran Signore, essendosi osservati certi inditii li quali denotavano la sua morte, o almeno pericolosissima infermità ... medesimamente il suo fratello ha havuto ancora lui le varole et dicono che stia fuori di pericolo." Also see Richard Knolles, *The Generall Historie of the Turkes* (London: Adam Islip, 1610; second edition), 1217, about Ahmed's sickness.

30 Hasan Beyzade, 3: 811: "*Erkān-ı devletün akılları başlarından gitti ve aʿyān-ı hazretün gumūm u hümūm cānlarına yitdi. Kulūb-ı müslimīn havf-ı firāk-ı şāh-ı güzīn ile toldı. İnkılāb-ı devlet-i Osmāniyye ihtimāli ile ıztırāba ve aʿdā-yı dīn istīlāsı vehmi ile iltihāba düşdiler.*"

31 For instance, Hasan Beyzade, 3: 811, notes that Ahmed did not attend the official ceremonies held at the palace to celebrate the first day of the Ramadan festival, which should have been taken place on March 3, 1604.

32 ASVe, SDC, filza 59, 81r (dated April 13, 1604): "per li molti discorsi et per le continue

At this point, one particular question comes to mind: From which type of smallpox did Ahmed and his brother suffer? Was it a benign (*Variola minor*) or a virulent (*Variola major*) one? The brief testimonies of the Venetian *bailo* and a few Ottoman authors unfortunately do not allow us to answer this question with any certainty. Yet given that both brothers were contracted with the disease at the same time (suggesting the disease was airborne in the harem) and that Ahmed was seriously ill for weeks as well as that signs of pox was still visible on his face even some five years later, the pathogen in question looks like the virulent one (*V. major*), which is known to be highly contagious and deadly. However, the possibility of chickenpox should also be considered here, for it is often confused with smallpox due to similar symptoms.[33]

A Young Sultan with a Delicate Constitution

If Ahmed's health was an issue of deep concern for the continuity and stability of the Ottoman dynastic establishment, his age and actions were just as serious a concern for the functioning of the royal court and the imperial government. He was barely fourteen years old, and except for the short first reign of Mehmed II some 150 years before, the Ottomans had never had such a young and inexperienced ruler.[34] Ahmed inherited an empire that had been at war for nearly twenty

---

mormorationi che si facevano da più condizioni di persone intorno la salute, et la vita del Gran Signore, che veramente è stata in qualche pericolo, ha convenuto sua Maestà lasciarsi vedere nella camera dell'audienza anticipatamente da quello si haveva dissegnato, con la qual occasione dentro al serraglio si sono più volte veduti, et sentiti segni di allegrezza, con fuochi, et suoni di gnacchere, et di trombette. La prima uscita sua del serraglio è stata alla Moschea di Santa Soffia, et il giorno seguente per Constantinopoli a visitare alcune Moschee, dove sono sepolti alcuni loro santi, et si è veduto alquanto segnata la faccia dalle varole."

33 On the history and different types of smallpox, see Alfred W. Crosby, "Smallpox," in *Cambridge World History of Human Disease*, ed. Kenneth F. Kiple (Cambridge: Cambridge University Press, 1993), 1008-13; Ann G. Carmichael and Arthur M. Silverstein, "Smallpox in Europe before the Seventeenth Century: Virulent Killer or Benign Disease," *Journal of the History of Medicine and Allied Sciences* 42, no. 2 (1987): 147-68; Ana Duggan et al., "17th century *Variola* Virus Reveals the Recent History of Smallpox," *Current Biology* 26 (2016): 1-6. According to Knolles, *The Generall Historie*, 1297, the signs of smallpox on Ahmed I's face were somewhat visible even around 1609–10.

34 Although there are some conflicting accounts about the actual date of Ahmed's birth, most sources agree that he was born in April 1590. For instance, Contarini writes that he was assured that the sultan was fourteen years old. He also mentions an interesting detail about how Ahmed's age was previously rumored to be sixteen while he was only twelve. ASVe, SDC, filza 58, 256r (dated January 3, 1604): "et si sparge voce che sia di sedici fino de disotto anni il Signore per apportarle maggio riputazione, et per avantaggiar il beneficio

years with the Habsburg Empire in the west and the Shiite Safavid Empire of Iran in the east while facing localized military uprisings in its central lands. The teenaged sultan thus needed guidance in the business of rule. Although there was no institutionalized tradition of regency at the Ottoman court, his mother, Handan Sultan, and the royal tutor, Mustafa Efendi, acted as *de facto* regents. These two powerful figures, until their deaths in 1605 and ca. 1608, respectively, were not only Ahmed's chief mentors, guiding the inexperienced ruler in selecting and controlling his viziers and military officers, but they also played crucial roles in securing the well-being of the young sultan.

However, ensuring Ahmed's safety and well-being was not an easy matter, given his eagerness to play the role of a warrior sultan. Since the beginning of his reign, Ahmed repeatedly announced that he would personally lead a military campaign just as his great-grandfather, Süleyman I, and his father, Mehmed III, had done soon after their successions. For instance, at his first public appearance on January 3, 1604, the day he visited the shrine of Abu Ayyub Al-Ansarî on the Golden Horn so as to be girded a sword by the mufti, Ahmed summoned his viziers en route to the palace in order to discuss the current state of governmental affairs. After this council (*dîvân*) meeting on horseback, according to the Venetian *bailo*, it was "decided that it would be proclaimed in the following days by the ministers delegated to the four usual places of the city that the same Grand Seigneur would go to Hungary and that he would declare war against the King of Persia."[35] In this context, it should be noted that at a time when expectation was mixed with uncertainty and centered on the young sultan's ability to continue the dynastic rule at a most difficult time, Ahmed's first public appearance was clearly designed to emphasize that he possessed the martial and religious virtues of his ancestors; that he was eager to go to war and determined to eliminate the Celâli rebels; and that the Islamic and dynastic legitimacy of the new sultan was fully established.[36]

dell'Imperio, ma per quello che tocca all'età mi viene affirmato assicurantemente che habbia finito li quattordici anni." In sum, Ahmed was definitely in his fourteenth year at the time of his enthronement; thus he must have been born in 1590.

35 ASVe, SDC, filza 58, 294r (dated January 17, 1604): "quel giorno divano a cavallo, cioè il Gran Signore intese il parere delli Visiri, chiamati a dirlo uno alla volta, secondo l'antico costume, et fu deliberato quello che si publicò li giorni seguenti dalli ministri deputati nelli quattro luoghi soliti della città, che il Gran Signore istesso anderà in Ongaria et che si dichiarava la guerra contra il Re di Persia."

36 What appears to have begun as Ahmed's attempt to portray himself as a warrior sultan would set a precedent and create the last essential element in the Ottoman ceremonies of accession, as almost all future Ottoman sultans would be girded with a sword at the shrine of Abu Ayyub upon their enthronement. Previously, sultans visited the shrine before setting out

But Ahmed had to wait for his circumcision to realize his war plans. His circumcision took place in late January and it took him a few weeks to fully recover. Then, in early March 1604, an official announcement was made in the capital that the sultan would go to war in Hungary. At the time, the viziers were divided into those supporting the idea that the young sultan should lead a campaign against the Habsburgs and those opposing it.[37] In any case, the young sultan's illness, which triggered fears of dynastic extinction as described above, halted this debate for some time.

A few months later, concerns about the future of the dynasty were finally allayed by the birth of Ahmed's first son on November 3, 1604. The birth of a prince naturally created much joy and excitement in the court and the capital as it proved that the young sultan was able to father children. Ahmed named his son Osman, after the eponymous founder of the Ottoman dynasty, and ordered public celebrations for seven days and nights in all corners of the empire. The birth of Prince Osman (later Osman II, r. 1618–22) was such an important event that Ahmed appeared on the throne the next day so that the members of his government and other grandees of the court could kiss his hands and congratulate him,

on campaign in order to seek blessing from the soul of Abu Ayyub, a companion of Prophet Muhammad, who fell during the first Arab siege of Constantinople in the late seventh century C.E. However, some scholars still mistakenly believe that this ceremony first took place not at Ahmed's enthronement but at that of his successor, his brother Mustafa I. For instance, see Colin Imber, "Frozen Legitimacy," in Hakan T. Karateke and Maurus Reinkowski, eds., *Legitimizing the Order*, 104. Notwithstanding, in addition to several Ottoman contemporary chronicles, one of the unpublished dispatches of the Venetian *bailo* and an hitherto unexamined Ottoman archival register leave no doubt that this ceremony was inaugurated by Ahmed I: ASVe, SDC, filza 58, 256r (dated January 3, 1604): "La prima uscita che ha fatto il Gran Signore fuori del Serraglio dopo il donativo dato alle militie, del quale dirò nelle seguenti, è stato alla sepoltura del padre, et hoggi è andato a Invasteri [i.e., El-Ansari] luoco poco discosto dalle Mura di Constantinopoli dove è un corpo honorato da Turchi, et dove ha cinto la spada secondo l'uso de suoi processori." The archival register in question, TSMA, D. 34, 234a, mentions the event in passing: "[el-vāki' fī sene 1012 ... ta'rīhün bin onikisinde] māh-ı şa'banü'l-mu'azzamun gurresinde [January 4, 1604] sa'ādetlü pādişāh Eyyüb-i Ensārī'ye kılıç kuşanmağa buyurduklarında." This register (originally titled *filori defteri*) provides convincing evidence that Ahmed I inaugurated this tradition of sword girding at Abu Ayyub. From the reign of Selim II to that of Ahmed I, the register was used to record the gold florins distributed from the sultan's personal treasury at various court ceremonies. Murad III, Mehmed III, and Ahmed I took the register with them wherever they went. The register notes details of all these sultans' enthronement ceremonies but mentions sword-girding only in the case of Ahmed's. There is a one-day discrepancy between all these Ottoman sources and the Venetian *bailo*'s report regarding the date of Ahmed's sword-girding ceremony, as in the case of Ahmed's enthronement. For further details, see Börekçi, "Factions and Favorites," 111–14.

37 ASVe, SDC, filza 59, 3r (dated March 9, 1604).

just as they would on a religious holiday. The birth of the prince was immediately announced to the representatives of foreign states resident in the capital.[38]

After his second son, Prince Mehmed, was born on March 11, 1605, Ahmed finally got the chance to take some concrete steps toward joining the ongoing war in Hungary.[39] In early October 1605, he made a spontaneous trip to Edirne, the former Ottoman capital. This was his first long journey outside the capital, by means of which he apparently wanted to test his readiness for a campaign march, as Edirne was the first major Ottoman military halting station on the imperial campaign route westwards. According to Ottaviano Bon, who replaced Contarini as *bailo* in late 1604, Ahmed's original plan was to spend part of the winter of 1605–6 in Edirne hunting like Süleyman I. He would then gather an army and proceed to Belgrade, where he would join the imperial army under Lala Mehmed Pasha, fighting in Hungary at the time. With this larger army, he could put pressure on the Habsburgs to sign a peace treaty.[40]

38 Mustafa Safi, *Zübdetü't-tevārīh*, ed. İbrahim Hakkı Çuhadar, 2 vols. (Ankara: Türk Tarih Kurumu, 2003), 2: 23–24; ASVe, SDC, filza 60, 151r (dated November 14, 1604): "È nato alli 3 del presente un figliolo al Gran Signore, il quale in dimostratione del contento ricevuto ha ordinato pubbliche feste da farsi per 7 giorni continui in Constantinopoli et in Pera, il che si è immediate esseguito con solene aparato di tuttte le botteghe adornate di panni d'oro, et altri adobamenti che per la varietà et richezza loro renderanno bella et sontuosa vista in particolare nel tempo di note secondo venivano tenute aperte con quantità di lumi accesi essendo anco il Gran Signore medesimo uscito frequentemente a riveder la città. Il giorno susseguente al parto comparve Sua Maestà in pubblico nel proprio seraglio dove è solito sedere al tempo del Bairano, et anderono a baciarli la mano li Visiri, Cadileschieri et altri grandi contra quello che si sia più accostumato di fare per simile occasione. Et ci fu mandato medesimamente una polizza dal Cheslaragassi cioè Agà maggiore della Regina Madre, che sarà acclusa nella presente con la traduttione per dar conto di questo nascimento, havendo anco fatto il medesimo il Bassà luogotenente con un suo huomo particolare." The name of Prince Osman's mother is still not certain, though later Ottoman sources refer to her as Mahfiruz Hadice Sultan (d. 1610). See Tezcan, "Searching for Osman," 335n64, for details.

39 According to the Venetian *bailo* Bon, Prince Mehmed was born on March 11, whereas Safi, *Zübde*, 2: 24–25, claims that he was born on March 8. Bon's date should be credited here as he was in the capital at that time and had a wide network of informants inside the palace, whereas Safi had no such personal knowledge of harem events during this period. Bon further reveals that in-between his two sons' births, that is between November 1604 and March 1605, Ahmed had his firstborn daughter. ASVe, SDC. Filza 61, 19v (dated March 14, 1605): "È nato un figliolo a sua Maestà già 3 giorni, et fin hora sono doi maschi, et una femina." Although the names of two of Ahmed's (at least) five daughters, Ayşe and Gevherhan, are known, their birth dates remain unclear. Kösem Sultan was the mother of both Prince Mehmed and Ayşe Sultan. For further information on Ahmed's daughers and their marriages to high-ranking viziers, see Tezcan, "Searching for Osman," 334n58.

40 ASVe, SDC, filza 62, 90v–91r (dated October 8, 1605): "Quello che più si crede è che

Ahmed undertook this trip in a very unusual and even dangerous way. According to contemporary sources, while he was hunting in Çatalca, a town close to Istanbul, he secretly gathered a few of his servants and, without informing anybody in the government or palace, headed to Edirne, a ride of at least five or six days. This impromptu departure naturally worried the sultan's regents, viziers and other grandees back in the capital, who were concerned about the young sultan's safety since he was traveling without sufficient guards or logistical support. Notwithstanding, Ahmed completed the journey in only three days without any problem and was welcomed by the townspeople.[41] Eight days after his arrival, however, he received a message from Istanbul urging him to return: Nasuh Pasha, who was recently entrusted with the command of the government forces against the Celâlis under the leadership of Tavil Halil, had just suffered a crushing defeat near Bolvadin close to Bursa.[42] Furious, Ahmed cancelled his war plans and started back. Although he ordered an ostentatious military procession to accompany his re-entry into the capital, as if he had been on a real campaign, the number of soldiers present in Istanbul was, as the Venetian *bailo* Bon reports, insufficient since most were deployed to various fronts.[43] Hence Ahmed re-entered the capital with only a limited number of troops on October 17, 1605.[44]

---

il Re come giovine dissegni di goder parte di questo verno la campagna di Andrinopoli abbondantissimo di caccie de tutte le sorti, come faceva Sultan Suliman, né che hora ha per ritornarsene. Questi dicono che havendo mandato a pigliar li padiglioni da campagna sia per passare sino a Belgrado per chiarirsi nel ritorno che farà lo essercito di Ongaria del numero et della qualità di esso con pensiero quando non segua pace di fermarlo per ingrossarlo, et esser l'anno venturo molto per tempo et potente in campagna."

41 Ahmed I's arrival in Edirne is depicted in a unique miniature included in the poetry collection of Ganizade Nadiri, who was the judge of Edirne during Ahmed's visit: *Dîvân-ı Nâdirî*, TSMK, ms. H. 889, 10a. Noteworthy here are Ahmed's youthful, beardless face, the small number of attendants surrounding him, and his extra horse apparently for speed, as well as the presence in the crowd of numerous people waving petitions.

42 Mehmed bin Mehmed, *Nuhbetü't-tevârîh ve'l-ahbâr*, in Abdurrahman Sağırlı ed., "Mehmed b. Mehmed Er-Rumî (Edirneli)'nin Nuhbetü't-tevârîh ve'l-ahbâr'ı ile Târîh-i Âl-i Osmân'ının Metni ve Tahlilleri," PhD diss., Istanbul University, 2000, 644.

43 Interestingly, both Ottoman and Venetian sources refer to this impromptu trip as a campaign. See Safi, *Zübde*, 2: 148–49; and ASVe, SDC, filza 62, 90r–91r (dated October 8, 1605).

44 Mehmed bin Mehmed, *Nuhbe*, 644; and ASVe, SDC, filza 62, 104r (dated October 20, 1605): "Il Re alli 17 il lunedì fu di ritorno nella città et volse far l'intrata sollene, perciò due giorni prima fu pubblicato che tutti li stipendiati et ogni altro dovesse uscire della porta di Andrinopoli ad incontrarlo con le loro armi et ben all'ordine, così l'entrata principiò da terza, et durò fino a mezo giorno, perché entrorno prima le cucine, li padiglioni, le cacie, et la guardaroba, ma perché la Città è vuota di militia, non è riuscita questa entrata né pomposa né frequente."

Ahmed was so determined to go to war that even his mother's death on November 9, 1605, could not stop him.[45] Without waiting for the end of the traditional seven-day mourning period, he re-issued his order for swift preparations for a campaign against the Celâlis who were still in the vicinity of Bursa as reported to him in person by Nasuh Pasha. The young sultan sailed to Mudanya on a war galley owned by Grand Admiral Cıgalazade Sinan Pasha, then he traveled to Bursa on horseback in the cold, accompanied only by his court and a small army. However, a few days later, he once again fell ill, probably either from the cold or from drinking contaminated water, and was forced to cancel his campaign when it had barely begun.[46] Ahmed thus had no choice but to compromise with the Celâlis, just as his father had done a few years earlier. Before he returned to the capital in early December 1605, he allowed some of the most prominent rebel leaders and their followers to enter the ranks of the Ottoman army.[47]

Ahmed's second episode of illness at a critical moment rekindled concerns about the health and actions of the sultan, thus the future of the dynasty. He found it difficult, however, to come to terms with his delicate health and the issues of dynastic continuity. In a short time, he aspired to go to war again, this time against Shah ʿAbbas I, his Shiite archenemy, but his regent Mustafa Efendi managed to change his mind. His Bursa campaign would remain his sole official military undertaking, yet he never gave up the idea of campaigning in person as long as his empire was at war. Only with the conclusion of the Long War in 1606 and the elimination of the Celâli rebels by Grand Vizier Kuyucu Murad Pasha by 1610, Ahmed gave up his idea of leading a campaign in person. In the following years, he would instead keep up the image of the warrior and active sultan by frequently going on hunts and trying to emulate Süleyman I in other ways such as by founding the Ahmediyye, his own imperial mosque complex in Istanbul styled after Süleymaniye.

---

45 Mehmed bin Mehmed, *Nuhbe*, 645; and French ambassador Salignac's report (dated November 24, 1605), in *Ambassade en Turquie de Jean de Gontaut Biron, Baron de Salignac, 1605 à 1610: Correspondance diplomatique & documents inédits*, ed. Comte Théodore de Gontaut Biron (Paris: [NP], 1889), 6.

46 Ahmed's Bursa campaign lasted only two weeks. For details, see Safi, *Zübde*, 2: 41–44; and ASVe, SDC, filza 62, 174r-178r (dated November 25, 1605) and 196r-197v (dated December 12, 1605).

47 Griswold, *Great Anatolian Rebellion*, 53–55; and Finkel, *Osman's Dream*, 184–85.

Conclusion

Ahmed I's enthronement in December 1603 marked the beginning of a new period in seventeenth-century Ottoman dynastic history. Most importantly, with the succession of this inexperienced, childless teenager in questionable health came the threat of genealogical extinction that would loom over the House of Osman for many years to come. Although the Ottoman custom of fratricide was not applied to Ahmed's only surviving brother, four-year-old Prince Mustafa, lest the dynasty's continuity be thrown into jeopardy, the fragility of the Ottoman male line was soon demonstrated when both Sultan Ahmed and Prince Mustafa contracted smallpox in March 1604, just when multi-front wars and rebellions were shaking the empire's military and financial foundations.

Although Ahmed I quickly demonstrated his ability to father children, the problem of dynastic continuity remained a major concern for the Ottomans for many years to come. At the beginning of his reign, Ahmed I's brother and his two young sons, Osman and Mehmed (born in November 1604 and March 1605, respectively), were all underage and were therefore not viable candidates for the throne. Throughout Sultan Ahmed's fourteen-year reign, in fact, none of his ten known sons reached an age at which he could be considered out of danger from illnesses such as smallpox.[48] Moreover, not only the sultan's sons but virtually all members of the dynasty lived under the constant threat of diseases, particularly epidemic diseases such as the plague, which frequently afflicted the capital, including the palace, during this period.[49]

For instance, the Venetian *bailo* Bon recorded the details of one such plague outbreak in the capital between early October 1607 and late January 1608. According to his reports, in its initial phases, the plague killed thousands of people in the capital proper and in Galata, and at least one-third of the residents of Topkapı and the Old Palace, which should have meant hundreds, if not thousands. Several grandee households also fell victim; for instance, the Mufti Hocazade Mehmed Efendi lost his son, while Nakkaş Hasan Pasha's sixty servants vanished. The dan-

48 Baki Tezcan provides the birth order of Ahmed's known sons as follows: Osman (November 1604), Mehmed (March 1605), Selim (June 1611), Murad (July 1612), Bayezid (ca. September-October 1612), Hüseyin (November 1613), Hasan (ca. 1615), Süleyman (?), Kasım (?) and İbrahim (ca. October 1617). For details, see Baki Tezcan, "The Debut of Kösem Sultan's Political Career," *Turcica* 40 (2008): 347–59 and idem, "The Question of Regency in the Ottoman Dynasty: The Case of the Early Reign of Ahmed I," *Archivum Ottomanicum* 25 (2008): 185–98 [published in 2009].

49 See ASVe, SDC, filza 65, 39r (dated October 4, 1607); 59r (dated October 20, 1607); 79v (dated November 4, 1607); 132r and 144r (dated December 6, 1607); 160r (dated December 23, 1607); and 218v (dated January 28, 1608).

ger posed by the plague was such that the sultan and the royal household had to reside elsewhere during this four-month period.

Overall, it can be argued that such constant threats posed by communicable diseases to the dynastic continuity of the House of Osman eventually became a decisive factor in the two separate enthronements of Ahmed I's brother Mustafa I (r. 1617–8; 1622–3) and in the introduction of a new principle to the Ottoman dynastic establishment. When Ahmed died in 1617 due to a stomach ailment, he left several sons, the eldest being thirteen-year-old Osman, who, along with Ahmed's brother Mustafa, was eligible to rule. A court faction then secured the enthronement of Mustafa instead of Osman, thus further solidifying the end of royal fratricide and confirming a new principle of seniority in succession.

Günhan Börekçi (gunhanborekci@sehir.edu.tr) is Assistant Professor of History at İstanbul Şehir University. After completing his BA and MA studies at Boğaziçi University (1991-1999), Börekçi received his PhD degree in history from the Ohio State University in 2010. His main areas of research and teaching include early modern Ottoman political, dynastic, and social history, the seventeenth-century crisis, military history, and traditional archery. In addition to numerous articles and encyclopedia entries on Ottoman history, he has published with Ahmet Arslantürk a facsimile edition of Feridun Ahmed Bey's illustrated chronicle, *Nüzhet-i Esrârü'l-Ahyâr der Ahbâr-ı Sefer-i Sigetvar* (Topkapı Palace Museum Library, ms. Hazine 1339), on Suleyman the Magnificent's last Hungarian campaign in 1566 (2012) and more recently, his study on the Ottoman imperial campaign against the Habsburgs in 1596 came out under the title *Macaristan'da Bir Osmanlı Padişahı: Sultan III. Mehmed'in Eğri Seferi Rûznâmesi – 1596* (An Ottoman Sultan in Hungary: Sultan Mehmed III's Eger Campaign Diary – 1596) (2016).

EPILEPSY AS A "CONTAGIOUS" DISEASE IN THE LATE MEDIEVAL AND EARLY MODERN OTTOMAN WORLD

ÖZGEN FELEK*
Yale University

IN A STORY narrated by the hagiographer of Shaykh Üftāde (d. 1580), an Ottoman mystic, a man visited the Shaykh and asked him to pray for his epileptic wife. Thus did the Shaykh. The man visited the Shaykh a few more times; yet his wife's condition worsened day by day. In despair, when he eventually brought his wife to the Shaykh, hoping that the "weak" woman's illness could be removed, the Shaykh gave him a piece of paper, told him to take that "honored guiding paper" to a certain location, and instructed him to draw a circle and sit inside it. The man did as he was told. While sitting inside the circle, he saw a mighty monarch approaching with numerous soldiers. The monarch reined his horse, stopped, and asked the man what his wish was. After conveying the greetings of the Shaykh, the man submitted the paper to this "Shah." Having read the message, the latter commanded his soldiers to investigate the matter and to bring the "harasser" to him at once. The soldiers said that the harasser must be the ruthless black cripple (*jinn*), who resided in Mount Kaf. After they brought the "black-faced" *jinn,* the Shah ordered him to stop harassing the man's wife. Yet the *jinn*'s response was that it was impossible to renounce her due to his passion for her. When the *jinn* resisted, the Shah ordered his soldiers to kill the unruly *jinn*. Upon witnessing this, the woman's husband lost his mind in awe of that gathering only to wake up next morning with a dead snake, which was the remnant of the *jinn*.[1] His wife had recovered from her illness.

---

* My interest in epilepsy started while researching the claims made in some Ottoman chronicles about Sultan Murad III (r. 1574–95)'s being an epileptic. I would like to thank Nükhet Varlık for inviting me to expand my interest in epilepsy to a wider perspective. I am grateful to her for our conversations on epilepsy in the Ottoman world as well as for her careful reading of and suggestions for the article. I also would like to thank Gottfried Hagen for his insightful suggestions on the final version of the article.

1 *Menākıb-ı Hazret-i Üftāde*, ed. Abdurrahman Yünal (Bursa: Celvet Yayınları, 1996), 29–31. Since I have not been able to locate the original manuscript, I used Abdurrahman Yünal's edition along with the copy of the text in the private library of Mustafa Kara of Uludağ University. I would like to thank Dr. Kara, Nihat Azamat, and the librarians at the İnebey Library in Bursa for their help in searching for the manuscript. On Shaykh Üftāde, see Nihat Azamat, "Üftâde," *Türkiye Diyanet Vakfı İslam Ansiklopedisi*, electronic edition.

For those who work with Ottoman hagiographical narratives (*menāḳıbnāme*), this story will hardly sound unusual. As a biographical genre that aimed to create a moral portrait of mystics by providing accounts of their noble deeds, hagiographies (or hagio-biographies) are full of such stories of miraculous healing offered by Sufi figures, including those about epileptics who could supposedly not receive help elsewhere. In these accounts, it is emphasized that mystics often treated people who suffered from epilepsy, plague, leprosy, stroke, and disabilities such as blindness.[2] In its essence, the hagiographical account of Üftāde serves to strengthen his sainthood and establish his spiritual authority in both the visible and invisible world. Moreover, a close reading of this story reveals important clues about the perception of epilepsy in early modern Ottoman society.

In today's world, cancer is one of the most frightening and challenging illnesses. Even though many advances have been made in cancer research, there are still many unknowns. The etiology of cancer is complex, involving nutritional habits, exposure to chemicals, heredity, and lifestyle choices. Hence different methods of prevention and treatment are suggested. Like cancer, epilepsy continues to be a poorly understood disease throughout history and across cultures. Although it has been identified as a disorder for at least four thousand years,[3] the research on the causes of and treatment for epilepsy has not been able to establish authoritatively its complex etiology. Even though research identifies numerous causes of epilepsy, ranging from heredity to birth defects, it is commonly understood as a seizure disorder and described as a neurological condition originating in the human brain.[4] Although superstitions about it are still prevalent in many societies, epilepsy is not considered a contagious disease in the contemporary world.[5]

---

2 For a discussion of how Ottoman hagiographical sources can be used to study the history of the plague and other epidemic diseases, see John J. Curry, "Scholars, Sufis, and Disease: Can Muslim Religious Works Offer Us Novel Insights on Plagues and Epidemics among the Medieval and Early Modern Ottomans?" (27–55).

3 Marten Stol, *Epilepsy in Babylonia* (Groningen: STYX Publications, 1993); M. J. Eadie, "Epilepsy—from the Sakikku to Hughlings Jackson," *Journal of Clinical Neuroscience* 2 (1995): 156–62.

4 See, for example, Ramon Edmundo D. Bautista, "Racial Differences in Coping Strategies Among Individuals with Epilepsy," *Epilepsy and Behavior* 29, no. 1 (2013): 67–71; G. M. Tedrus, L. C. Fonseca, F. De Pietro Magri, P. H. Mendes, "Spiritual/Religious Coping in Patients with Epilepsy: Relationship with Sociodemographic and Clinical Aspects and Quality of Life," in *Epilepsy and Behavior* 28, no. 3 (2013): 386–90.

5 The causes of epilepsy remain to be a mystery, ranging from genetic factors, congenital abnormalities, antenatal and perinatal injury, the effects subsequent to prolonged febrile convulsions, trauma, and craniotomy, as well as infections, immunization, vascular causes, cerebral tumors, toxic causes, metabolic causes, Alzheimer's disease, and other dementias.

Through an analysis of a wide range of texts from the late medieval and early modern periods, the present paper will demonstrate that Ottoman society imagined epilepsy not only as a disorder caused by physical conditions but also as a contagious disease, which could be transmitted by the *jinn* and evil spirits. Thus, its treatments targeted these causes. It should be emphasized that what is meant by "contagious" here is not infectious diseases that can be transmitted by pathogenic microorganisms; this particular notion of contagion was not fully articulated until the laboratory revolution of the late nineteenth century.[6] Here "contagious" is defined rather loosely to refer to a disease that is "transmissible" or "communicable."[7] In this sense, epilepsy was understood to be similar to the plague (or other such transmittable diseases), which was also explained as being caused by "the sting of a *jinn*."[8] This perception of epilepsy was largely informed by the Islamic medical tradition, which entailed a complex system of disease etiology, prevention, and therapeutic methods.

In what follows, I first explore discussions of epilepsy in the early Ottoman medical texts, namely İshak bin Murad's *Edviye-i müfrede*, Hacı Paşa's *Müntahab-ı şifā*, İbn Şerif's *Yādigār*, and the *Ebvāb-ı şifā*, whose author is unknown to us.[9]

See Anthony Hopkins, ed., *Epilepsy* (London: Chapman and Hall, 1987), 115–24; Jerrold E. Levy, "Epilepsy," in *The Cambridge World History of Human Disease*, ed. Kenneth F. Kiple (Cambridge: Cambridge University Press, 1993), 713–18.

6 For further discussion of the laboratory revolution in medicine, see for example, Andrew Cunningham and Perry Williams, eds., *The Laboratory Revolution in Medicine* (Cambridge: Cambridge University Press, 1992).

7 For notions of contagion and the contagious in the late medieval and early modern Mediterranean world, see Justin K. Stearns, *Infectious Ideas: Contagion in Premodern Islamic and Christian Thought in the Western Mediterranean* (Baltimore: Johns Hopkins University Press, 2011); Vivian Nutton, "The Seeds of Disease: An Explanation of Contagion and Infection from the Greeks to the Renaissance," *Medical History* 27 (1983): 1–34. Also see Nükhet Varlık, "Contagious Metaphors: Ideas of Disease Transmission in Early Modern Ottoman Society," presented at Second International Congress on the Turkish History of Medicine, December 10–13, 2012, Istanbul, Turkey. I am grateful to Nükhet Varlık for sharing her unpublished paper with me.

8 Nükhet Varlık, "From '*Bête Noire*' to '*le Mal de* Constantinople': Plagues, Medicine, and the Early Modern Ottoman State," *Journal of World History* 24, no. 4 (2013): 741–70; Ahmed Taşköprizade, *Risālah al-shifā' li-adwā' al-wabā'*, Süleymaniye Library, ms. Aşir Efendi 275, 61a; and Manfred Ullmann, *Islamic Medicine* (Edinburgh: Edinburgh University Press, 1978), 4–5.

9 İshak bin Murad, *Edviye-i Müfrede: Metin-Sözlük* (Ankara: Türk Dil Kurumu, 2007); Celalüddin Hızır (Hacı Paşa), *Müntahab-ı Şifâ*, ed. Zafer Önler (Ankara: Türk Dil Kurumu, 1990); Tabîb İbn-i Şerîf, *Yâdigâr, 15. Yüzyıl Türkçe Tıp Kitabı*, eds. Ayten Altıntaş, Yahya Okutan, Doğan Koçer, Mecit Yıldız (Istanbul: Yerküre, 2004); and Özen Yaylagül, *Ebvâb-ı şifâ: Metin Dilbilimsel Bir İnceleme* (Ankara: KÖKSAV, 2010).

In addition, works of prophetic medicine and medieval Islamic medicine will be briefly discussed in order to demonstrate their influence on the perception of epilepsy in the Ottoman medical tradition. This will be followed by a survey of the social context of epilepsy and popular perceptions of epileptics as depicted in the hagiographical narratives, namely that of Shaykh Üftāde, Shaykh İsa of Akhisar, and Sadreddin Konevi. The travel account of Evliya Çelebi, a well-known seventeenth-century Ottoman traveler and storyteller, also provides interesting details about epileptics and their struggle to receive the right treatments.[10] Finally, the implications of epilepsy as a source of stigma and political device will be examined through a medieval Islamic hagiography, namely that Shaykh al-Kirmānī (d. 1021), and the assertions relating the epilepsy of the Ottoman sultan Murad III (r. 1574–95).

Epilepsy in the Early Modern Ottoman Medical Literature

Epilepsy has been long imagined as a spiritual disease. It was first Hippocrates (ca. 410 BCE) who refuted the connection between epilepsy and the Divine in his discourse on the "Sacred Disease," arguing that epilepsy is not "any more divine or more sacred than other diseases, but has a natural cause, and its supposed divine origin is due to men's inexperience, and to their wonder at its peculiar character."[11] However, despite Hippocrates' attempt to separate the beliefs of prophetic and mystical powers attributed to epileptic individuals, popular belief in a divine cause behind the disorder persisted, and so did remedies outside "standard" medicine.[12] Not surprisingly, significant religious figures, such as Jesus, were seen as healers of epilepsy.[13] Likewise, biographers of Christian saints narrated numerous

10 *Menâkıb-ı Hazret-i Üftâde*; *İlyas İbn-i Isa-yı Akhisari Saruhani, Akhisarlı Şeyh İsa Menakıbnamesi (XVI. Yüzyıl)*, eds. Sezai Küçük and Ramazan Muslu (Sakarya: Aşiyan Yayınları, 2003); *Şeyh Evhadü'd-din Hamid el-Kırmânî ve Menâkıb-nâmesi*, ed. Bayram Mikâil (Istanbul: Kardelen Yayınları, 2005); Şeyh Musa Es-Sadrî, *Regâyibü'l-Menâkıb Sadreddin Konevî'nin Menkıbeleri*, ed. Emin Agar (Istanbul: Anka, 2002); and Evliyâ Çelebi, *Evliyâ Çelebi Seyahatnâmesi Topkapı Sarâyı Kütüphanesi Bağdat 307 Numaralı Yazmanın Transkripsiyonu-Dizini*, eds. Yücel Dağlı, Seyit Ali Kahraman, and İbrahim Sezgin (Istanbul: Yapı Kredi Yayınları, 2001).

11 Hippocrates, "The Sacred Disease," in *Hippocrates with an English Translation by W. H. S. Jones* (Cambridge, MA: Harvard University Press, 1923), 139.

12 Orrin Devinsky and George Lai, "Spirituality and Religion in Epilepsy," *Epilepsy and Behavior* 12, no. 4 (2008): 636–43; Lawrence I. Conrad, Michael Neve, Vivian Nutton, Roy Porter, and Andrew Wear, *The Western Medical Tradition: 800 B.C.–1800 A.D.* (Cambridge: Cambridge University Press, 1995), 16.

13 Luke, who was a physician, recounted how Jesus casted out the evil spirit from a boy with epilepsy who had just had a seizure, thereby curing him. See, the gospels of Mark (9:14–29),

stories about healer-saints who cured possessed individuals. In France alone, for example, between the years 1200 and 1400, over 80 saints were considered to have been healers of mental disorders and epilepsy. Of particular interest was the shrine of St. Willibrord at Echternach (Luxembourg), a popular place often visited by epileptics.[14]

The Islamic tradition also recognized epilepsy as a disorder, as testified in the hadith collections of al-Bukhari (d. 870) and Muslim (d. 875), which are accepted among the most reputable sources about the Prophet in the Sunni tradition. According to a hadith narrated in both collections, an epileptic "black" woman is reported to have sought help from the Prophet:

> Ibn ʿAbbas once said to me, "Shall I show you a woman of the people of Paradise?" I said, "Yes." He said, "This black lady came to the Prophet and said, 'I get attacks of epilepsy and my body becomes uncovered; please invoke Allah for me.' The Prophet said (to her), 'If you wish, be patient and you will have (enter) Paradise; and if you wish, I will invoke Allah to cure you.' She said, 'I will remain patient,' and added, 'but I become uncovered, so please invoke Allah for me that I may not become uncovered.' So he invoked Allah for her."[15]

Regardless of whether the hadith was authentic or not, the recognition of epilepsy as a disorder is noteworthy. Likewise, the prophetic medicine (*al-ṭibb al-nabawī*) corpus, a specific genre that collects the Prophet's sayings and deeds regarding health and disease, treats epilepsy along similar lines. These works combined hadith with "elements of Greek medical learning (in Arabic dress) and religious elements specific to Islam with pre-Islamic Arabian practices" along with the authors' interpretations based on their knowledge on medicine, whether academic or folk-based.[16] For example, the work of Ibn Qayyim (d. 1350), one of the

---

and Luke (9:37–43) in *The New Oxford Annotated Bible with the Apocrypha: Revised standard version, containing the second edition of the New Testament and an expanded edition of the Apocrypha*, eds. Herbert G. May, Bruce M. Metzger (New York: Oxford University Press, 1977).

14 In such places, medical and religious therapies co-existed with bathing and special foods. Conrad, Neve, Nutton, Porter, and Wear, *Western Medical Tradition*, 186. For a comprehensive study on the perception and history of epilepsy in the West, see also Owsei Temkin, *The Falling Sickness: A History of Epilepsy from the Greeks to the Beginnings of Modern Neurology, Second Edition, Revised* (Baltimore: Johns Hopkins University Press, 1979).

15 Translation of *Sahih Bukhari*, book 70, 7, no. 555: www.usc.edu/org/cmje/religious-texts/hadith/bukhari/.

16 Peter E. Pormann and Emilie Savage-Smith, *Medieval Islamic Medicine* (Washington, DC: Georgetown University Press, 2007), 74. Al-Bukhari, the compiler of the *Sahih al-Bukhari*,

most well-known texts of prophetic medicine, recognizes two kinds of epilepsy. The first one is caused by the earthly evil spirits; the second is a psychosomatic disorder that originates from physical aggravation of humors in the human body. He even stresses that while the first kind is recognized only by the more spiritually enlightened physicians, the heretical doctors only confirm the kind of epilepsy that results from physical causes.[17]

As Paula Jolin, whose "Epilepsy in Medieval Islamic History" stands as the only deep analysis of epilepsy in the early modern Islamic tradition, rightly noted, "Medieval Islamic understandings and treatment of epilepsy were undeniably influenced by Greek medicine and the Middle Eastern cultural milieu: nonetheless, they represent a distinct cultural interpretation of the disease."[18] Jolin's study places four preeminent Muslim scholars' views on epilepsy in the wider context of a medieval Islamic cultural milieu through their medical treatises. According to Jolin, the works of preeminent medieval Muslim authors, such as Ibn Sīnā (d. 1037), al-Rāzi (d. 1209), Ibn Qayyim, and Sanawbarī al-Hindī (d. 1412) show that their perception of epilepsy was "both porous and flexible."[19] The doctrine of humors, the physiology of metabolism, the theories of the three digestions and of the movement of the blood proposed by Galen (d. ca. 210) highly influenced Arabic medicine and Islamic medical tradition. An imbalance of the humors would cause sickness, and the mixing of others into the black bile would cause epilepsy.[20] While medical encyclopedist al-Tabari (d. 870) lists epilepsy in his chapter on the thirteen mental illnesses, including despair, madness, delirium, damages to the imagination and intelligence, forgetfulness, insomnia, lethargy, roaring in the head, vertigo, and swelling, another medical author, Thabit ibn Qurra (d. 901),

---

dedicated two chapters to the hadith accounts on medicine, under the titles *Kitab al-ṭibb* ("The Book of Medicine") and *Kitab al-marda* ("The Book of the Sick"); and Abu Dawud (d. 889), another prominent hadith scholar, collected such hadith accounts under the title, *Kitab al-ṭibb.* Likewise, other significant hadith scholars al-Tirmidhi, Ibn Majah, Muslim, al-Nasa'i, Aḥmad ibn Ḥanbal, and Malik ibn Anas included in their work hadith accounts on medicine. On prophetic medicine, see Pormann and Savage-Smith, *Medieval Islamic Medicine*, 71–75.

17 Muḥammad ibn Abī Bakr Ibn Qayyim al-Jawzīyah, *Ṣaḥīḥ al-ṭibb al-nabawī fī ḍawʾ al-maʿārif al-ṭibbīyah wa al-ʿilmīyah al-ḥadīthah* (ʿAjmān: Maktabat al-Furqān, 2003), 113–14.

18 Paula Jolin, "Epilepsy in Medieval Islamic History," MA thesis, McGill University, 1999, 2.

19 Ibid., iii.

20 According to the Galenic understanding, health is rooted in a balance of the following four humors: blood bile (or the sanguine humor) which is hot and wet, phlegm (or the phlegmatic humor) which is cold and wet, black bile (or the melancholic humor) which is cold and dry, and yellow bile (or the choleric humor) which is hot and dry. These four humors are associated with air, water, fire, and earth. Temkin, *The Falling Sickness*, 60–65.

places it among the hereditary diseases along with leprosy, vitiligo, consumption, phthisis, melancholy, and gout.[21] Likewise, al-Razi, who is influenced by Galen's understanding of the contagious nature of epidemic diseases, recognizes epilepsy among the inherited diseases along with leprosy, tuberculosis, and hemorrhoids.[22]

While there is a vast literature on epilepsy in the Western world, the perception of epilepsy in the Islamic context has hitherto not been thoroughly examined. Discussions of epilepsy can be found in a wide variety of genres and forms outside the medical literature, ranging from hagiographical narratives to travel accounts, and to chronicles. The large corpus devoted to the subject in the premodern Islamicate world testifies to the significance of the problem. What follows is a preliminary exploration of the perception of epilepsy in the Ottoman world. Before immersing into a detailed analysis of the Ottoman corpus on the subject, however, I should state that my goal here is not to downplay the importance of Galenic medicine, which has a systematic, coherent, and rational approach to disease. On the contrary, I acknowledge that Galenic medicine was central to Ottoman medicine, which also embraced folkloristic and religious elements. As Miri Shefer-Mossensohn aptly observes, "The Ottoman medical system was based on several traditions—Galenic humoralism, folkloristic medicine, and religious medicine."[23] The present article will demonstrate that texts on epilepsy follow this pluralistic model which also included religious and folk medicine.

As early as the fourteenth century, Turkish medical texts began to flourish in Anatolia, under the support and patronage of Ottoman and other sovereign households.[24] The Ottoman medical corpus included works translated from Arabic and those composed in Turkish, which benefited from the earlier texts produced in Arabic and Persian. As a living testimony of that tradition, there are about three thousand medical treatises that are preserved in the manuscript libraries of Turkey alone.[25] A comprehensive study of epilepsy and its perception in

---

21 ʿAlī ibn Rabbān al-Ṭabarī, *Firdaws al-hikmah fī al-ṭibb*, ed. M. Z. Siddiqi (Berlin, 1928), 138; Max Meyerhof, "The 'Book of Treasure', an Early Arabic Treatise on Medicine," *Isis* 14 (1930): 55–76, 60–61.

22 Abū Bakr Muḥammad Ibn Zakariyya al-Rāzī, *al-Ḥāwī fī al-ṭibb* (Beirut, 2002), 8: 3823–3824.

23 Miri Shefer-Mossensohn, *Ottoman Medicine: Healing and Medical Institutions 1500-1700* (Albany: SUNY Press, 2009), 12.

24 Adnan Adıvar, *Osmanlı Türklerinde İlim* (Istanbul: Remzi Kitabevi, 1970), 13; Mustafa Canbolat, "XIV. Yüzyılda Yazılmış Değerli Bir Tıp Eseri, *Edviye-i Müfrede*," *Türkoloji* 5, no. 1 (1973): 21–48.

25 Yaylagül, *Ebvâb-ı şifâ*, 5.

the Islamicate tradition is obviously beyond the limitations of a short article. In exploring epilepsy in these medical texts, I shall thus limit the discussion to four early examples of medical texts composed in Turkish, written in the fourteenth and fifteenth centuries. Of these, the *Edviye-i müfrede*, written in 1387 by İshak bin Murad, of whom we know nearly nothing, is generally credited as the first medical text composed in Turkish.[26] The *Müntahab-ı şifā*, a fifteenth-century medical compendium by Celalüddin Hızır bin Ali (Hacı Paşa),[27] and the *Ebvāb-ı şifā,* whose author is unknown, are particularly important for our purposes for they provide Qur'anic chapters and numerology as well as different types of remedies originating from herbs and animals. The last text used here to explore epilepsy is İbn-i Şerīf's *Yādigār*, a fifteenth-century medical compendium. The existence of several copies of the *Yādigār* and numerous references given to it attest to its popularity in the Ottoman medical tradition.

In defining epilepsy, these texts use a wide range of vocabulary, from the Arabic word "*sarʿa*" to several Turkish words, including "screaming on waking up" (*uykuda belk olma*), "ache in the brain" (*dimağ ağrısı*), "madness" (*cünunluk*), "insanity" (*uçuk*), and "possessed" (*dutarık*). In terms of organizational structure, these medical works generally follow a consistent order in discussing diseases, starting with ailments related to the head and gradually continuing toward those of the feet. In the *Edviye-i müfrede,* epilepsy appears only in a brief statement that "epilepsy is insanity," suggesting that the author perceived epilepsy to be possession by madness. The only mention of the disease is in the section where remedies are introduced.[28] In the *Müntahab-ı şifā*, *Yādigār,* and *Ebvāb-ı şifā*, however, epilepsy is clearly discussed "together with maladies of the head due to its relationship with the brain where the seizures originate," as generally treated in Ottoman medicine.[29] The *Müntahab-ı şifā* and *Ebvāb-ı şifā* list epilepsy in the same category as dizziness, depression, and madness.[30]

---

26 İshâk bin Murâd, *Edviye-i müfrede*, 9. Also see Ayşegül Demirhan Erdemir, "Geredeli İshak," *Türkiye Diyanet Vakfı İslam Ansiklopedisi*, electronic edition.

27 For Hacı Paşa and his intellectual milieu, see Sara Nur Yıldız, "From Cairo to Ayasuluk: Hacı Paşa and the Transmission of Islamic Learning to Western Anatolia in the Late Fourteenth Century," *Journal of Islamic Studies* 25, no. 3 (2014): 263–97.

28 İshâk bin Murâd, *Edviye-i müfrede,* 41.

29 For the treatment of diseases related to the head in Ottoman medical tradition, see Vildan Taşkıran Demirsoy, "Analysis of a Manuscript: *Risāla-i Ṭibb bi't-Turkî*: Treatment of Head Diseases in Ottoman Medicine," in *Journal of the International Society for the History of Islamic Medicine* 12–13, nos. 23–26 (2013–2014): 8–20.

30 Celalüddin Hızır, *Müntahab-ı şifâ,* 40; Yaylagül, *Ebvâb-ı şifâ*, 99.

In the medieval period, the *jinn* were believed to cause illnesses, "especially fever, epidemics, epilepsy, etc. and disturb their sexual functions (causing impotence in man, sterility or miscarriage in a woman)."[31] It was believed that epilepsy had "a divine cause that was implemented by the *jinn*, and the effects of their possession might be considered analogous to the behavior of the deranged."[32] Similarly, the *jinn* appear as a major cause of epilepsy in three of these four Ottoman medical texts. While the *Edviye-i müfrede* does not mention any causes of epilepsy, the other three texts propose different causes. The *Müntahab-ı şifā* recognizes epilepsy as caused by phlegm,[33] yet the methods of treatment it recommends suggest that its author also recognizes the *jinn* as a major cause of this disorder. Likewise, the *Ebvāb-ı şifā* includes remedies against the *jinn*, even though it does not specify the causes of the disorder. Unlike the other texts, the *Yādigār* states that epilepsy originates in the brain, but it is sternly related to nightmares, which are thought of as precursors to epilepsy. According to the *Yādigār*, both nightmares and epilepsy are caused by the *jinn*.[34]

These four texts provide little information on the symptoms of epilepsy.[35] The briefness and lack of information regarding the symptoms suggests that either the authors were not quite familiar with the symptoms of the disease, or there was a common image of epilepsy known and recognized by everyone; the authors, thus, did not see a need to repeat or to further describe it; nor did they provide detailed information regarding its symptoms. They did however offer a wide range of remedies to avoid and cure it. The wide array of treatments listed suggests that they showed great effort to cure a disease that had not been clearly identified yet.

---

31 Since people considered the *jinn* causing mental disorders as well, the word *majnūn* (madman), literally meaning "possessed by the *jinn*," has been repeatedly used for epileptics. For a thorough research concerning the beliefs in the *jinn*, see Joseph Henninger, "Beliefs in Spirits among the Pre-Islamic Arabs," in *Magic and Divination in Early Islam*, ed. Emilie Savage-Smith (Aldershot: Ashgate, 2004), 1–53; Michael W. Dols, *Majnūn: The Madman in Medieval Islamic Society*, ed. Diana E. Immisch (Oxford: Clarendon Press, 1992), 211–23.

32 Dols, *Majnūn*, 219.

33 Although the author does not categorize the types of epilepsy, a close reading of his suggestions demonstrates that he recognizes different types of epilepsy based on the condition of the patients. Celalüddin Hızır, *Müntahab-ı şifâ*, 49.

34 İbn Şerîf, *Yâdigâr*, 241, 244.

35 For example, the *Müntahab-ı şifâ* warns its readers that when a person is possessed by epilepsy, it is dangerous when the patient falls down and produces foam. This indicates that its author recognized the grand mal seizure and distinguished it from other types of seizures. Celalüddin Hızır, *Müntahab-ı şifâ*, 49. The *Yâdigâr* mentions other symptoms, though briefly, such as that the patient's eyes become dull, and the five senses of the body have reduced function. İbn Şerîf, *Yâdigâr*, 241.

As significant sources for the early modern folk medicine as well as religious healing in the Ottoman realm, these texts offer a variety of remedies: Herbal and animal-based remedies, magical remedies, and recitation of prayers and Qur'anic verses. As examples of herbal remedies, it is mentioned that sedatives, such as jasmine and lotus are to be used for preventing epilepsy and convulsions. In addition, a number of herbal substances (e.g., violet, sesame, anise, water lily, red rose, and cucumber seeds) are recommended for preparing remedies. As for animal-based remedies, beaver, weasel, billy goat, tinamou, and donkey were praised for their curative powers. It is recommended that a mix of herbs be rubbed on the patient's head with the testicle of a beaver. Epileptic patients were advised to eat the breast of a billy goat, a donkey, or a tinamou.[36] Similarly, drinking turtle or rabbit blood mixed with vinegar, or eating water buffalo's burnt and crushed hoof, burnt bloodsuckers, and licking bear blood were among recommended methods of treatment. Some remedies mixed different types of subtances. For example, pills made from a mixture of turtle blood, honey, and barley flour was to be taken every sunset and sunrise.[37]

Ottoman medical texts also build a strong link between nutrition and epilepsy. Certain types of food are listed as safe for the consumption of epileptics, such as chicken, partridge and quail, the red flesh of sparrows and baby sheep, and zucchini cooked with chickpea, cinnamon, tinamou, francolin, pheasant, red part of lamb meat, soup with chickpeas, cumin, anise, and coriander, as well as vegetables and pennyroyal. Epileptics are advised to refrain from "disgusting food," such as black pepper, mustard, onion, lentil, and dairy.[38] In particular, they are warned about eating, smelling, and even having celery at home, since it was believed to trigger epileptic seizures.[39] The strong emphasis on dietetic prescriptions was in line with general principles of classical Islamic medicine. It also suggests the difficulty in identifying the causes of epilepsy.

As epileptics have been widely associated with the Divine, demonic, and supernatural forces, religious and magical treatments of epilepsy predominated throughout the medieval and early modern eras.[40] In his *Sacred Disease,* Hippocrates argues that epilepsy was attributed a "sacred character" by those who "concealed and sheltered themselves behind superstition, and called this illness sacred, so that their utter ignorance might not be manifest," for they were at a loss

---

36 In this regard see, for example, Celalüddin Hızır, *Müntahab-ı şifâ*, 50–51.

37 Yaylagül, *Ebvâb-ı şifâ*, 104–5.

38 İbn Şerîf, *Yâdigâr*, 240–41; Yaylagül, *Ebvâb-ı şifâ*, 104–6; İshâk bin Murâd, *Edviye-i müfrede*, 41.

39 İshâk bin Murâd, *Edviye-i müfrede*, 45.

40 Devinsky and Lai, "Spirituality and Religion in Epilepsy," 636.

with no treatment for this malady.[41] According to the author of the *Yādigār*, however, the evidence that these diseases are caused by the *jinn* and evil spirits is that they can be cured by means of magic.[42] In addition to herbal and animal-based remedies, the *Ebvāb-ı şifā* recommends wearing necklaces made of chrysolite, gold, and emerald, and carrying on one's body remedies based on animal products, such as fox's molar tooth, and the head of a hedgehog cut with a sword that had killed a human being before. If an epileptic carries around one's neck common peony (*Paeonia officinalis*) cooked with wine, the author guarantees that he or she would never have an epileptic seizure again.[43]

The most enduring of these remedies are perhaps prayers and Qur'anic verses, which have been consistently recommended for protection from evil spirits and the *jinn*, along with numbers and letters in certain orders. Based on the Qur'anic statement that the Qur'an itself is "a healing,"[44] and advice of the Prophet, the tradition holds that reading certain Qur'anic quotations over the sick provides protection and healing. The *Yādigār*, according to which nightmares are a precursor to epilepsy caused by the *jinn*, recommends that Qur'anic chapters are read over children three times. After each time, the reciter should also spit over the children.[45] The author of the text claims that he has witnessed many times that this prayer worked for children. Yet he warns that this prayer would not work for those who are inclined to evil and have intimacy with evil spirits. Otherwise, they would benefit little from it, since evil spirits cause this disease. Nevertheless, not every nightmare is regarded as a precursor to epilepsy. Nightmares could trigger epilepsy only for those without a gentle personality, who eat heavily, and drink excessively. He continues:

> Nightmares that occur to children and people with a gentle and polite personality usually result from steam and bad spirits. These are immediately cured via prayer, incense, and other remedies, and are not a precur-

41 Hippocrates, "Sacred Disease," 141.

42 İbn Şerîf, *Yâdigâr*, 244.

43 Yaylagül, *Ebvâb-ı şifâ*, 105.

44 The Qur'an, 17: 82, and 41: 44. It is reported in the hadith collections that when the Prophet became sick, he would recite *al-Muʿawwidhatayn* (the Qur'anic chapters *al-Falaq* and *al-Nās*) and then blow his breath over his body. See *Translation of Sahih Bukhari, Virtues of the Qur'an*, vol. 6, book 61, no. 535; and vol. 6, book 61, no. 536.

45 İbn Şerîf, *Yâdigâr*, 243. The *al-Muʿawwidhatayn,* which is recommended for epilepsy, means "the two (verses) for seeking refuge [in God]," referring to the 113th and 114th chapters of the Qur'an, and entitled chapters al-Nās (The Mankind) and al-Falaq (The Daybreak). Chapter Ikhlas (The Unity; Purity) is the 112th chapter of the Qur'an.

> sor to epilepsy. And most of the physicians do not believe in evil spirits and the *jinn*, yet our knowledge is [good] enough [that] some diseases, such as nightmares, *ummu sibyan*,[46] epilepsy, and gripes, are caused by the *jinn* and evil spirits, that is Satan, and by the *jinn* who are infidels, Jews, or Zoroastrians.[47]

Listing epilepsy among the illnesses caused by Satan, and by the *jinn* who are infidels, Jews, or Zoroastrians reflects the belief that the *jinn* have religions and their freedom to choose their religion. Moreover, such diseases, not surprisingly, come from non-Muslim *jinn*, stressing their dreadful nature.

For protection from and remedy for epilepsy and evil spirits, the *Müntahab-ı şifā* suggests writing down the "Throne Verse" (verse 255 of the second chapter of the Qur'an) five times along with the names of the *jinn* that attack epileptics. It further recommends to write down the Throne Verse on a piece of paper to be carried on the body of the patient or to recite it over a piece of paper along with the prayer, "There is neither power nor ability save by Allah," crush and put it in water to be drunk by the patient for a few days.[48] Likewise, the *Ebvāb-ı şifā* suggests reading certain Qur'anic verses, especially the Throne Verse, prayers, and magical numbers to cure and prevent epilepsy:

> for the trouble of epilepsy, may [one] write the Throne Verse for five times, and then write down these [following] names: *Istidfā*, and *Mermāremer, Revfa, Behūçārā, Ehyuca*. And then, again write the Throne Verse under that [list of the names] five more times. If that epilepsy is from the *jinn* or fairy, it will be removed, and he will never have epilepsy again.[49]

The names mentioned in the above passage are most likely the names of certain *jinn* who were thought to have been responsible for epilepsy, and perhaps some other similar diseases, such as the plague, for which a clear physical cause had not been identified. These same names also appear in the *Müntahab-ı şifā*, indicating that these *jinn* were perceived to have specialized in causing epilepsy in human beings.[50] The *Ebvāb-ı şifā* then suggests other Qur'anic verses, emphasizing the importance of reciting the Qur'an for epilepsy:

---

46 "Ummu Sibyan" was the name given to the specific *jinn* that was believed to have targeted pregnant women, causing miscarriages.

47 İbn Şerîf, *Yâdigâr*, 244.

48 Celalüddin Hızır, *Müntahab-ı şifâ*, 51.

49 Yaylagül, *Ebvâb-ı şifâ*, 105.

50 Assigning specific diseases to specific *jinn* was not unique to the *Ebvâb-ı şifâ* and *Müntahab-ı şifâ*, as we learn from Arius al-Rumi, a Byzantine author who wrote books on

> The physician says if the *Havvās-ı Qur'an*, which is helpful for any epileptic who is possessed by the *jinn*, is recited to the ears of an epileptic, the patient is healed. If it is recited every day and night, his *jinn*[51] does not bother him anymore with the permission of God Almighty.[52]

A close examination of the chapters on epilepsy in the Ottoman treatises indicates that late medieval Ottoman magical concepts of illness belong to the same Islamic tradition as medical and religious ones, showing a pluralistic understanding of epilepsy. These four early medical texts reveal that the Ottoman physicians understood epilepsy as a disease related to the head and caused by humors and the *jinn*, reflecting and re-producing the various approaches presented in Islamic medical literature produced in Arabic.

While these texts provide significant information about how some late medieval Ottoman physicians understood epilepsy as a disease, its causes and remedies, they also hint at the perception of epileptics as individuals afflicted by the *jinn*. However, the hagiographical literature, travel writings, and chronicles provide an understanding of personal and social aspects of epilepsy.

Epilepsy in Hagiographical Narratives and Other Non-Medical Literature

The analysis of medical texts demonstrates that the *jinn* were considered as one of the major causes of epilepsy, yet these texts do not touch upon the social perceptions of this disorder. Hagiographical narratives can be used to complement the medical texts, especially to fill in such missing aspects. These accounts often contain both identified and anonymous epileptics and their relatives who take them to certain Sufi figures, seeking a cure for them. The perception of epilepsy as a contagious disease transmitted by the *jinn* seems to have been commonly accepted in medieval and early modern societies. In the opening story, for example, Shaykh Üftāde cures an epileptic woman by expelling the *jinn* that harasses her. As a cause of epilepsy, the *jinn* also appears in another sixteenth-century

---

magic, that the *jinn* specialized in diseases. Dols, "The Theory of Magic in Healing," in *Magic and Divination in Early Islam*, 92–93.

51 The author's expression "his *jinn*" draws parallel with the pre-modern common belief that every human being had a personal *jinn*. See Dols, *Majnūn*, 33.

52 Yaylagül, *Ebvâb-ı şifa*, 106. These Qur'anic verses recommended in the *Ebvâb-ı şifâ* to be recited over the epileptics can be listed as 3: 84–85, 1: 1–7; 61: 1; 7: 54–56; 23: 1; 23: 116; 113: 1; 114: 1; and 72: 1–3, the first verses of chapter *Jinn*, which was believed to enable meetings with the *jinn* by some.

hagiography, the *Regāyibü'l-Menākıb*, dedicated to Sadreddin Konevi (d. 1274).[53] According to the story, during the time of one "Sultan Alaeddin," there is a man who has plentiful possessions in addition to his property, and thus is called "the master of the world." He has a son who is possessed by epilepsy. He thus spends much of his property to find a solution for his son's problem, yet he cannot succeed and becomes helpless. One day, he supplicates Konevi to find a remedy for his helpless son. Having heard of his complaint, Konevi asks him his son's and wife's name. The man replies, "His name is Ali; his mother's is İsmihan." Konevi then writes an "honorable" prayer, recites it over the hat of the man's son, and gives it back to him, saying:

> After sealing this prayer with wax and spreading over a [piece of] green taffeta, attach it to this hat, and put it on your son's head. God Almighty will save your son from that disease.

The man does as Konevi orders. When his son is cured from that disease, he donates his house to the mystic. Later on, as the story continues, that prayer becomes famous as the prayer written by Konevi, who said, "May this prayer be a remedy for whatever disease it is written, and may the need be fulfilled for whatever need it is written."[54]

Although the main role of these two significant anecdotes is to establish their protagonist's saintly identity as a purveyor of miracles and an effective saintly figure that is powerful over invisible creatures and demons, the stories also reflect

53 For Konevi, see Şeyh Musa Es-Sadrî, *Regâyibü'l-Menâkıb*, 14–15.

54 Şeyh Musa Es-Sadrî, *Regâyibü'l-Menâkıb*, 28–30. The prayer is given as follows: "I take refuge in God who knows and hears everything. In the name of God, who is most merciful and compassionate. In the name of God with whose name nothing in the skies and on Earth can harm. He is the One who knows and hears everything. With all the names of God, ask God for protection from his [wrath], His punishment, the bad doings of His servants, and the bad doings of Satan. O my Lord, I also seek protection from You against the presence of *İrkāş, Kāiş, Merkāş, İstittāf, İstitfāf, Hutūf, Hattāt, Şefdās* and *Firdās* [the names of the *jinn*]. God is the Lord of Might. O, *tā sīn he lām vav* [the Disjoined/Opener Letters in the Qur'an] *subbūh, erkah, şunūh, ermū, hasīsā* [not clear]. He is the Beginningless, the Eternal, the Endless. There is Hell as a punishment for those who try to turn the faithful men and women from their religions, and refuse to repent for that. The punishment [called] *Harik* is for them, too. I refer the situations of the *jinn* to God who is Mighty and Overwhelming. He is the one who forces away and protects. He is the word of God that carries the name of Sulayman ibn Dawud (peace be upon him). May He not abandon İsmihan and her son who carry this [prayer] on themselves, and may He take them under His safekeeping and protect them. For the sake of Prophet Muhammad. Power and Might only belong to God who is Almighty and All-knowing. 332 83 1151 11 11 11."

the perception of epilepsy and the epileptic individuals who are possessed by the *jinn*. Furthermore, these anecdotes serve to draw a strong line between epilepsy and the moment of *jadhba* (Sufi experiences of spiritual ecstasy).

It is worth noting that in these narratives, epileptic patients are not always women and children who are traditionally portrayed as weak and helpless. Adult male patients also appear to seek cures for their epilepsy as in the hagiography of Shaykh İsa of Akhisar, a sixteenth-century master of the Bayramiyye order. According to his hagiographer, who is also his son, during Shaykh İsa's travel to Aleppo, a Persian man approaches him to ask for help with his epilepsy, which causes three seizures every day. Although he has visited many physicians and tried many different types of syrups, as he tells the Shaykh, he has been unable to find remedy for his illness. Eventually he is recommended to visit a shaykh who would be coming to Aleppo from Anatolia. When Shaykh İsa arrives in the city, the epileptic man says, he immediately knew that Shaykh İsa was the one who has been recommended to him. Having listened to the epileptic man, the Shaykh tells him to do his ablution, perform his night prayer, and lie down in his bed facing the direction where the Shaykh stays, saying, "Let's see what will be seen to you." Thus does the man. In the morning, he comes and throws himself at the feet of the Shaykh with twenty golden coins as a gift for the Shaykh, saying:

> O, my sultan! I had a dream last night. Your majesty told me, "Open your mouth!" When I opened my mouth, you stuck your hand down my mouth, grabbed my heart, and wrung it. Then you pulled out your hand filled with clotted blood. And you said, "From now on, may you be free from epilepsy!" And then, I woke up, and came to [throw myself to] the dust of your feet.[55]

According to the hagiographer of Shaykh İsa, the epileptic man does not have any epileptic seizures during the Shaykh's seventeen-day stay in Aleppo. This anecdote is striking for it reminds a hadith in which Prophet Muhammad put his hand on an epileptic boy's chest, and something black came out of the boy's mouth:

> A woman came to the Prophet with her son and said: This son of mine has madness, it attacks him during the day and night. The Prophet gently put his hand on the boy's chest and prayed for him. The boy choked and something black came out of his mouth.[56]

---

55 İbn-i Isa-yı Akhisari, *Akhisarlı Şeyh İsa Menakıbnamesi*, 84.

56 Musnad Imam Aḥmad, 1: 268, quoted in Abū al-Fidā' Ismā'īl ibn Kathīr, *Book of Evidences: The Miracles of the Prophet (P.B.U.H.)*, trans. Ali Mwinyi Mziwa and Ibn R. Ramadhan (Al-Mansoura, 2004), 76.

Through this anecdote, Shaykh İsa's hagiographer strengthens the sainthood and saintly abilities of his protagonist not only via miraculous healing for which he is presented to have been known in a vast geographical area, but also via a direct link and resemblance to the Prophet. More interestingly, the story gives clues about the influence and recognition of the story about the Prophet's approach to the phenomena of epilepsy and epileptics in sixteenth-century Anatolia.

As stated above, not only women and children, but also adult male figures are depicted as epileptics, indicating that epilepsy was not seen as specific to those who were traditionally presented as physically weak. The only exceptions to this are the prophets and the friends of God, *walī*. Just as prophets are described as physically and mentally perfect, mystics, as the carriers of the prophetic line, are also seen in the same way. This suggests that epilepsy is viewed as an imperfection and weakness in holy persons, and thus experienced only by common and unholy human beings. Furthermore, since prophets and Sufi masters are able to exorcise the *jinn* from the epileptics, it is not surprising that they themselves would never be possessed by the *jinn* or demons.

This perception of epilepsy in medical texts and hagiographical narratives also overlaps with the writings of Evliya Çelebi, a seventeenth-century Ottoman traveler. The travel writings of Evliya Çelebi show that the approach to epilepsy as narrated in the sixteenth-century hagiographical literature was still in circulation during his time. What is more striking about his account is that he expresses his observations drawn from different regions, stretching from northern Iran to southern Anatolia and Egypt, indicating how epilepsy was perceived in the same way over a vast area.

As in the late medieval medical texts, Evliya Çelebi presents epilepsy as a mental disorder that results from one's body being possessed by the *jinn*. He refers to epilepsy under different names, such as "possessed" (*dutarık*), "*jinn*" (*ecinne*), and "epileptic" (*masrūʿ*). Even though he does not discuss the causes of epilepsy, he pays great attention to the remedies suggested in folk medicine. He claims that wolves, sheep, camels, cows, and dogs are enemies to the *jinn*. Relating a saying of Prophet Shuʿayb, he narrates that if an epileptic eats a fork-antlered ram, he will not have an epileptic seizure again.[57] Likewise, on the banks of the Nile, he writes, the liver of alligators was used for curing epilepsy. This remedy is particularly interesting for it indicates how solutions for the illness varied by what was locally available. In addition, Evliya Çelebi mentions that it was beneficial for epileptics to visit sacred places, such as the shrine of Monla Kasım, and the cities of Kum in northern Iran, and Nusaybin in southern Anatolia, from which the *jinn*

57 Evliyâ Çelebi, *Seyahatnâme*, 4: 318.

are believed to have been banned by Prophet Muhammad. According to the belief, not only were all *jinn* removed from the city of Kum, but also none would survive there. Thus, the people of Kum are not afflicted by epilepsy. If a person gets epilepsy outside this city as a result of being possessed by the *jinn*, and is brought to Kum, he would be relieved from it.[58] Yet visiting Kum is not a final solution, as Evliya Çelebi emphasizes, because the *jinn* can possess the patients once again when they leave the city.[59]

Another shrine visited by epileptics was Şeyh Sinan Efendi's tomb located outside Yenikapı in Istanbul. Not only visiting the Sufi figures' tombs, but even the rain drops collected in those places where a Sufi figure or powerful person, namely Mehmed II, touched previously were seen as remedy for the desperate epileptics.[60] As we learn from Evliya, such remedies were also common among the non-Muslims in the empire. Our traveler also notes that for the non-Muslim epileptics, *Ziyaret-i Sicn-i Hazret-i İsa*, where Jesus was believed to have been imprisoned for forty days, was a well-known pilgrimage site among Christian patients; especially those who suffered epilepsy stayed there overnight.[61]

Along with visits to sacred places, Evliya also mentions visits to prominent religious figures seeking relief from epilepsy. For example, Kemalpaşazade (d. 1536), a leading religious scholar and Chief Jurisconsult, is described as having powers over the *jinn* and demons. For this reason, he was visited by hundreds of epileptics every Saturday morning.[62] Although Evliya Çelebi is known for his exaggerated reports, his emphasis on the numbers of the epileptics that visit Kemalpaşazade may suggest an abundance of epileptics or cases somehow confused with epilepsy. Kemalpaşazade's being reported as healing epileptics is a good example that certain religious figures were famed as specialists on healing certain illnesses.[63]

58 Ibid., 4: 211.

59 Ibid., 4: 313, 321. The same healing properties are also attributed to Nusaybin.

60 Ibid., 8: 145.

61 Ibid., 9: 214. The Christian tradition holds that Jesus was not in prison for forty days, but only for an evening or possibly a few nights. The location of this visiting site mentioned by Evliya Çelebi is unclear. Based on the narration in the Gospels, the location is known as "The Mount of Olives," which is believed to be Gethsemane. See "Gethsemane," in David Noel Freedman, ed., *Eerdman's Dictionary of The Bible* (Grand Rapids, MI: William B. Eerdmans Publishing Company, 2000), 499. For stories regarding Jesus's being imprisoned by the Jews in the Islamic tradition, see "Christ in Mohammedan Literature," in *Dictionary of Christ and the Gospels*, ed. James Hastings (New York: Charles Scribners' Sons, 1908), 882–86.

62 Evliyâ Çelebi, *Seyahatnâme*, 1: 166.

63 Visiting certain Sufi shrines in the hope of finding relief from epilepsy still continues in some places in Turkey. For such shrines, see Yaşar Kalafat, "Diyanet İşleri Başkanlığı Arşivine

The fact that healing epileptics was employed as a motif that challenges and strengthens the saintly power of mystics indicates the difficulty to cure it. Furthermore, talismanic artists carved certain prayers on silver seals and rings to be carried on epileptics, indicating that treating epilepsy developed economic opportunities for artists.

Epilepsy as Social Stigma

All the sources we have looked at so far relate to the efforts of epileptics and their families seeking help as well as the difficulty of defining epilepsy as a disease, without touching upon the social aspects of epilepsy and public perceptions of epileptics. There are hagiographical accounts and chronicles that include anecdotes indicating a strong social stigma attached to the disease. The fact that a husband looks for a remedy for his epileptic wife in one of the aforementioned anecdotes is a clear indication that epileptics were not isolated from social life, at least in certain cultures and time periods. They could be married and integrated into their communities.

However, epileptics occasionally appear to have been isolated and even abused, presumably for the purpose of removing the *jinn* that had possessed their bodies. This approach is vividly depicted, for example, by the hagiographer of Shaykh al-Kirmānī (d. 1021), a preeminent Ismaili theologian and philosopher of the Fatimid period. According to the story, al-Kirmānī's uncle, who does not approve his nephew's dedication to the Sufi path, harshly criticizes and belittles him for abandoning the family trade business and joining in "the perverted, gluttonous, fraudulent, and faithless people," and implores him to remove "these vicious ideas and satanic delusions" from himself. In response to his uncle's words, when al-Kirmānī insists in remaining in the spiritual path no matter what, his uncle commands his men to tie al-Kirmānī's hands and feet, saying he is possessed by epilepsy. Al-Kirmānī is beaten by his uncle's men for days and nights. He is eventually released, when his uncle realizes that his nephew's condition can not be cured

---

Göre Horasaneri Olarak Bilinen Anadolu Yatırları –I," *Ankara Üniversitesi İlahiyat Fakültesi Yayınları* 40, no. 1 (1999): 511–35; Ülkü Kara Düzgün, "Giresun Adak Yerlerinde Tespit Edilen Çeşitli Uygulama, İnanış ve Efsaneler," *Uluslararası Sosyal Araştırmalar Dergisi* 2, no. 7 (2009): 133–53; Doğan Kaya, "Sivas'ta Yatmakta Olan Horasan Merkezli Anadolu Erenleri," *I. Uluslararası Türk Dünyası Eren ve Evliyaları Kongresi Bildirileri* (1998), 265–80; İskender Oymak, "Elazığ Merkez ve Çevresinde Ziyaret Yerleri ile İlgili İnanç ve Uygulamalar," *Fırat Üniversitesi İlahiyat Fakültesi Dergisi* 14, no. 2 (2009): 29–61; Mustafa Bayar, "Şebinkarahisar Yöresinde Ziyaret Yerleri ile İlgili İnanç ve Uygulamalar," *Karadeniz Araştırmaları* 41 (2014): 180–207.

by beating or advising.[64] Another story from al-Kirmânî's hagiography is about a college professor who is suddenly possessed by an unidentified psychological situation. Since he is escaping from people and wandering on the streets aimlessly day and night, people finally assume he has been afflicted by epilepsy. The narrator relates the stories about how local children are gathering around him and bothering him until he feels powerless and falls down on the street.[65]

These anecdotes are remarkable for they demonstrate not only the perception of Sufis as "perverted, gluttonous, fraudulent, and faithless people" by some, but that of epileptics—or those who were denounced as epileptics—in medieval Islamicate society in which they could at times be isolated and treated unfavorably.[66] This harsh perception from the tenth-century Fatimid society is somewhat hinted at in the stories regarding the rumors about the epilepsy of an Ottoman sultan, Murad III, from the late sixteenth-century.

Sultan Murad III is one of the most controversial Ottoman sultans in terms of his skills and credentials as a ruler. While he is portrayed as a devout Sufi by some chronicles,[67] he is castigated by others for corruption, injustice, impotency, sex addiction, and bribery. Furthermore, he is reported to have had epilepsy, secluded himself from interactions with his subjects, isolated himself in his palace, and is criticized for abandoning the leadership of military campaigns and expeditions.[68] What is even more interesting for our purposes here is that he was also reported as an epileptic by at least two of his contemporaries: Mustafa Ali (d. 1600), an Ottoman bureaucrat and historian, and Salomon Schweigger (d. 1622), a German Lutheran theologian and minister in the Habsburg embassy to Istanbul.

In *Künhü'l-ahbār* ("The Essence of History"), while introducing Murad III, historian Mustafa Ali states that the Sultan never led a military campaign. He then brings up rumors that epilepsy is the reason for Sultan Murad's seclusion. Although he ends the topic by stating no matter how much he has investigated the

---

64 Mikâil, *Şeyh Evhadü'd-din Hâmid El-Kirmânî ve Menâkıb-nâmesi*, 212–13.

65 Ibid., 121–22.

66 Epileptic phenomena are still interpreted negatively and demonologically in some communities. See for example Graham Scambler, "Sociological Aspects of Epilepsy," in Hopkins, ed., *Epilepsy*, 497–510.

67 Nevʿizade ʿAtāʾi, *Hadāʾikü'l-hakāʾik fī tekmileti'ş-şekāʾik: Zeyl-i şekāʾik* (Istanbul: [1852]), 364.

68 See, for example, Mustafa Âlî, *Gelibolulu Mustafa Âlî ve Künhü'l-ahbâr'ında II. Selim, III. Murat ve III. Mehmet Devirleri*, ed. Faris Çerçi (Kayseri: Erciyes Üniversitesi Yayınları, 2000), 2: 225, 250–51; İbrahim Peçevi, *Tarih-i Peçevi, cild-i sani* ([Istanbul]: Matba'a-yi Âmire, 1283 [1866]), 2: 5.

subject, the soundness of this assertion is not traceable; he leaves an image of an epileptic sultan behind him:

> Although it never happened in his whole life that the late [Murad] went on campaign or went anywhere other than his coming from Manisa to Istanbul for the fortunate event of his accession, no matter how much he inspired his viziers to take the path of Holy War and battles for the Faith, his noble nature was not seriously inclined [in this direction]. According to some, he was afflicted by epilepsy. They say that, from this perspective, in cases of activity and travel, fear of revealing [this secret] was an impediment to [his] asserting claims [about this unwillingness]. However, this servant of God's [Murad's] being healthy is well known and no matter how much I investigated [it], the soundness [of this assertion] is not perceptible. So, according to this poor author, his being silent [on this subject] is obligatory from the perspective that supposition about his aims and campaigning is over and done with.[69]

Since chroniclers place their focus not only on the events but also the individuals, they often provide information about their protagonists' health issues. These details not only embellish their stories with colorful details regarding the private life of their protagonists, but also turn into an effective strategy that empowers their reliability and sovereignty over the events, details, and figures they report. They can either conceal or highlight some private health details of individuals in order to shape their readers' view of certain historical figures and events in sculpting their protagonist in the best way that fits their perception of these figures. Mustafa Ali's preference to highlight Murad's epilepsy is thus a striking effort despite his closing comments that "the soundness [of this assertion] is not perceptible."

The rumors that Mustafa Ali reported only in passing were also repeated by Salomon Schweigger, another contemporary of Murad. Schweigger arrived in Istanbul in the Habsburg embassy entourage on January 1, 1578, and stayed until March 3, 1581. Later on, he published his notes and observations that contain interesting remarks on the city, the daily life in Istanbul, and Sultan Murad III and his courtiers.[70] As can be gleaned from his writings, he did not have a good impres-

---

69 Mustafa Âlî, *Künhü'l-ahbâr*, 2: 225. Mustafa Ali is a difficult author to translate. I am grateful to Walter G. Andrews for editing my translation of this passage.

70 The original title, *Ein newe Reiss Beschreibung auss Teutschland nach Constantinopel und Jerusalem*, was published by Johann Lantzenberg in Nuremberg in 1608. The first part of the book is dedicated to Schweigger's journey from Vienna to Istanbul; the second part describes his experiences in Istanbul from January 1578 to March 1581, including three years during Murad's reign. In the last section, he relates his pilgrimage to Jerusalem.

sion about either Murad or his courtiers. He exclusively describes the sultan as a poor looking, chubby man, whose "face was pale and colorless like suet. His long, Roman nose gave his face an angry demeanor." This unappealing and unhealthy image of Sultan Murad is further embellished with the assertion of epilepsy:

> In fact, he was an unhealthy man. He was possessed by terrible epilepsy, and therefore preferred a silent, calm life, far from people's view.[71]

Other than these two reports, there is no known report on the Sultan's epilepsy. Nevertheless, the comments of these two authors have been circulated up until today. I discuss elsewhere the claims about Murad's epilepsy in greater detail;[72] what is most interesting for the purposes of the present study is that both of these two authors were unhappy with Murad being the sultan. While Mustafa Ali was dissatisfied with Murad's skills and performance as a sultan, for Schweigger, Murad was the head of the archenemy and the rival empire.[73] In these two anecdotes, epilepsy appears to have been an essential device in establishing Murad as a defective ruler figure.

It should be emphasized here that Murad's story stands as a unique case different from the stories of the epileptic women, boys, and adult male figures presented in the aforementioned hagiographical narratives. In the case of a male ruler, epilepsy seems to have served as a political device in order to weaken an unwanted ruler's impact over his subjects by bringing up questions about his credentials as a sovereign. The fact that epilepsy was employed as a defect to emphasize an individual's imperfection further indicates the misperception of epilepsy in the early modern mind, both within and outside the Ottoman Empire.

Conclusion

Although the etiology of epilepsy remains complex, it is commonly discussed in modern medicine as a neurological disorder originating in the human brain. It is generally agreed upon that it is not a contagious disease. However, as the present

---

Salomon Schweigger, *Sultanlar Kentine Yolculuk, 1578–1581*, ed. Heidi Stein, trans. S. Türkis Noyan (Istanbul: Kitap Yayınevi, 2004), 159–60.

71 Ibid.

72 For more discussion on the topic, see the author's article in progress, entitled, "Did Sultan Murad Have Epilepsy?"

73 In his *Bureaucrat and Intellectual in the Ottoman Empire,* historian Cornell Fleischer explains in detail the reasons behind Mustafa Ali's disappointments. Cornell H. Fleischer, *Bureaucrat and Intellectual in the Ottoman Empire: The Historian Mustafa Ali (1541–1600)* (Princeton: Princeton University Press, 1986).

study attempts to demonstrate, despite medical discussions of epilepsy as a disease that occurred due to the problems in brain, the pre-modern Ottomans commonly perceived epilepsy as a contagious/transmissible disease that passed from the *jinn* to humans, and thus the methods of treatments developed accordingly. The literature on epilepsy is extensive, yet a close examination of the chapters on epilepsy in late medieval and early modern Ottoman medical texts, hagiographical narratives, and travel accounts demonstrates that Ottoman medical, religious, and magical concepts of the illness were largely informed by the Islamic tradition, which allowed humoral medicine and folk medicine to diagnose epilepsy in their own ways.

Evliya Çelebi's notes on epilepsy and epileptics are significant for reflecting the seventeenth-century perception of the disease and those afflicted by it in the popular imagination. In particular, his assertion about epilepsy being caused by "the sting of a *jinn*" was still common long after the composition of the medical treatises discussed above. What can be gleaned from his writings is that the perception of epilepsy did not undergo a drastic transformation in Ottoman society from the late medieval to the early modern era. Although epilepsy had been already classified as a brain disease, both etiology and treatment involved supernatural powers. In addition to myriad remedies suggested in medical texts, people visited saints, religious figures, and healers in the hope of receiving treatment. The hardship of treating epilepsy may have channeled health-seekers to find solutions outside classical medicine.

Furthermore, the fact that hagiographical narratives relate stories of epileptics from different genders, ages, social, ethnic, and economic classes, as well as from different geographical areas, demonstrates that epilepsy was not perceived as an illness unique to some people. It was seen as an illness that might afflict anybody, any time, without a specific, known reason. Apparently, it was this mystery that made it even more frightening and challenging to people. As the stories of Shaykh al-Kirmānī and Sultan Murad display, this mystery caused epilepsy to be misunderstood, leading to an unfavorable perception of the disease as a destructive quality that occasionally brought isolation to epileptics either by force or voluntarily in late medieval and early modern Islamicate societies.

Özgen Felek is the coordinator of the Turkish Program, and the lector of Ottoman and Modern Turkish in the Department of Near Eastern Languages and Civilizations at Yale University. She holds two PhD degrees. She received her first PhD from Fırat University in Turkey and second PhD from the University of Michigan. Before joining Yale, she was a Postdoctoral Research Fellow at the Graduate Center of the City University of New York (2013-2016), and a Mellon Postdoctoral Fellow in the Department of Religious Studies at Stanford University (2011-2013). Felek specializes in religion, gender, and visual representations in the Ottoman Empire. She has published a diplomatic edition of Ottoman Sultan Murad III's dream letters, titled *Kitābü'l-Menāmāt: Sultan III. Murad'ın Rüya Mektupları* (The Book of Dreams: The Dream Letters of Sultan Murad III) (Tarih Vakfı Yurt Yayınları, 2014). She is also co-editor of *Dreams and Visions in Islamic Societies* (SUNY, 2012), and *Victoria Rowe Holbrook'a Armağan* (Festschrift to Victoria Rowe Holbrook) (Kanat Kitap, 2006).

PART THREE

RESPONSES TO EPIDEMIC DISEASES

RELIGION AND OTTOMAN SOCIETY'S RESPONSES TO EPIDEMICS IN THE SEVENTEENTH AND EIGHTEENTH CENTURIES

YARON AYALON
Ball State University

AT DAWN ON August 29, 2005 Hurricane Katrina made landfall in New Orleans. Despite initial reports that the storm would cause little damage,[1] Katrina turned out to be one of the deadliest natural disasters and the costliest one in US history. The storm raged for several hours, wreaking devastation of unprecedented measure on the city. Nearly 2,000 people lost their lives; thousands became homeless. "We've lost everything, and it's a city that's doomed. I don't think we could go back," one victim said. "I have no idea where to go from here ... yesterday I felt flush. Today I got nothing," said another, in despair.[2]

Katrina and a few other recent disasters, such as the Asian Tsunami of 2004, the Sichuan Earthquake of 2008, the Haiti earthquake of 2010, and the east Japan earthquakes and tsunami of March 2011, have spurred a very impressive volume of literature on natural disasters.[3] The interdisciplinary field of Disaster Studies

---

1 "A blast of rain but little damage as hurricane hits South Florida" and "Hurricane drenches Florida and leaves seven dead," *New York Times*, August 26, 2005, A10; August 27, 2005, A8.

2 "Astrodome a step up from the New Orleans Chaos," ibid., September 2, 2005, A19; for more on Hurricane Katrina, see Danielle Hidalgo and Kristen Barber, eds., *Narrating the Storm: Sociological Stories of Hurricane Katrina* (Newcastle: Cambridge Scholars, 2007).

3 See, for example: Ronald Daniels et al., eds., *On Risk and Disaster: Lessons from Hurricane Katrina* (Philadelphia: University of Pennsylvania Press, 2006); David Brunsma et al., eds., *The Sociology of Katrina: Perspectives on a Modern Catastrophe* (Lanham: Rowman & Littlefield, 2007); Shireen Hyrapiet, *Responding to a Tsunami: a Case Study from India* (Saarbrücken, Germany: VDM Verlag, 2007); Hillary Potter, ed., *Racing the Storm: Racial Implications and Lessons Learned from Hurricane Katrina* (Lanham: Lexington Books, 2007); Harry Richardson et al., eds., *Natural Disaster Analysis After Hurricane Katrina: Risk Assessment, Economic Impacts and Social Implications* (Cheltenham, UK: Edward Elgar, 2008); Philip Steinberg and Rob Shields, eds., *What Is a City?: Rethinking the Urban After Hurricane Katrina* (Athens, GA: University of Georgia Press, 2008); Stanley Weeber, *Post-Rita Reflections: a Sociological Journey* (Lanham: Hamilton Books, 2009); Seiko Sugimoto et al., "Sociocultural Frame, Religious Networks, Miracles: Experiences from Tsunami Disaster Management in South India," in Pradyumna Karan et al., eds., *The Indian Ocean Tsunami: The Global Response to a Natural Disaster* (Lexington: University Press of Kentucky, 2011), 213–35; Joshua Miller, *Psychosocial Capacity Building in Response to Disasters* (New York:

has existed for several decades. But those recent events have brought more scholars—mostly social scientists—to the study of disasters not in order to understand their causes and reduce future occurrences, but rather to explore "aspects of social structures and processes that are hidden in everyday affairs" through gathering evidence that provides "rich data for addressing basic questions about social organization—its origins, adaptive capacities, and survival."[4] Parallel to this growing interest in contemporary disasters, historians too have devoted more attention to historical calamities. Recent studies have taught us not only about the effect of disasters on past societies, but also much about their structure, relationships between different elements in society, behavioral patterns, and people's perception of state and local authorities.[5]

In this study, I examine a commonly recurring natural disaster in the pre-nineteenth century Ottoman Empire, plague epidemics.[6] I argue that, unlike what previous scholarship has suggested, there was little connection between responses to plagues and religious belief, and that the latter was not the main factor to determine people's responses to life-threatening situations. As I shall show, this suggests that religious boundaries—but not *religious identity*—were looser and not

Columbia University Press, 2012), 1–31; Jennifer Duyne Barenstein and Esther Leemann, *Post-Disaster Reconstruction and Change: Communities' Perspectives* (Boca Raton, FL: CRC Press, 2013).

4 Robert Stallings, "Weberian Political Sociology and Sociological Disaster Studies," *Sociological Forum* 17, no. 2 (2002): 283.

5 For historical works dealing with natural disasters and the responses to them (mostly those issued by state authorities), see: David Arnold, *Colonizing the Body: State Medicine and Epidemic Disease in Nineteenth-Century India* (Berkeley: University of California Press, 1993); William Jordan, *The Great Famine: Northern Europe in the Early Fourteenth Century* (Princeton: Princeton University Press, 1996); Lillian Li, *Fighting Famine in North China: State, Market, and Environmental Decline, 1690s-1990s* (Stanford: Stanford University Press, 2007); Alan Mikhail, *Nature and Empire in Ottoman Egypt: an Environmental History* (Cambridge: Cambridge University Press, 2011); Sam White, *The Climate of Rebellion in the Early Modern Ottoman Empire* (Cambridge: Cambridge University Press, 2011); William Summers, *The Great Manchurian Plague of 1910–1911: The Geopolitics of an Epidemic Disease* (New Haven: Yale University Press, 2012); Xun Zhou, *The Great Famine in China, 1958–1962: A Documentary History* (New Haven: Yale University Press, 2012); and the many studies on the Black Death, such as Ole Benedictow, *The Black Death, 1346–1353: The Complete History* (Woodbridge, Suffolk, UK: Boydell Press, 2004).

6 For plague as a frequent disaster in the Ottoman Empire, see White, *Climate*, 85–91. Because plague was a disease whose causes people in the Ottoman Empire did not understand, I define it here as natural, as I do with other disasters elsewhere (see: Yaron Ayalon, "Ottoman Urban Privacy in Light of Disaster Recovery," *International Journal of Middle East Studies* 43, no. 3 (2011): 513–28.

as significant in Ottoman society as historians had previously thought. I do so by looking at the question of flight, one among several common responses to epidemics, which also included confinement at one's home, supplication to God and mass prayers, wearing protective amulets, or simply going on with life as usual. Of these, flight has so far attracted the most historiographical attention because of its implications for the understanding of religious boundaries in Muslim society. Early modern European observers and modern historians have hitherto assumed that flight was a typical response to plagues for Jews and Christians but not for Muslims, whose tradition allegedly prohibited leaving plague-stricken areas. In recent years, historians exploring plague in an Ottoman context have moved away from an explanation that focuses exclusively on religiously based responses. Some even argued that flight from plague was a rather common reaction. Reviewing the different approaches, I maintain that flight was in fact a choice few people made, but for reasons that had little to do with religious beliefs. Instead, I offer an explanation for human behavior under life-threatening situations in the Ottoman Empire that incorporates economic, psychological, as well as religious considerations. This, I claim, reflected broader characteristics of Ottoman society, where religious boundaries did not play as central a role in people's everyday experiences as we used to assume.

The Question of Flight

Was there a correlation between the religious arguments provided in plague treatises, which mostly called on Muslims to refrain from fleeing plague-infected areas, and people's actual responses? So far, historians who have visited this question have concluded that Muslim scholars overwhelmingly condemned flight, and that most people followed this advice and refrained from taking action that might have saved their lives. Recently, Justin Stearns has shown that Muslim scholars debated the question of contagion, and hence whether flight would be an appropriate reaction to plague, up to the Black Death of the fourteenth century. Henceforth, the debate waned, with Muslim authors mostly rejecting the idea of contagion,[7] believing plague was God's ordained form of punishment (or blessing), from which there was no point in seeking refuge at another location. Three decades earlier, it was Michael Dols who, in the first major study of Muslim soci-

7 Justin Stearns, *Infectious Ideas: Contagion in Premodern Islamic and Christian Thought in the Western Mediterranean* (Baltimore: Johns Hopkins University Press, 2011), 69–76, 85–89. For a good summary of the different approaches to flight among Muslim scholars, see Stearns, "New Directions in the Study of Religious Responses to the Black Death," *History Compass* 7, no. 5 (2009): 1363–75.

ety's response to plague, argued for a direct link between the interdictions against flight found in the plague literature, and people's behavioral patterns. During epidemics, he noted, there was great social chaos in Egyptian cities, city streets were filled with beggars and the bodies of the dead, and funerals constantly took place. The Muslim inhabitants of cities were obsessed with ritual purity, attending prayers at the mosque daily, where they confronted updated lists of those who had died the previous day, and prepared their own wills for their imminent death. Supplications for lifting the plague were held everywhere, either in mosques or outside in the streets or the desert.[8] Dols acknowledged some people fled epidemic areas, but claimed they were a small minority. Overall, the question if we could "really explain the apparently pacific, collective and controlled Muslim reaction ... as largely the result of theoretical theological principles" was a clear yes: "we are struck by the fact that the interpretations and arguments of the Muslim jurists take fuller cognizance of the beliefs and practices of their community" than comparable arguments made in Christian-European plague treatises. In other words, Dols believed that in the Muslim world religion was a very potent force in determining people's reactions to the plague.[9]

Later works did little to challenge Dols's conclusions. In his study of plague in the Ottoman Empire in the eighteenth and nineteenth centuries, Daniel Panzac maintained that religion was a key component in people's conduct during natural disasters. Thus Muslims accepted the plague with utter fatalism, whereas Christians and Jews fled cities when they felt it was no longer safe to remain.[10] Panzac did not overlook other factors that might have affected people's reactions to plague, such as their economic situation. Yet he found that economic factors were secondary to religious ones: the poor among Christians and Jews, who were inclined to flee, usually stayed behind. The same could not be said about Muslims, who believed in predestination rather than contagion, and thus took no precautions regardless of their material fortunes. For Panzac, therefore, religious identity was the primary factor dividing a city's population during catastrophes as in any other time.[11]

Heath Lowry also discussed the link between religion and people's attitude to epidemics. He argued that Ottoman attitudes toward flight changed sometime

---

8 Michael Dols, *The Black Death in the Middle East* (Princeton: Princeton University Press, 1977), 236–54, 22–25, 172–75, 292–93.

9 Ibid., 298–99.

10 Daniel Panzac, *La peste dans l'empire ottoman, 1700–1850* (Leuven, Belgium: Peeters, 1985), 283–86, 300–1.

11 Ibid., 301–11.

between the reigns of Mehmed II (r. 1451–81) and Süleyman I (r. 1520–66). The former avoided plague-ridden areas by rerouting his campaign trail; the latter refused to abandon the palace or allegedly let others flee the capital, even when members of his household were dying of plague. Although the Muslim tradition clearly distinguished between entering a plague-infected area and refusing to leave one,[12] Lowry understood the supposedly different approach to flight by the Empire's changing religious orientation of the early sixteenth century. It was the conquest of the Arab world (1516–17), thus Lowry, that had changed the Empire from being a pluralistic polity that integrated several cultures and faiths, to a Muslim empire. In their new form, the Ottomans adopted a rather fatalistic approach to disease, so flight was no longer an acceptable option.[13] Lowry thus saw religion as a key to explaining people's responses to plague even though other political or social considerations could have led Ottoman rulers to change their minds about flight. This was clearly evident in the testimony of Busbecq from sixteenth-century Istanbul—the source upon which Lowry relies for Süleyman's period—where the same sultan first denounced flight but later condoned it, due to changing political circumstances.[14]

Historians' conclusion about Muslim society's attitude toward plague, namely that most people did not flee plague-affected areas, made some sense given the sources they used: plague treatises, chronicles, and reports by Europeans visiting the Middle East. Treatises reflected theoretical, normative responses to plague rather than actual reactions. The Muslim authors of treatises and chronicles in Arabic and Turkish—jurists, physicians, or historians—by virtue of their literacy, belonged to a small group of educated men, who until the nineteenth century received their training in religious schools (*madrasa*). A pious outlook informed their writing, and that was also true when discussing plagues and responses to them: it would not be unreasonable to assume they emphasized measures taken during epidemic outbreaks that were consonant with the faith, while being dismis-

12 Most Muslim jurists argued choosing not to enter a place already infected by plague – unlike leaving one – was permissible (Stearns, *Infectious Ideas*, 25–36).

13 Heath Lowry, "Pushing the Stone Uphill: The Impact of Bubonic Plague on Ottoman Urban Society in the Fifteenth and Sixteenth Centuries," *The Journal of Ottoman Studies* 23 (2004), 93–132, especially 128–30. There was a fundamental difference between Mehmed II's response to the plague and that of Süleyman, which Lowry did not draw attention to: while Süleyman proscribed escaping from the plague, Mehmed II merely avoided entering plague-stricken cities.

14 Ogier Ghiselin de Busbecq, *The Turkish Letters of Ogier Ghiselin de Busbecq, Imperial Ambassador at Constantinople, 1554–1562, translated from the Latin of the Elzevir Edition of 1663* by Edward Seymour Forster (Baton Rouge: Louisiana State University Press, 2005), 182–83.

sive toward acts that could not, in their view, improve one's chances of survival, such as flight.[15] The reports in Arab chronicles about religious measures, such as mass prayers, do not necessarily indicate that religious identity dictated response to plague. They merely suggest that piety played a major part in the reactions of many, not that it was the sole principle dictating how people would behave when facing a major epidemic. Furthermore, since the accounts in chronicles deal primarily with Muslims, they do not reveal whether Muslims were more inclined, or less so, to participate in religious rituals than non-Muslims. For all we know, during plague epidemics Christians and Jews took part in interfaith prayers and other ceremonies as often as Muslims.[16] Thus the testimonies found in such sources do not allow us to conclude what part religious beliefs played in shaping people's decision whether to flee a plague-ridden area. Participating in mass prayers and demonstrations, caring about ritual purity, or registering wills and dedicating *waqf*s, were common measures that did not exclude other forms of reaction: one could follow such rituals and yet flee the city, his or her departure having little to do with religious identity.

Europeans writing about Ottoman society often betrayed their scorn for Muslims, typically seeing them as uneducated religious bigots with strange, if fascinating, manners and customs. Short-term visitors to the Empire often resorted to sweeping generalizations about the societies they described, which were based on their brief experiences and previous knowledge they had acquired about Islam and the Middle East, often from reading accounts of earlier travelers.[17] Thus, learning that Islam in general proscribed flight from plague and unaware of debates among Muslim jurists on the issue, they were prone to ascribe a fatalistic behavior to all Muslims in times of plague. And as they were usually unable to tell Muslims from non-Muslims,[18] European observers were likely to refer to all those who did

---

15 See Ibn Taghri Birdi and al-Maqrizi's description of the Black Death as quoted by Dols (Dols, *Black Death*, 241–50), and comparable eighteenth-century descriptions of plague epidemics in Aḥmad al-Budayrī, *Ḥawādith dimashq al-yawmiyya* (Cairo: Al-Jamʿiyya al-Miṣriyya, 1959), 34, 49, 180, 186, 222–3; and Muḥammad ibn Kannān, *Yawmiyyāt shāmiyya* (Damascus: Dār al-Ṭabbaʿ, 1994), 54, 61–64, 197, 299.

16 Dols provided an account of Muslims, Christians, and Jews in Cairo conducting a mass public prayer during the Black Death (Dols, *Black Death*, 251); for another example, see Bernard Heyberger, *Les chrétiens du Proche-Orient au temps de la réforme catholique: Syrie, Liban, Palestine, XVIIe–XVIIIe siècles* (Rome: Ecole Française de Rome, 1994), 527–28.

17 For more on European travelers and how they engaged with Middle Eastern society, see: Sonja Brentjes, "The Interests of the Republic of Letters in the Middle East, 1550–1700," *Science in Context* 12, no. 3 (1999): 435–68.

18 Abraham Marcus showed that differences between Muslims and non-Muslims, although

not flee (or seek confinement) as one, and to attribute such immobility to Islam. Knowing most inhabitants of Ottoman cities were Muslims, the logical conclusion for a European visitor with a patently superficial notion on Muslim society in general and its attitudes to plagues in particular would be that Muslims facing plague did not take meaningful measures such as preemptive steps as one would take in Europe. Examples for such understanding of plague among Muslims abound.[19] Especially revealing of the lack of understanding of Muslim society among European travelers is the seventeenth-century visitor Jean du Mont's testimony, which borrowed Christian motifs to explain why Muslims did not flee plague areas: "when God designs to execute the fury of his vengeance on obstinate sinners, he sends an army of black angels to destroy 'em. They [Muslims] add, that every angel receives a bow and two sorts of arrows, to inflict either death or sickness, with orders to shoot their mortal arrows at those whom they find under the power of sin, and to direct the others at such who are only tainted with some pollution." Du Mont ascribed the relatively high survival rates to "white angels" who fought on behalf of the believers against the "black angels."[20] Overall, therefore, such perspectives are of little value to the historian trying to probe the question of flight from plagues.

Testimonies of foreigners who for years or even decades resided in the Empire, however, may be quite credible for our purpose. Diplomats, missionaries, and merchants who stayed in the Empire long term learned local languages, interacted with the indigenous population, developed ties with provincial governors and urban notables, and even assimilated into Muslim society. Their insights into Ottoman society would therefore be more complex. Laurent d'Arvieux (1635–1702), a French traveler and diplomat who spent over three decades in North Africa and

clear to Ottoman city inhabitants, were often too subtle to be noticed by the outside observer (Abraham Marcus, *The Middle East on the Eve of Modernity: Aleppo in the Eighteenth Century* (New York: Columbia University Press, 1989), 41–48).

19 See, for example: George Sandys, *A Relation of a Journey Begun An. Dom. 1610* (London: Ro. Allot, 1632), 38; Corneille Le Bruyn, *Voyage au Levant: c'est-à-dire, dans les principaux endroits de l'Asie Mineure, dans les isles de Chio, Rhodes, Chypre, &c.* (Paris: Jean-Baptiste-Claude Bauche, 1725), 1: 447; Edward Brown, *The Travels and Adventures of Edward Brown, Esq.* (London: J. Applebee, 1739), 405–6; H. G. O. Dwight, *Memoir of Mrs. Elizabeth B. Dwight Including an Account of the Plague of 1837* (New York: M. W. Dodd, 1840), 7.

20 Jean du Mont, *A New Voyage to the Levant Containing an Account of the Most Remarkable Curiosities in Germany, France, Italy, Malta, and Turkey* (London: M. Gillyflower, 1696), 258–59. For a discussion of this belief in Ottoman sources, see Nükhet Varlık, *Plague and Empire in the Early Modern Mediterranean World: The Ottoman Experience, 1347–1600* (Cambridge: Cambridge University Press, 2015), 237–38.

the Levant in the seventeenth century,[21] and the English brothers and physicians Alexander and Patrick Russell, who in the eighteenth century lived in Aleppo for 14 and 18 years respectively, are obvious examples.[22] Yet even a much shorter stay of eight years was sufficient to obtain a closer view. John Covel (1638–1722), an English priest who traveled extensively in the Empire and served as interim ambassador in Istanbul, knew Islam prohibited flight from plague. But witnessing an epidemic in Edirne, he admitted reality was more complex than certain religious expectations:

> The best sort of people fled to other places, as the Turkes likewise themselves did from Adrianople to their houses here, for that same is a story that they are not afraid of the plague, because their fortunes are wrote "in their forehead;" for all fled, but such as were poor, or had offices about Court, and could not get away. There dyed that year about 100 persons out of the Vizier's own house; and really, those that are forc't to stay by it value it no more then we do an ague. But this is the same amongst Jewes, Greeks, Armenians, and every body else ... All slaves and poor people, so soon as they are dead, are wrapt in some pittiful covering (perhaps nothing but an old mat), and so laid upon a Hamal's or porter's back, and caryed away to his grave, without any more adoe. Infinites of Turkes came out of the Town and lived in Tents, as well as we; yet many Turkes came or sent out their women to their countrey houses there.[23]

Covel thus suggested one's economic status and various other commitments determined reaction to plague more than one's faith. Similar depictions of fleeing people of all faiths, including many Muslims, are found in other European and Ottoman sources.[24] European historians of the Empire also shared this perspec-

---

21 D'Arvieux's memoirs were published posthumously in six volumes: Laurent d'Arvieux, *Mémoires du chevalier d'Arvieux* (Paris: C. J. B. Delespine, 1735).

22 For the Russell brothers, see: Maurits van den Boogert, *Aleppo Observed: Ottoman Syria through the Eyes of Two Scottish Doctors, Alexander and Patrick Russell* (Oxford: Oxford University Press, 2010).

23 J. Theodore Bent, *Early Voyages and Travels in the Levant* (London: Hakluyt Society, 1893), 244.

24 Evliya Çelebi's ten-volume travelogue that spans over fifty years cites many instances of Muslims and non-Muslims fleeing plague and other disaster areas (Evliya Çelebi, *Evliya Çelebi Seyahatnâmesi* (Istanbul: Yapı Kredi Yayınları, 1994–2007), 1: 187, 7: 50, 189, 234, 8: 97, 137, 154, 162, 301, 9: 59, 95). Other examples include a report on Muslims arriving in Damascus in 1632 after leaving Aleppo during a plague (Ferdinan Tawtal, *Wathāʾiq taʾrīkhiyya ʿan ḥalab* (Beirut: al-Maṭbaʿa al-Kathulikiyya, 1958–63), 1: 11–14); and a French diplomat's observation of people from many cities and faiths deserting their homes during a famine in

tive. In 1686, historian and diplomat Paul Rycaut (also Ricaut, 1629–1700), who worked in the British embassy in Istanbul and later as consul in İzmir, argued that well-off Turks usually ignored the advice to stay, and left the city for their vacation homes in the countryside, to return only after the plague subsided.[25] A century later, the French historian Elias Habesci explained that if in the past Muslims would not flee the plague, in his time many in fact did, especially those who had the means.[26]

Such testimonies do not conclusively prove that faith and religious expectations were not factors in determining people's behavior during life-threatening situations. They suggest, however, that the link between religious theory and practice was rather weak, and that we need to consider other explanations for people's responses to plagues. In addition, they indicate that flight was not a form of response reserved almost exclusively for non-Muslims. This conclusion in itself is not new: Sam White has noted in a recent article that many "Ottomans did often take active measures to confront infection,"[27] namely flight. Yet I mention this conclusion here because it still leaves two questions unresolved: Muslims fled plague epidemics, but how common such a reaction was? And, what were the motivations for abandoning one's home and town beyond religious beliefs or possible economic considerations?

One way to address these questions is to assume that Muslims indeed fled from plague more than we had previously thought, but that the connection between the advice given in plague treatises and people's actions remained relatively strong. That is, people had mostly followed the advice of Muslim jurists regarding desired conduct in such situations, but it was the advice that had changed over the years. For example, Nükhet Varlık suggested an increase in the number of works by Ottoman jurists who justified flight from plague areas on Islamic legal grounds in the fifteenth and sixteenth centuries.[28] Even though the concurrent change in Muslim jurists' opinions and people's responses to plague might have been coincidental—after all, most Ottoman subjects did not read those legal opinions—it is not entirely unlikely that popular perceptions with regard to plague had changed

1757 (Marseille, Archives de la Chambre de Commerce et d'Industrie (ACCM), J 914, report dated 1 September 1757). See also the cases discussed in White, *Climate*, 178–79, 254–58.

25 Paul Rycaut, *The History of the Present State of the Ottoman Empire* (London: Charles Brome, 1686), 219–21.

26 Elias Habesci, *The Present State of the Ottoman Empire* (London: R. Baldwin, 1784), 417–18.

27 White, "Rethinking Disease in Ottoman history," *International Journal of Middle East Studies* 42 (2010), 4: 553–61, quotation from 561.

28 Varlık, *Plague and Empire*, 242–45.

over time. Plague treatises must have reflected common notions about disease to some degree.[29] Yet they do not offer conclusive evidence of the type that would enable us to argue that flight was "the most common precaution people took in the Empire to ward off plague" or that "most Ottoman subjects understood plague as a naturally occurring phenomenon that required a physical response; namely, leaving the area," as one historian has recently suggested.[30]

In fact, judging by evidence found in Ottoman documents, flight seems to have been the resort of a small segment of a typical city's population. For example, in 1699 plague killed most of the people in Edirne's Cisr Mustafa Pasha neighborhood; only a few fled from there.[31] A report from the same year regarding plague that had hit the province of İpsala (about 120 km south of Edirne), accounted for 18 individuals who would not be able to pay their taxes, of whom only 5 had fled.[32] A letter sent from Ormenio, a village in the *sanjak* of Çirmen (on the Greek-Bulgarian-Turkish border) in 1708, asked for reassessment of taxes because most of the people in the *sanjak*'s villages had died of plague; of the survivors, only a small share had fled to other places.[33] Petitions written by provincial *qadi*s and sent to Istanbul also create the impression that during plague epidemics most people did not flee. A 1660 petition sent from Boyalıca, a village in the province of Göynük, asked for tax adjustment, as most of the village's residents had died in a plague, while those who had remained were too poor to pay their tax bill; very few managed to leave the area.[34] Another petition from 1712 reported that most of the inhabitants of villages in the vicinity of Ankara had died in a plague epidemic, while very few escaped.[35] A similar account was sent to Istanbul about a plague and famine that had hit the area of Adana some time before 1763.[36] Admittedly, there were reports of mass flight from plague areas. Yet these were far and few

29 For more on this, see Varlık, "From '*Bête Noire*' to '*le Mal de* Constantinople': Plagues, Medicine, and the Early Modern Ottoman State," *Journal of World History* 24, no. 4 (2013): 741–70.

30 Birsen Bulmuş, *Plague, Quarantines and Geopolitics in the Ottoman Empire* (Edinburgh: Edinburgh University Press, 2012), 23–24.

31 Başbakanlık Osmanlı Arşivi (Prime Ministry's Ottoman Archives), Istanbul (BOA), İbnülemin Sıhhiye (İ.E. SH.), 138.

32 BOA, İ.E. SH., 107.

33 BOA, İ.E. Ensab, 737. For other examples, see: İ.E. SH., 134 (Erikli, 1652); İ.E. SH., 149 (Şehirköy, 1703); and Cevdet Askeriye, 37877 (Livadiye and İzdin, 1789).

34 BOA, Cevdet Sıhhiye, 1204.

35 BOA, İ.E. SH., 150.

36 BOA, Cevdet Dahiliye (C. DH.), 3112.

and were often instigated by external factors that prompted people to leave, such as riots or raids by Bedouins.[37] It therefore appears that flight, overall, was one among several common responses to plague, but probably not the one used by the majority of people.[38] Analyzing the different motivations for reactions to plague will further clarify why.

Factors Determining Response to Plague

Religious interdictions alone could not account for all responses to plague epidemics. As I mentioned earlier, economics significantly affected people's actions when facing danger. Studies on medieval and early modern European society have shown that the poor were always exposed to greater risks during disasters, suffered the most, and overall had fewer options facing plague than those who were better off.[39] For instance, during the Black Death of the mid-fourteenth century, the indigent were more susceptible to the outbreak of epidemics than others: they resided in filthy and unventilated houses, washed their clothes rarely, and did not frequent public baths. The plague ravaged poor neighborhoods first, and those living in them had no means to escape.[40] Quarantine, which became popular as a prevention method in European Mediterranean port cities by the fifteenth century, had a devastating effect on day laborers. Disrupting routine commercial activity by cutting off cities from the outside world, it reduced many to begging.[41] In later centuries, epidemics prompted authorities to enact regulations that limited the poor's prospects of earning a living, as was the case in Venice, where beggars were not allowed within city limits.[42] The connection between economic condition and

37 See, for example: BOA, Topkapı Sarayı Müzesi Arşivi Defterleri, 6955/0001/01 (1650s); Ali Emiri, Mustafa II, 350 (1699); Cevdet Maliye (C. ML.), 2005 (1706); İ.E. SH., 182 (1720); C.ML., 12456 (1783); and C. ML., 3047 (Perkuki and Rusçuk, 1795).

38 White, *Climate*, 1, 6, 11, 84–91; See also Mikhail, *Nature and Empire*, 75, 224, 283.

39 Jean-Noël Biraben, *Les hommes et la peste en France et dans les pays européens et méditerranéens* (Paris: Mouton, 1975), 1: 65, 158, 235–36, 244, 2: 83–84, 145–49; Joël Coste, *Représentations et comportements en temps d'épidémie dans la littérature imprimée de peste (1490–1725): contribution à l'histoire culturelle de la peste en France à l'époque moderne* (Paris: Honoré Champion, 2007), 499–555.

40 Michel Mollat, *The Poor in the Middle Ages: An Essay in Social History* (New Haven: Yale University Press, 1986), 193–97. See more on the connection between plague and the poor in Ann Carmichael, *Plague and the Poor in Renaissance Florence* (Cambridge: Cambridge University Press, 1986), 121–31.

41 Robert Jütte, *Poverty and Deviance in Early Modern Europe* (Cambridge: Cambridge University Press, 1994), 22–23.

42 Pullan, *Rich and Poor*, 249–51.

people's ability to withstand plague was apparent elsewhere too, such as in Ming and Qing China, Tokogawa Japan, and Mughal India.[43] Similarly, examples from the Middle East prove there was much correlation between one's economic status and his or her chances of surviving a plague epidemic.[44]

That economics affected responses to plagues is not in itself surprising. Panzac has already demonstrated the effects of people's economic status on their ability or willingness to flee plague areas.[45] There were other factors, however, that further suggest religious expectations or beliefs had little effect on people's reactions to plague. Sociologists and social psychologists studying human behavior during disasters have pointed to recurrent patterns of individual and collective reactions and have offered some illuminating explanations for them. Derived mostly from twentieth-century cases, their findings and observations may prove valuable for explaining responses to plagues in the Ottoman period as well.

Flight and Human Psychology

Until recently, the widely accepted understanding of human behavior under life-threatening situations relied on four basic assumptions, which also supports an interpretation of religious beliefs as a major force determining people's reactions to plague. The four assumptions were: "1. The typical response to danger is self-preservative aggression or flight ... 2. Flight is directed toward an objectively safe place, away from danger ... 3. Physical dangers are more disturbing or stressful than other kinds of events. 4. Flight is prevented from occurring in danger situations by social control."[46] The last point is of particular interest to us, because it implies that religion, as a form of social control, can hinder people from fleeing

43 Jennifer Downs, "Famine Policy and Discourses on Famine in Ming China, 1368–1644," PhD diss., University of Minnesota, 1995, 45–46; Li, *Fighting Famine*, 34–36; Maren Ehlers, "Poor Relief and the Negotiation of Local Order in Early Modern Japan," PhD diss., Princeton University, 2011, 274–75; C. M. Agrawal, *Natural Calamities and the Great Mughals* (Bodh Gaya, India: Kanchan Publications, 1983), 90–116.

44 European and Arab sources attribute behaviors considered to provide some protection from plague, namely confinement at home or flight, to wealthy individuals. Furthermore, the rich lived in sanitary quarters, and could afford to subsist without income for a while and hire servants to perform tasks on their behalf. See Ibn Kannān, *Yawmiyyāt*, 172–73; al-Budayrī, *Ḥawādith*, 54–55, 64–65, 155; ACCM, J 914, letter dated 3 March; Patrick Russell, *A Treatise of the Plague* (London: G. G. & J. Robinson, 1791), 336, 359–60; Alexander Russell, *The Natural History of Aleppo* (London: G. G. & J. Robinson, 1794), 2: 383–84.

45 Panzac, *Peste*, 303–10.

46 Anthony Mawson, *Mass Panic and Social Attachment: The Dynamics of Human Behavior* (Aldershot, UK: Ashgate, 2007), 236–37.

a plague-ridden area. It fits with earlier conclusions about plague in the Middle East, whereby Muslims usually followed the rules and norms of the social (i.e., religious) group, which explicitly precluded succumbing to a sense of danger. Thus panic was not likely, and neither was self-preservative aggression, or flight. Accordingly, the increase in the popularity of flight from plague, which recent studies have pointed to, could only have happened if religious attitudes toward flight changed as well. In light of recent developments in the field of disaster studies, however, such an interpretation is no longer sustainable.

Social scientists now largely reject the four assumptions mentioned above, offering explanations of attachment instead. The "attachment theory," originally developed by John Bowlby in the 1950s and 1960s, focuses on the instincts that drive people to establish strong bonds with particular others during childhood and the effects of these bonds throughout adulthood. Such ties are meant to address the needs, both physical and psychological, of securing protection for survival, especially in dangerous situations.[47] Accordingly, scholars have argued that human conduct under life-threatening situations is marked not by aggression or an urge for physical safety (as the first assumption above states), but rather by seeking social affiliation. Disaster studies have found that imminent danger boosted rather than reduced people's concern for their loved ones—the objects of their attachment—and the urge to protect them before fleeing. Psychologists have discovered that those who did flee a disaster-stricken area were either foreigners not attached to the place or individuals without families.[48] This pattern fits the testimonies of Patrick Russell, the physician who worked for the Levant Company in Aleppo in the mid-eighteenth century. In several cases, when one came down with the plague, family, servants, or students took care of the sick person and continued even when the disease spread to some of them. Only when the situation was clearly beyond control, or after the death of that person, did the family abandon the house.[49] In one instance, when the wife of a wealthy European Jew

47 John Bowlby, *Attachment and Loss* (New York: Basic Books, 1969); for more recent interpretations of attachment theory, see Joan Woodward, "Introduction to Attachment Theory," *Attachment and Human Survival*, Marci Green and Marc Scholes, eds. (London: Karnac, 2004), 7–20; Mario Mikulincer and Phillip Shaver, *Attachment in Adulthood: Structure, Dynamics, and Change* (New York: Guilford Press, 2007), 3–28.

48 Mawson, *Mass Panic*, 237–38; Beverley Raphael, *When Disaster Strikes: How Individuals and Communities Cope with Catastrophe* (New York: Basic Books, 1986), 47; Ronald Perry, "Disaster Preparedness and Response among Minority Citizens,"in Russell Dynes et al., eds., *Sociology of Disasters: Contribution of Sociology to Disaster Research* (Milan: Franco Angeli, 1987), 147.

49 Russell, *Plague*, 64, and the appendix, 3–7, 13–15, 68–69.

became ill, household members immediately fled, but her husband and a few of the personal servants refused to go.[50]

Regarding the second assumption—flight being directed toward an objectively safe place—scholars have shown that people often choose to leave for familiar places that are subjectively perceived to be safe rather than to remote and hence patently safe ones. The need for social affiliation (which increases one's sense of security) sometimes superseded the drive to escape to a remote place. People left along with other familiar persons, or sought them immediately upon arrival in the new location.[51] Examples from the Ottoman period suggest these findings are applicable to earlier periods as well: in sixteenth-century Damascus, and possibly also later, it was customary for some to leave the city in convoys when plague struck, and to reside in groups in neighboring villages.[52] People from Denizli resettled in the town's provinces, while others built temporary housing in its gardens after an earthquake shook the area in 1717.[53] Similarly, the earthquake that shattered that city in 1759 led Jewish, Christian, and Muslim families and friends to regroup in the gardens around the city.[54] And in 1822, after Aleppo was all but destroyed in a powerful quake, its fleeing residents gathered in one area on the city's outskirts, where they set up a temporary tent city.[55]

As for the third and fourth assumptions, regarding physical dangers and social control, observations of human conduct in dangerous or stressful situations have shown that physical threat was perceived as less distressing than separation from one's family, home, or neighborhood. Exploring issues of mental health (an intricate matter to study, let alone in an Ottoman context), scholars have found that physical damage was sometimes less detrimental to a victim's health than disruption of family bonds. This led to the understanding that a familiar environment, rather than some form of social control (such as religion), can potentially calm even the severest apprehension, while being alone or with strangers could worsen one's anxiety.[56] In view of these observations, Anthony Mawson has suggested that since most people are in familiar surroundings when disaster occurs, their

50 Ibid., 50–51.

51 Mawson, *Mass Panic*, 238.

52 Yoshiyah Pinto, *Nivḥar mi-kesef* (Aleppo: A. Sasson, 1869), 125.

53 BOA, C. ML., 31320.

54 Mīkhā'īl Burayk, *Ta'rīkh al-shām* (Damascus: Dār Qutayba, 1982), 78-80.

55 BOA, Hatt-ı Hümayun, 753, 753B; C. DH. 2619. For a similar response, particularly among the Jews of Aleppo, see Avraham ʿAntebi, *Sefer yoshev ohalim* (Jerusalem: Mekhon ha-Ktav, 1981), author's introduction.

56 Mawson, *Mass Panic*, 239–40.

expected behavior should be "affiliated bunching" rather than flight, that is, even when people do escape, they do so as a group. The only exception would be strangers or those without friends and family, who would be inclined to flee, seeking faraway familiar people and places. Thus, Mawson concluded, people's behavior during disasters tends to disregard societal conventions one would normally feel committed to follow.[57] In our context this may be a bit confusing, because a religious framework was sometimes one's only "familiar environment." Where this was so, one would expect to see a behavior compatible with religious expectations. Yet since communities were not segregated and many people were members of several, often competing social circles,[58] one cannot assume that the religious community was everyone's "familiar environment" in the psychological sense.

The "attachment theory" offers a possible interpretation of human behavior during plagues. Like other explanations, it does not account for all cases. One difficulty with using this theory to explain responses to plagues is that by definition the object of attachment itself may be an abstract idea rather than a person. Psychologists have noticed that for some people belief in God and a routine of religious practices formed bonds of relationship equivalent to those people have with each other.[59] One scholar has suggested that God could be perceived as a protective and caring parent, an "adequate attachment-figure."[60] "God 'really' is an attachment figure for many believers," Lee Kirkpatrick has argued,[61] suggesting that God offered believers a secure base that was always there even when other attachment figures were gone. Research has shown a rise in mental and physical wellbeing and a drop in anxiety among those who sought attachment with God during times of hardship.[62] Unlike bonds formed with God, believers did not usually develop comparable attachment to the clergy, as attachment by definition is formed with a *person*, not with the *role* the person fulfills; or to groups such as a religious congregation, which could not serve as objects of attachment.[63] Such

57 Ibid., 240–42.

58 Uriel Simonsohn, *A Common Justice: The Legal Allegiances of Christians and Jews under Early Islam* (Philadelphia: University of Pennsylvania Press, 2011), 5–10. Although this study covers the early Islamic period, one may assume its findings apply to Ottoman times as well.

59 Andrew Greeley, *The Religious Imagination* (Los Angeles: Sadlier, 1981), 18.

60 Gordon Kaufman, *The Theological Imagination: Constructing the Concept of God* (Philadelphia: Westminster Press, 1981), 67.

61 Lee Kirkpatrick, *Attachment, Evolution, and the Psychology of Religion* (New York: Guilford Press, 2005), 55.

62 Ibid., 61–74.

63 Ibid., 93–6; quotation from 94–95.

observations do not negate our basic view of Ottoman society as one in which nearly everyone believed in God, the omnipresent and the source of all natural phenomena. This was true of people from all religious groups. The level of trust in God and hence of attachment to Him obviously varied among Ottoman subjects; there were those whose deep attachment to God led them to avoid any action in the face of a looming danger. For the latter, this attachment, not religious principles, was the main factor that informed their behavior. It was plain and pure belief in and link with God that prompted some people to react the way they did, not a sophisticated analysis of ideas about epidemics discussed in scholarly works, to which most people had little exposure.

Some historians may wonder if the attachment theory, developed in the twentieth century and used to study twentieth-century cases, is applicable for Ottoman society. After all, human psychology is a function of social settings, cultures, ecologies, and environments as these affect the ways attachments are formed, and their quality.[64] One cannot help but wonder: were there factors that affected reaction to fear, the development of panic, or the formation of attachments that were universal and that characterized humans (and other mammals) in the centuries prior to the period of this study? It is hard to tell. Studies at the juncture of neuroscience and evolutionary biology indicate that attachments, in Bowlby's widely accepted definition, had existed among mammals, including humans, for millennia. Essentially all mammals share the basic neural systems supporting attachment-related behavior, which have evolved over millions of years.[65] But such findings only prove attachments were there from the very beginning, not how they were formed. Different people experience stress and fear differently. It is hard to say what situations triggered attachment-related behaviors among Ottoman urbanites.

One may reasonably assume, however, that the thought of imminent death or loss of relatives and friends was difficult for people living in a seventeenth- or eighteenth-century Ottoman city just as it is for us today. Patrick Russell's testimony of responses to quick and multiple deaths in Aleppo seems to confirm such sentiments: in June 1762, as deaths from plague in the city increased in intensity, the streets became deserted except for funeral processes, and "in the nights, the shrill voices of the women deploring their departed friends, were heard from all hands."[66] A *qadi* in Aleppo, who apparently understood the impact of such loud

---

64 Eliot Smith and Diane Mackie, *Social Psychology* (Philadelphia: Taylor & Francis, 2000), 3–13.

65 Jean Decety, "The Neuroevolution of Empathy," *Annals of the New York Academy of Sciences* 1231 (2011), 36–37.

66 Russell, *Plague*, 52.

cries of despair on public morale, instructed women following funeral processions to refrain from screaming, so people would not be "alarmed by the noise of frequent burials."[67] Likewise, the Italian traveler Giovanni Mariti reported cries of agony in the plague-ridden city of Aleppo coming out of houses.[68] It thus appears quite plausible, even with the meager historical evidence at hand, that the presence of disease and death would yield similar emotional reactions to those found among communities in the twentieth century. At the same time, it is equally likely that the frequent occurrence of disasters—plagues, as well as famines, earthquakes, floods, and fires—enhanced cohesion and a sense of "togetherness" among Ottoman urbanites. Thus with each calamity, attachments grew stronger and prompted people to stay and care for the sick, wounded, and homeless. Even when people did leave, they did so not only as detached individuals but also, as often, in groups that stuck together. This fits well with recent attachment explanations for disaster-induced behavior. Such theories supporting the relatively few cases of flight from plague would seem sounder than the one relying on the Muslim belief in predestination, or on the evolution of religious precepts to reject it.

Wider Implications for Ottoman Society

What insights may one gain from this new understanding of responses to plague? Historians have characterized Ottoman society as one in which religious identity was "the primary organizing principle."[69] Generally, this assessment holds. Muslims fulfilled all key political and judiciary positions, from the sultan down to provincial governors and judges. Serving in the army was also limited to Muslims, as was, with some variations over time and place, access to services such as public baths, soup kitchens, and hospitals. Non-Muslims thus seem to have been, in many aspects, second-class subjects.[70]

If the exclusion of non-Muslims from positions of power reflected conventions of social division within Ottoman society, one would expect similar findings

67 Ibid., 49.

68 Giovanni Mariti, *Travels Through Cyprus, Syria and Palestine: with a General History of the Levant* (Dublin: Messrs. P. Byrne and A. Grueber, 1792), 284.

69 M. Şükrü Hanioğlu, *A Brief History of the Late Ottoman Empire* (Princeton: Princeton University Press, 2008), 25; see also Marcus, *Eve of Modernity*, 39–48; Gül Akyılmaz, "Osmanlı Devletinde Reaya Kavramı ve Devlet-Reaya İlişkileri," in Güler Eren, ed., *Osmanlı* (Ankara: Yeni Türkiye Yayınları, 1999), 4: 40–54.

70 For an overview of the status of non-Muslims in the Ottoman Empire, see Bruce Masters, *Christians and Jews in the Ottoman Arab World: the Roots of Sectarianism* (New York: Cambridge University Press, 2001), 16–40.

when examining the state's handling of natural disasters, from plague epidemics to earthquakes. Accordingly, the state would prioritize Muslims in food allocation, reassessing of taxes, or rebuilding a city destroyed in a fire or earthquake in ways that would primarily benefit Muslims. Evidence, however, suggests otherwise. In a study about the earthquakes and plagues that hit Ottoman Syria in 1759–62, I have shown that the state's intervention, primarily its plans to rebuild sections of the city, reflected an array of interests that had little to do with a Muslim–non-Muslim dichotomy or with emphasizing the Islamic character of the state. The preservation of sultanic patronage and prestige, as well as a concern for privacy, were the values driving the state to take action; in most cases, Jews and Christians were eligible to receive support from the state just like Muslims were.[71] Admittedly, a religious agenda did at times prompt the state to act in the aftermath of disasters, such as after the Great Fire in Istanbul of 1660, when the evacuation of Jews from Eminönü allowed for the building of the New Mosque (*Yeni Cami*).[72] Yet such actions seem to have been the exception rather than the norm in Ottoman post-disaster recovery efforts, as many other cases demonstrate.[73]

To be sure, Islamic principles were always at the background of state action in the face of calamities, and it was so even when these actions were motivated by practical or pragmatic concerns unrelated to religious matters. It is difficult to explain Ottoman state activities in the seventeenth and eighteenth centuries without reference to Islam. Yet an Islamic identity, which led to occasional harassing of non-Muslims, did not necessitate systematic discrimination against them, or prevent Jews and Christians from being well integrated into Ottoman society. The ability to rule in the name of Islam while assimilating members of other religious groups was part of the heritage of tolerance and inclusiveness the Ottomans had developed in the fourteenth and fifteenth centuries, when there was still a Muslim minority governing Christians.[74] The various considerations that dictated individ-

71 Ayalon, "Ottoman Urban Privacy," 513–28.

72 Marc Baer, "The Great Fire of 1660 and the Islamization of Christian and Jewish Space in Istanbul," *International Journal of Middle East Studies* 36, no. 2 (2004): 159–81.

73 Reassessing taxes after a plague or famine hit an area was common practice, and when it happened, Muslims and non-Muslims alike benefitted from the lower rates. For examples of such cases, see Coşkun Yılmaz and Necdet Yılmaz, eds., *Osmanlılarda Sağlık* (Istanbul: Biofarma, 2006), 2: 218–29. Similarly, food distribution to the poor during famines did not usually target only Muslims (e.g., Aleppo, 1696, *Kāmil bin Ḥusayn al-Ghazzī, Kitāb nahr al-dhahab fī taʾrīkh ḥalab* (Aleppo: Dār al-Qalam al-ʿArabī, 1992), 3: 229; Damascus, 1757, ACCM, J914, letter dated 1 September 1757).

74 Heath Lowry, *The Nature of the Early Ottoman State* (Albany: SUNY Press, 2003), 66–67, 93; and Lowry, *The Shaping of the Ottoman Balkans, 1350–1550: The Conquest, Settlement*

ual and state reactions to plague and other disasters only exemplify wider trends in the relatively inclusive society the Ottomans had created: one in which religious identity was important, but for many people not the central defining principle.

Yaron Ayalon (yayalon@bsu.edu) is Assistant Professor of History at Ball State University in Muncie, Indiana. He is a historian of the Ottoman Empire and the early modern Middle East in general. He is the author of *Natural Disasters in the Ottoman Empire: Plague, Famine, and Other Misfortunes* (Cambridge University Press, 2015) and several other articles, and has served as an editor for *The Encyclopedia of Jews in the Islamic World.*

and Infrastructural Development of Northern Greece (Istanbul: Bahçeşehir University Publications, 2008), 16–64, especially 35–39.

PLAGUE IN EIGHTEENTH-CENTURY CAIRO: IN SEARCH OF BURIAL AND MEMORIAL SITES

EDNA BONHOMME
Princeton University

Unmarked Site, Epidemics and Mass Burial: Fieldwork of the Dead

"Utopias are sites with no real place."— Michel Foucault[1]

In March 1791, a plague outbreak that "exceeded all limits of excess" in Cairo and its surrounding towns resulted in an "uncounted number of babies and boys, and girls, maidservants and slaves, Mamluks and soldiers, inspectors and amirs died from it."[2] As the disease waxed and waned within the city, the cities of Cairo and Giza had a mortuary problem where some groups were memorialized and others lacked commemoration. An eyewitness to the epidemic, ʿAbd al-Raḥmān al-Jabartī (d. 1825), the author of the renowned chronicle *ʿAjāʾib al-āthār fī al-tarājim wa al-akhbār*, remarked: "Likewise marines and Albanians stationed in Bulaq, Old Cairo, and Giza [died], so that they were digging pits for those in Giza near the mosque of Abū Hurairah and throwing them in it."[3] Within his chronology, al-Jabartī listed a range of epidemics and natural disasters, including but not limited to fevers, floods, and fires.[4] He proclaimed that thousands and thousands died from the plague by walking us through their life and death. His contemporary al-Khashshāb estimated that approximately 1,000 to 2,000 people died daily during the 1791 outbreak, which would mean that approximately 30,000 to 60,000 of Cairo's 600,000 inhabitants perished.[5] Whether one accepts these figures or

1 Michel Foucault, "Of Other Spaces," *Diacritics* 16, no. 1 (1986): 22–27, quote on 24.

2 ʿAbd al-Raḥmān al-Jabartī, *ʿAjāʾib al-āthār fī al-tarājim wa al-akhbār* (Cairo: Lajnat al-Bayān al-ʿArabī, 1958), Microfilm from Dār al-Kutub al-Miṣriyya.

3 Ibid.

4 For a thorough account of eighteenth-century references to biological and natural disasters in Egypt, refer to Alan Mikhail, *Nature and Empire in Ottoman Egypt: An Environmental History* (Cambridge: Cambridge University Press, 2011).

5 Al-Jabartī, *ʿAjāʾib al-āthār*; Ismāʿīl al-Khashshāb, *Khulāṣat mā yurād min akhbār al-amīr Murād* (Cairo: Al-Maktaba al-Taʾrīkhiyya, 1992 [1801]). In addition to al-Jabartī's reference, I referred to the following records stating that there was an outbreak. Archives Nationale de France, Alexandrie, BI 114, 28 avril 1791. For a secondary account of the demographics of the plague, see Daniel Panzac, *La peste dans l'empire ottoman, 1700–1850* (Leuven: Peeters, 1985).

not, they are a marker for aggregating the "extraordinary" through numbers and venerating a disease as an epidemic.

In addition, the year 1791 was exceptional because it points to the fragility of burial practices during an epidemic. Yet what makes the aforementioned excerpt unusual is that al-Jabartī catalogued the fractures in the bereavement during a moment of crisis. Understanding the author, the event, and the society can allow one to problematize eighteenth-century Egyptian hierarchy of memorialization. I argue that plague is an integral part of understanding that discourse. The plague has a metaphorical and practical function in that it offers a cultural, demographic, and political history of death in eighteenth-century Egypt.[6] The soldiers, Albanians, and slaves who were dumped in the pit do not have a plaque commemorating their death. In contrast, one of the more famous plague victims of 1791, the governor of Cairo Ismail Bey, and his colleagues had special forms of memorialization. These men were provided with elaborate memorial sites including a mausoleum at al-Qarafa (most commonly referred to by non-Egyptians as the City of the Dead).[7] I would like to use this isolated reference to understand the ways that history of science can incorporate the "losers" of burial practices by delving into textual depictions of the urban poor, and then move on to the "winners" of the history that are documented through material history.

For the sake of transparency, I seek to make clear that my decision to explore this topic emerges from a minor, "unimportant" detail and constructing a narrative around the events. I seek to layer al-Jabartī's reference to the pit by considering how the memorialized like Ismail Bey, and the forgotten like the unnamed in the pit, exist within Egypt's imaginary sphere. One way to grasp this history is to examine the ways that historians and literary scholars have generated narratives for the voiceless.[8]

---

6 Various scholars have looked at the bubonic plague in Egypt. See Michael Dols, *The Black Death in the Middle East* (Princeton: Princeton University Press, 1977); Mikhail, "The Nature of Plague in Late Eighteenth-Century Egypt," *Bulletin of History of Medicine* 82, no. 2 (2008): 249–75; Mikhail, "Plague and Environment in Late Ottoman Egypt," in *Water on Sand: Environmental Histories of the Middle East and North Africa*, ed. Alan Mikhail (Oxford: Oxford University Press, 2012), 111–31; Panzac, *La peste*; André Raymond, "Les grandes épidémies de peste au Caire aux XVIIe et XVIIIe siècles," *Bulletin d'études orientales* 25 (1972): 203–10.

7 For more information on al-Qarafa, see Hani Hamza, *The North Cemetery of Cairo* (Cairo: The American University in Cairo Press, 2001); D. Sims, *Understanding Cairo: The Logic of a City Out of Control* (Oxford: Oxford University Press, 2011); Jeffrey A. Nedoroscik, *The City of the Dead: A History of Cairo's Cemetery Communities* (Westport, CT: Greenwood Publishing, 1997).

8 Gayatri Chakravorty Spivak, "Can the Subaltern Speak?," in *Marxism and the Interpretation of Culture*, ed. Cary Nelson and Lawrence Grossberg (Urbana: University of Illinois Press, 1988).

As such, I will work more deeply with the sources I accessed to lay out the built environment and the people who came to witness mass death during the 1791 epidemic. Thus the intervention in the historiography is multifold; it will outline (1) the relationship between social status and memorialization; (2) how officials and everyday people adjust to epidemics; and (3) the ways that death rituals are a methodological practice.

Historians of the Ottoman Empire and Egypt have tackled the ways that plague impacted the demographic, environmental, and geopolitical elements of the region.[9] Nükhet Varlık suggests that the changing perceptions of the disease that emerged during the sixteenth century were part of a burgeoning conception of "public health."[10] Auxiliary to this point, discovering the ways that pre-modern actors understand health and medicine is incorporating a multitude of sources and perspectives into the Ottoman history of medicine. In a recent article, Sam White provides a revisionist approach to the historiography and argues that historians should provide an interdisciplinary perspective on the history of medicine in the Ottoman Empire. If one is to accept this trend to re-interpret the sources and use more material, then the 1791 event can be an opportunity to further understand how one traces the fine line between plague and death so as to reflect on the non-elite people who were often consigned to the backdrop of history.

By looking at the relationship between plague and burial practices of its named and unnamed victims in Egypt, one can begin to re-conceptualize memorialization at such moments of crisis. The soldiers, Albanians, and slaves who were dumped in the pit do not have a plaque commemorating their death. Although they are only known through a fleeting reference from a late eighteenth-century Egyptian historian, their current invisibility opens room for a new historical interpretation. What would it mean if the local residents reclaimed this space and made the invisible visible? This matters because we can begin to create an archive for the poor and develop a "banquet for the dead" that not only lists the Egyptian pashas or the Ottoman beys but also explicates the urban poor who were stricken with plague.[11]

---

9 Raymond, "Les grandes épidémies de peste"; Birsen Bulmuş, *Plague, Quarantines and Geopolitics in the Ottoman Empire* (Edinburgh: Edinburgh University Press, 2012); Mikhail, "The Nature of Plague."

10 Nükhet Varlık, *Plague and Empire in the Early Modern Mediterranean World: The Ottoman Experience, 1347–1600* (Cambridge: Cambridge University Press, 2015), chapter 8.

11 I am using the term "banquet of the dead" in the manner that Walter Benjamin uses it in his *The Arcades Project*. In this particular way, he sought to make a clear connection between history and its reverence for people who have died.

The History and the Historiography Unearthed

"We have called history 'the science of men.' That is still far too vague. It is necessary to add: 'of men in time.' The historian does not think of the human in the abstract. His thoughts breathe freely the air of the climate of time."— Marc Bloch[12]

Late eighteenth-century Cairo was a political nucleus of the Ottoman Empire, and plague was interwoven within the empire's commercial and political matrix.[13] By the time the 1791 plague broke out, Sultan Selim III (r. 1789–1807) ruled over the empire and delegated governors to regulate various provinces.[14] Beys and pashas were de-facto tax collectors and planners who could develop land or order people to move at will; they accomplished this by regulating tax farms (*iltizām*) and coordinating land tenure.[15] Given the power of these officials their potential to disrupt local configurations was quite great. The Ottoman Egyptian political climate "brought about a diffusion of power at the centre, at the court of the sultan, while matters that did not affect the entire empire directly would increasingly be left to the local elites."[16] The late eighteenth-century was a moment when denizens were vying for the coveted governor position. As historian Zeinab Abul-Magd remarks, "with the plague and Mamluk oppression in Upper Egypt, the subaltern rebellion became a daily practice of the inhabitants of towns, villages, and mountains, in the deserts."[17] Her study shows how the urban and rural poor were challenging their local leaders through coordinated and spontaneous political actions. One act of resistance was refusing to pay taxes or demanding the resignation of their leaders. The 1780s were a period of revolts between various *agha*s and the pashas that resulted in the internal exile of Murad and Ibrahim Bey who were Mamluk beys vying for power during the late eighteenth century.[18] In a letter dated 25 August

---

12 Marc Bloch, *The Historian's Craft* (Manchester: Manchester University Press, 1992), 23.

13 Nelly Hanna and Raouf Abbas, eds., *Society and Economy in Egypt and the Eastern Mediterranean, 1600–1900* (Cairo: The American University in Cairo Press, 2005), 11. Also see Zeinab Abul-Magd, *Imagined Empires: A History of Revolt in Egypt* (Berkeley: University of California Press, 2013), 40.

14 Stanford J. Shaw, *Between Old and New: The Ottoman Empire under Sultan Selim III, 1789–1807* (Cambridge, MA: Harvard University Press, 1971).

15 Lars Bjørneboe, *In Search of the True Political Position of the 'Ulama: An Analysis of the Aims and Perspectives of the Chronicles of Abd al-Rahman al-Jabartī (1753–1825)* (Aarhus: Aarhus University Press, 2007), 19.

16 Ibid., 18.

17 Ibid., 40.

18 Daniel Crecelius, *The Roots of Modern Egypt: A Study of the Regimes of Ali Bey al-Kabir*

1786, from British diplomat Robert Ainslie to the French administrator Marquis Carmarthen, they discussed the dissension among some of the Mamluk beys.[19] In particular, they pointed to the rebellion of a political surrender of Ibrahim Bey and Murad Bey and the eventual ascension of Ismail Bey to local power. Although plague was not the only issue that people were wrestling with, it was a concern for foreigners living in Egypt.

The plague outbreaks of the 1780s and 1790s had commercial and political consequences for the country. British and French administrators and travelers documented their accounts in Alexandria and Cairo by pointing to the intensity of the disease. John Antes, a British traveler had the following to say about the plague: "In the year 1781, the plague broke out about the middle of April, and increased with such rapidity and virulence, that sometimes one thousand people died of it in one day at Grand Cairo."[20] A French consular letter from March 1784 stated: "Le fléau de la peste...fait des ravages ici [Alexandrie] et à Rossette commence dit-on à faire du mal au Caire."[21] By the end of the year, the French consul was concerned about another outbreak and commented, "La maladie dure jusqu'en juin sans qu'on puisse juger de sa violence qui semble avoir été assez élevée, du moins au Caire."[22] In another instance of plague, British merchant George Baldwin writes: "From the very best authority it appears that, on the Captain Pasha's arrival at Alexandria, he found that the troops collected at Damascus, the different parts of Syria had been delayed in their march to Egypt by the severe ravages of the contagion; that only a few of the transports with the troops collected from his expedition."[23] These accounts strongly suggest that the plague occurred at multiple times and with negative results. This dovetails with al-Jabartī's claims about power and rule in eighteenth-century Egypt.

---

and Muhammad Bey Abu al-Dhahab, 1760–1775 (Minneapolis: Bibliotheca Islamica, 1981).

19 British Library, India Office of Records G/17/6.

20 John Antes, *Observations on the Manners and Customs of the Egyptians, the Overflowing of the Nile and Its Effects; with Remarks on the Plague, and Other Subjects* (London: J. Stockdale, 1800), 44.

21 Lettre de Martin et Pelletier à Roux du 29 mars 1784, Archives National de France, ACCM, L IX 761.

22 Lettre du consul de France du 4 décembre 1784, Archives Nationales Affaires étrangères, B 113.

23 British Library, India Office of Records, G/17/6, 25 August 1786. In other sources within the India Office of Records, Baldwin provides point by point analysis on the political affairs in Egypt, with focus on the rebel beys (Murad and Ibrahim), Ismael Bey, the Russians, the French, and trade within the Red Sea.

At the beginning of the 1791 epidemic, Ismail Bey, governor of Cairo, died of the plague. Shortly after his death, he was buried in the Masoleum of ʿAli Bey with Ibrahim Kathuda near the tomb of Imam al-Shafiʿi in al-Qarafa.[24] However, Ibrahim and Murad Bey were challenging Ismail Bey's rule over the Ottoman Egyptian province.[25] Upon his death, they left Asyut and headed for Cairo to acquire the governor position.[26] By 17 September 1791, George Baldwin commented, "The Beys have regained their power. If the Porte are determined to expel them they must yield and then what will be the Governance of Egypt."[27] Although these disputes were important, it was not until Ismail Bey's death that Ibrahim Bey and Murad Bey could truly challenge the configuration. In order to understand the significance of this moment and al-Jabartī's reference to the mass burial, we must turn to the author himself and the context in which he was writing.

ʿAbd al-Raḥmān al-Jabartī and the Chronicle Tradition

> "The very beauty of history lies in that messiness, the fact that unless two versions of the same set of events can be imagined, there is no reason for the historian to take upon himself the authority of giving the true account of what really happened."— Wendy Warren[28]

ʿAbd al-Raḥmān al-Jabartī (d. 1825) stands as one of the renowned Egyptian chroniclers of the late eighteenth and early nineteenth century. [29] Although he wrote at a time when the chronological tradition was diminishing as a practice in Egypt, he was an erudite who was engaged within a thriving academic community and had access to a myriad of human and textual resources. Al-Jabartī was a

24 Ismail Bey, al-Qarafa Cemetery, the tomb of Ali Bey al-Kabir and Ismail Bey al-Kabir.

25 Jane Hathaway, *Al-Jabarti's History of Egypt* (Princeton: Markus Wiener Publishers, 2009), 141.

26 Al-Jabartī, *ʿAjāʾib al-āthār*, 297. A lesser-known scholar of his time, Ismāʿīl al-Khashshāb described similar events to al-Jabartī following Ismail Bey's death. See al-Khashshāb, *Khulāṣat mā yurād*.

27 British Library, India Office of Records G/17/6.

28 W. A. Warren, "'The Cause of Her Grief': The Rape of a Slave in Early New England," *The Journal of American History* 93, no. 4 (2007): 1031–1049, quote on 1049.

29 This university was founded in the tenth century and has continued to educate scholars since then. For an extensive account on the ulema class and its internal structure, see Madeline C. Zilfi, *The Politics of Piety: The Ottoman Ulema in the Postclassical Age (1600–1800)* (Minneapolis: Bibliotheca Islamica, 1988). As the oldest existing university in Egypt, al-Azhar plays an important role in establishing and debating formal Islamic pedagogy and practice.

Hanafi Sunni Muslim who came from a lineage of educated ulema. Under the guidance of Muḥammad al-Murtaḍā al-Zabīdī, he was instructed at the preeminent al-Azhar University, which was the prominent Islamic university in the region.[30] Over time, al-Jabartī assisted his mentor in collecting biographical material and composing sections of al-Murtaḍā's manuscripts.[31] As a de-facto research assistant for his mentor, he gathered the experience and skills to eventually conduct his work independently.

When al-Murtaḍā died from the plague (April 1791), al-Jabartī began working on his own chronology, *'Ajā'ib al-āthār*, in which he adopted a standard biographical format.[32] Al-Murtaḍā's untimely death was al-Jabartī's opportunity to become a serious historian. He completed the first three volumes of the chronicle at the beginning of 1805–6 and the fourth volume was not completed until 1821.[33] Given the date of composition, al-Jabartī's three volumes mostly covered late eighteenth-century Ottoman rule, the three-year French Occupation of Egypt, and Muḥammad 'Ali's rule (r. 1805–48) over Egypt.[34] Because of his vehement attacks against Muḥammad 'Ali, the governor of Egypt in the early nineteenth century, al-Jabartī's text was initially banned in Ottoman Egypt.[35] Nevertheless, *'Ajā'ib al-āthār* has been critical for historians who study late eighteenth and early nineteenth-century Egypt because it takes into account everyday life and extraordinary events.[36]

30 For information on the history of al-Azhar University, see Meir Hatina, *'Ulama' Politics and the Public Sphere: An Egyptian Perspective* (Salt Lake City: University of Utah Press, 2010).

31 David Ayalon, "al-Dj̲abartī," *EI2.*

32 C. Brockelmann, "Muḥammad Murtaḍā." *EI2.*

33 Al-Jabartī is said to have passed away between 1822–1826. According to David Ayalon and Edward Lane, there is some controversy of al-Jabartī's death. He was supposedly buried at Turbat al-Sahra cemetery. See Ayalon, "The Historian al-Jabartī and His Background," *Bulletin of the School of Oriental and African Studies* 23, no. 2 (1960): 217–49.

34 Al-Jabartī's chronicle circulated before it was published and E. W. Lane, a nineteenth-century Orientalist, claims that he possessed a manuscript in 1837. Muḥammad 'Ali was an Albanian governor who ruled over Egypt. The standard narrative in the historiography is that he modernized Egypt. For an analysis and critique of that historiography refer to Khaled Fahmy, *All the Pasha's Men: Mehmed Ali, His Army, and the Making of Modern Egypt* (Cambridge: Cambridge University Press, 1997).

35 Some historians have claimed that al-Jabartī's work was banned because he criticized Muḥammad 'Ali and his regime. While this list is not exhaustive, some of the North American scholars who have used al-Jabartī's work include: Juan Cole, *Napoleon's Egypt: Invading the Middle East* (New York: Palgrave Macmillan, 2007); Mikhail, *Nature and Empire in Ottoman Egypt*; Nancy Elizabeth Gallagher, *Egypt's Other Wars: Epidemics and the Politics of Public Health* (Syracuse: Syracuse University Press, 1990); Hathaway, *Al-Jabarti's History of Egypt.*

36 Government and bureaucratic records were written in Ottoman Turkish. Late eighteenth-

Moreover, al-Jabartī's accounts about the plague complement the narratives of European travelers and merchants of the late eighteenth century. For example, British merchant George Baldwin's letters to Mr. Dunda on 4 July 1791 reads: "He has been confined for days on account of the Plague which still rages. It has almost annihilated the Mamluks, they have sought a reconciliation with the Porte which they will probably obtain till a fit opportunity presents to take Vengeance of their repeated revolts."[37] The juxtaposition of plague and revolt was a common theme in al-Jabartī's writing as well as the eighteenth-century British and French reports. Yet the element that set al-Jabartī apart was the scholarly tradition he adopted.

The purpose of the chronicle is multifarious and reflects a longstanding intellectual tradition that emerged under Mamluk rule in Egypt. As Dana Sajdi has noted, "The Arabic chronicle is about the establishment and legitimization of the Islamic order. Organized annalistically by the Islamic hijra date, the main subject of the chronicle is the accomplishments (and predicaments) of Muslim rulers whose very existence, and hence preservation, ensures the continuing existence of an Islamic polity."[38] At the same time, the chronologies were one type of memory-making that allowed a political dynasty to take shape and to legitimize it. Islamic historiography went through considerable evolution from the early Islamic period to the nineteenth century, however, by al-Jabartī's time historians within the religion had the practice of cataloguing in their chronicles the passing of every major figure at the end of every year.[39] By structuring different Arabic chronologies in the same fashion, the authors were entangled in a performance that outlined the "important" events while occasionally documenting the lives of the urban poor, slaves, and women. Accordingly, the chronology was a "trans-provincial biographical project"[40]

century sharia court records were composed in Arabic and have proven to be important in describing legal disputes and endowments of the period. André Raymond, Nelly Hanna, and other historians of eighteenth-century Egypt have made good use of these sources. Hanna, ed. *Money, Land and Trade: An Economic History of the Muslim Mediterranean* (London: I. B. Tauris, 2002).

37 British Library, India Office of Records, G/17/6.

38 Dana Sajdi, *The Barber of Damascus: Nouveau Literacy in the Eighteenth-Century Ottoman Levant* (Stanford: Stanford University Press, 2013), 6–7.

39 Although I do not wish to go into detail about the historical debates within Islamic historiography, there are various schools about the reliability of early Islamic historical writing. Skeptics such as Patricia Crone and Michael Cook have denounced early texts and sources. For a more nuanced view, see Fred McGraw Donner, *Narratives of Islamic Origins: The Beginnings of Islamic Historical Writing* (Princeton, NJ: Darwin Press, 1998).

40 Hathaway, *Al-Jabarti's History of Egypt*, xxi.

that collected the major political events in late eighteenth-century Egypt while making claims about natural disasters.

North African Ottoman provinces had a network of scholars and chroniclers who read and borrowed from each other's works. Some of those people included Abū al-Qāsim ibn Aḥmad Zayānī (d. 1833) and Moḥammad ibn al-Ṭayyib al-Qādirī (d. 1773). These two historians hailed from Morocco and complemented the political and social transformations during the late seventeenth and eighteenth century. Like his contemporaries, al-Jabartī occasionally borrowed entire passages from other historians who preceded him, such as Aḥmad Çelebi ibn ʿAbd al-Ghanī and Aḥmad Damurdashi.[41] These men differed in their country of origin but they had similar styles of writing. A standard practice for writing was that the texts began with a blessing (*basmala*), thanked their patrons, and described a series of events within their province and beyond. As per the custom, al-Jabartī composed his chronology by listing each hijra year with a description of major political events and ended each year with a necrology of the prominent men. This was a continuation of Arabic medieval historical genre and was quite common.[42]

Death was at the center of historical writing and the necrology took up a significant amount of space for it described the lives of the men who passed away via odes and poetry. A significant portion of the necrologies contained panegyrics praising amirs, pashas, and beys. The style was unique among the chroniclers of his time because it contained rhymed couplets that were part of a broader medieval classical style. By mixing the fantastical with an epidemic, I argue that al-Jabartī wanted to point to the fragility of ritual at a moment of crisis.

At the same time, his assemblage did have issues that contemporary historians have problematized.[43] Ottoman historian Jane Hathaway asserts: "As its title implies, *ʿAjāʾib al-āthār* consists of both narratives of events (*akhbār*, today the Arabic word for "news") and obituaries-cum-life historians (*tarājim*, literally

41 Ayalon, "The Historian al-Jabartī and His Background." Al-Damurdashi's seminal chronicle covers Egyptian history preceding the period that al-Jabartī covers. See *Al-Damurdashi's Chronicle of Egypt, 1688–1755: Al-Durra al-Musana fi Akhbar al-Kinana, translated and annotated by* Daniel Crecelius and *ʿAbd al-Wahhab Bakr* (Leiden: Brill, 1991).

42 For an extensive account of the Islamic intellectual tradition, see R. Stephen Humphreys, *Islamic History: A Framework for Inquiry* (Princeton: Princeton University Press, 1991). For an explanation of how that shifts, see Christopher S. Taylor, *In the Vicinity of the Righteous: Ziyāra and the Veneration of Muslim Saints in Late Medieval Egypt* (Leiden: Brill, 1999).

43 For more information on how al-Jabartī composed his piece, see Shmuel Moreh, "Reputed Autographs of ʿAbd Al-Raḥmān al-Jabartī and Related Problems," *Bulletin of the School of Oriental and African Studies*, 28, no. 3 (1965): 524–40.

"translations")."[44] Indeed, al-Jabartī was a master of allegory and his narrative provided hidden meanings for moral and political themes. In the necrology of 1791, al-Jabartī acknowledged that the biographers who preceded him "wrote many poems of substantial outpouring and unblemished words and brides of verses possessing beautiful designs."[45] At the same time, John Antes, challenged the Arabic intellectual tradition and wrote, "There are still Arabic writers of chronicles at Grand Cairo, who will give the most boasting accounts of a trifling and insignificant fight between the Egyptian Beys, where, perhaps, five or six out of several thousands were killed."[46] What we gather from this is comment is that European travelers were aware of the Arabic historical tradition and that their accounts did not always map on to al-Jabartī's history.

Al-Jabartī's chronology is one part of the many strands that weave an Egyptian history and his necrology lists the notables that died during the 1791 outbreak. Of the twenty-nine notables listed that year, twenty-one of them had died of the plague. Writers such as ʿUthmān ibn Muḥammad ibn Ḥusain al-Shamsī and Sidi ʿUthmān Efendi ibn Aḥmad al-Safaʿī al-Miṣrī could not avoid the wrath of the plague. In some cases, al-Jabartī mentions where people were buried. Amir ʿAli al-Sassani, a Mamluk, was buried in the al-Ḥusayni shrine (a place that was usually afforded to *qadis*). When Ismail Bey—the Governor of Egypt—died on the sixteenth of Shaban he was buried in al-Qarafa at the Mausoleum of ʿAli Bey with his former major Ibrahim Kathuda near the tomb of Imam at Shafiʿi. Given the number of people who died during the outbreak, the chronicle is an entry point to uncovering the events and sites that were revered and forgotten during the plague.

I return to the unmarked site in Giza to reflect on the power of epidemics in wiping out the memory of the poor. Yet epidemics are remarkable for preserving the memory of the ordinary and the cultural imagination. I will bring us back to the minor events by speaking of the unnamed individuals who died during the 1791 outbreak. They passed away in a scene entangled in a web of disposable bodies. Al-Jabartī wrote:

---

44 Hathaway, *Al-Jabarti's History of Egypt*, xxiv.

45 Al-Jabartī, *ʿAjāʾib al-āthār*, 338.

46 Antes, *Observations*, 12, 15. The author considered himself an Englishman with a father who was naturalized and working in the Americas. He admits that he spent most of his time among foreigners. He is particularly interested in geography and this was something he had been fond of since childhood. He goes on to say that Arabs have a natural disposition to boast. He challenges the accounts made by Mr. Volney and Mr. Bruce (in Nubia) by asserting that his twelve years living in Egypt go against the accounts that they assert. He says that Mr. Bruce spent four years in Abyssinia and had learned Arabic.

> People were returning from funerals, walking with the coffin or returning from the burial. Additionally, there were those who were busy preparing the dead and those who were crying in fear of getting the plague. The plague did not stop its course from the mosques nor the praying areas and also it was rare to see the symptoms.[47]

The first portion of the text points to the high volume of people consoling the dead and the ways that society had to reorganize itself to accommodate the sick and dying. The plague and its aftermath, according to al-Jabartī, produced a city of mourners. He evinced that the death toll was so great that the lives of the living were centered on the misfortune of the dead. The outbreak meant that people were mostly reflecting on funeral rites and the fear of death. For al-Jabartī, the plague was not only a medical crisis but it was a predicament for labor. Yet it is not clear just how many lives were lost. Unlike the unnamed people in the pit, Ismail Bey had a more elite form of memorialization by being included in the mausoleum at al-Qarafa. Cemeteries were sites where the dead and living could coexist, yet people who did not have enough resources could not be brought there. At the time, the main cemetery lay outside of the Cairo proper.

There is a corpus of Arabic juridical-medical texts on plague that documents epidemics along with information on treatment, yet al-Jabartī's text is distinct for bringing the reader to the practical concerns of an outbreak.[48] Within the necrology section, al-Jabartī listed the names of ulama, poets, and rulers who died for each successive year. In contrast, the names and lives of everyday people were not usually listed in the necrology. Yet these "events" and "data" provided some context to the social texture of the urban poor and their tragedy. In contrast, Ismail Bey and his fellow notables were individually exalted by al-Jabartī by being listed in his chronology. ʿAbd al-Raḥmān Bey, an Ottoman notable who commissioned to build the mosque of Abū Hurairah in Giza, died of plague during this outbreak.[49]

---

47 This translation is my own.

48 For a discussion on plague literature refer to Dols, *Black Death*; Justin K. Stearns, *Infectious Ideas: Contagion in Premodern Islamic and Christian Thought in the Western Mediterranean* (Baltimore: Johns Hopkins University Press, 2011).

49 Ibid. Also, ʿAbd al-Raḥmān Bey ʿUthmān built the mosque of Abū Hurairah in Giza and he built a palace beside it in the year 1188 H / 1774–5.

Cemeteries and Burial Sites: The Significance of Process and Place in the Death Industry

"The list is endless. Where exactly was the cemetery, and are the remains still there?"— Michel Trouillot[50]

The plague was not only intimately connected to broader political discourses but to a vibrant debate concerning memorialization within the Islamic tradition. Historians Oleg Grabar and Ira Lapidus have done extensive work on early Islamic commemorative structures yet what is missing is an analysis that tackles disease and death.[51] In particular, these historians reflected on the tenet that death, under Islam, is not the end of an individual's life but rather a transition into a new phase of existence. These scholars rightly noted the Islamic conversations and debates on the body and spirit of a person (*rūh*). There is a corpus of hadith that explores death and remembrance that can be traced to the early Islamic period.[52] One particularly important point about the body is the Muslim belief that it will be resurrected from their body and soul together, at the Day of Judgment. Thus, the life of the grave prefigures the coming Day of Judgment. Another wave of social scientists studying ritual, such as Clifford Geertz and Lila Abu-Lughod, have looked at the cultural aspects of burial under Islam. A recent work by Jane Smith and Yvonne Haddad, *The Islamic Understanding of Death and Resurrection*, harps over cemeteries as sites of habitation in the final abodes of recompense.

Within both the eighteenth- and twenty-first century Cairo, the al-Qarafa cemetery has pre-figured as a site of residence for the dead and the living. An early account of memorialization occurs in Ohtoshi Tetsuya's depiction of al-Qarafa as a meeting place for the lower echelon of society during the Mamluk period. Although my period is later, he highlights how important cemeteries and death rituals were for the living and dead in Cairo. It should also be noted that Basserine Cemetery, a Jewish Cemetery in Cairo, is near al-Qarafa. Ibn Tulun donated the site in the ninth century and it remains the second oldest functioning Jewish cemetery in the world after Mount Olives in East Jerusalem. A more recent work,

50 Michel-Rolph Trouillot, *Silencing the Past: Power and the Production of History* (Boston, MA: Beacon Press, 1995), 10.

51 Oleg Grabar, "The Earliest Islamic Commemorative Structures, Notes and Documents," *Ars Orientalis* 6 (1966): 7–46; Ira M. Lapidus, *A History of Islamic Societies* (Cambridge: Cambridge University Press, 2002).

52 For a history of the early Islamic death rituals and debates, refer to Leor Halevi, *Muhammad's Grave: Death Rites and the Making of Islamic Society* (New York: Columbia University Press, 2007).

Shane Minkin's "Simone's Funeral" explores Jewish burial rites in nineteenth- and twenty-first century Egypt. Additionally, the legal debates that spewed might be fruitful for thinking about epidemics and their exceptionality by people in the death industry.[53]

Eighteenth-century Cairene funeral rites can be examined through two vantage points—process and place—and these two vertices speak more broadly to the development of Islamic Sunni practice and Egyptian cultural memory. The funeral process was primarily based on hadith and the place extended to cemeteries such as al-Qarafa. Funeral rites vary according to one's financial means, social status, and religious affiliation.[54] During the first century that Islam developed, early observers crystalized practices by interpreting and debating over a set of Quranic verses and hadith.[55] The process originally emerged during the seventh century and broke away from pre-Islamic Arabian funeral practices such as cremation.[56] As Leor Halevi points out, these early rites were not only linked to economic and political factors but early observers of Islam wanted to distinguish themselves from Christian, Jewish, and Zoroastrian rites. Sunni Islamic funeral rites followed a particular rubric and counseled speediness and cleanliness for burial.

Outside of cremation, there were other pre-Islamic practices that had been frowned upon which included lamenting the dead for "too long" and paying women to wail during funeral processions.[57] By the eighteenth century, a broader layer of Hanafi religious scholars opposed these practices, however, up until the

---

53 There are various perspectives that are missing from this account. For one, Coptic Christian sources and Jewish sources are lacking and could provide a fruitful layer to late eighteenth-century burial practices. For an account of the nineteenth- and twentieth-century burial practices in Egypt, see Shane Minkin, "Simone's Funeral: Egyptian Lives, Jewish Deaths in Twenty-First-Century Cairo," *The Journal of Theory and Practice* 16, no. 1 (2012). Shane Minkin explores Jewish burial rights in Cairo and spoke of the political lengths that Egyptian Jews went to preserve the site and memory of Jewish funeral rites in contemporary Cairo.

54 Jane I. Smith and Yvonne Yazbeck Haddad, *The Islamic Understanding of Death and Resurrection* (Oxford: Oxford University Press, 2002); Grabar, "Earliest Islamic Commemorative Structures"; Lila Abu-Lughod, "Islam and the Gendered Discourses of Death," *International Journal of Middle East Studies* 25, no. 2 (1993): 187–205.

55 For a detailed account of the matter, see Halevi, *Muhammad's Grave*.

56 Ibid.

57 Ibid. Wailing for the dead was discouraged by some early Islamic scholars. Prior to the emergence of Islam in Mesopotamia, the practice of paying women to wail for the dead was one component of funeral rites. After a series of jurists' debates, scholars began to condemn this practice.

end of the twentieth century female wailers could still be found in Egypt.[58] The conditions and circumstances that women lament in public has taken on different meanings, however, anthropologist Lila Abu-Lughod has witnessed this practice amongst women in the Awlad ʿAli Bedouin community in Egypt.[59] The author argued that lamenting is on the one hand informed by Islamic law/piety and on the other hand it is also a reflection of the cultural traditions specific to the community. She further argued that women played a gendered role in lamenting that reproduced a hierarchy within this community. This religiously "subversive" act could be seen as a direct affront to a predominantly male religious authority. What this goes to show is that funeral practices are flexible even when there are core tenets guiding one's piety.

Funerals were a marker of one's religious and social status in Ottoman society.[60] The funeral process brought workers and mourners together.[61] During the rite, funeral biers helped to carry the casket. If bier carriers were not part of the family, they were compensated for their time. Upon arrival to the tomb, one person removed the corpse out of the casket, deposited it into a vault, and adjusted the body so that it could face Mecca. For the religiously reverent, the ritual was a virtue that allowed the spirit and the body to be cleansed from the pollutants of life in preparation for the purity of paradise.

There are practical and humanistic reasons for understanding the circumstances that people "were digging pits for those in Giza near the mosque of Abū Hurairah and throwing them in."[62] First, tombstones, cemeteries, and inscriptions could potentially provide an estimate of the number of people that were living and dying during a period. Because the census was not yet established in Egypt, the tombstone is one type of official record of generations of people who died. Second, an eighteenth-century Cairene cemetery was not merely a site for tombstones and mausoleums but this was a space where religious communities socialized. Third, burial is of utmost importance for indicating one's membership in a religious com-

58 Abu-Lughod, "Islam and the Gendered Discourses of Death."

59 Ibid.

60 For more information on funeral rites within the Ottoman Empire, see Edhem Eldem, *Death in Istanbul: Death and Its Rituals in Ottoman-Islamic Culture* (Istanbul: Ottoman Bank Archives and Research Centre, 2005); Eldem, "Death and Funerary Culture," in *Encyclopedia of the Ottoman Empire*, edited by Gábor Ágoston and Bruce Alan Masters (New York: Facts on File, 2009), 177–80; Godfrey Goodwin, "Gardens of the Dead in Ottoman Times," *Muqarnas* 5 (1988): 61–69.

61 Muhammad Qasim Zaman, "Death, Funeral Processions, and the Articulation of Religious Authority in Early Islam," *Studia Islamica* 93 (2001): 27–58.

62 al-Jabartī, *ʿAjāʾib al-āthār*.

munity. While these cenotaphs and memorabilia provide a broad sketch of the dead, we can also see how absence plays a role in historical construction. One of the stakes of this research is developing a method for resurrecting the banal and the inconspicuous from pre-existing sources and providing their commemoration with other possibilities.

Eighteenth-century cemeteries and tombstones in Cairo had several ingredients in their composition and the structure and the final product marked the social strata of the deceased. Cemeteries are microcosms of cities that can further elucidate the specter of plague; I see this operating in multiple ways.[63] As anthropologist Nadia Abu El-Haj has pointed out in her book, *Facts on the Ground,* memorials in a cemetery dictate sociality and formulate a particular collective memory.[64] The cemetery has been stratified along religious and social differences and has also served as a housing community for the urban poor. In the contemporary context, Cairo's Al-Qarafa cemetery—both a cemetery and a slum—is an entry point to understanding postcolonial conceptions of death and the metaphorical uses of plague. Amongst historians of the Ottoman Empire, Nicolas Vatin has mostly explored how tombstones are situated within Istanbul and the way it maps on to broader political events.[65] While this research speaks to geopolitical and practical concerns about the cemetery, it leaves out the role that memory plays in shaping the cultural capital of the cemetery.

Among scholars of the global south, there is a growing interest in examining the relationship between space and collective memory. Scholars such as Gyan Prakash have reflected on how the urban poor interact with their city's memory by engaging in a politics of survival.[66] Slums and their surroundings can be part of the collective memory especially when they are engulfed in a cemetery. Al-Qarafa's social configuration has a lot to do with the rise of slums in Egypt, but it is not entirely attributed to the contemporary economic situation.[67] Local Cairene residents engaged with the pre-modern and contemporary artifacts of memori-

63 Donald Flanell Friedman, *The Symbolist Dead City: A Landscape of Poesis* (New York: Garland, 1990).

64 Nadia Abu El-Haj, *Facts on the Ground: Archaeological Practice and Territorial Self-Fashioning in Israeli Society* (Chicago: The University of Chicago Press, 2001).

65 Nicolas Vatin, Stephane Yerasimos, *Les cimetières dans la ville: status, choix et organisation des lieux d'inhumation dans Istanbul intra muros* (Istanbul: Institut français d'études anatoliennes Georges Dumézil, 2001).

66 Gyan Prakash and Kevin Michael Kruse, eds., *The Spaces of the Modern City: Imaginaries, Politics, and Everyday Life* (Princeton: Princeton University Press, 2008).

67 Marwa A Khalifa, "Redefining Slums in Egypt: Unplanned Versus Unsafe Areas," *Habitat International* 35, no. 1 (2011): 40–49.

alization by walking next to the mausoleums and tombstones. Living in al-Qarafa was not a twentieth century invention but part of a long-standing process of living amongst the dead.

During the Mamluk period, residents in two major Cairene cemeteries—al-Qarafa al-Sughra and al-Qarafa al-Kubra—maintained a self-sustaining community with various centers including mosques, schools, and shops.[68] Tetsuya argued that cemeteries developed into public spaces where urban poor Egyptians gathered. In addition, these cemeteries were zones where religious practice could adjust outside of the strict boundaries of the Islamic jurists.[69] People could be found drinking and dancing. Thus, the cemetery was a place where living people could establish their own social norms. Al-Qarafa is a cemetery with transformative identity that emerged as a burial site for the elite, a celebratory space for commoners, and a slum for the urban poor. It also serves as a three-dimensional archive. The cemetery continues to serve as a microcosm of the city. It is a gateway to understanding other forms of memorialization. Second, the cemetery is malleable in its composition in that it was open in some contexts and closed in others. Al-Qarafa cemetery continues to be open to its residents who live there and occasionally cater to tourists who want to fawn over the tombstones. For the residents of al-Qarafa cemetery, the monuments are a living reminder of how the upper echelon of society was venerated.

While the cemetery is an important element to develop notions about memorialization, tombstones provide archival evidence about individuals. Their presence and absence captures the essence of the value people place on the dead. A modest tombstone can be oblong while a more elaborate site can be an erected mausoleum. Whatever the form, it is generally the case that the artifact stands upright and often bears inscriptions in Arabic, however, if the gravestone commemorates an Ottoman ruler, then it would also include Ottoman Turkish script. In general, writing can be plain or decorated. However, it generally contains the name of the deceased, their date of birth, and a quote from the Qur'an. If the person is an eminent scholar, then they had a modest building erected over their grave. Tombstones in Egypt varied in style from the seventh century to the eighteenth century but many of them contained similar styles of presentation, i.e., a raised stone marking an individual's life and death.

Within the framework of the pre-colonial city, cemeteries were part of social organization that permitted the privileged to sustain their memory beyond their

68 For a thorough account of the Cairene cemetery, see Tetsuya, "Cairene Cemeteries as Public Loci in Mamluk Egypt."

69 Ibid.

family and friends. Cemeteries were and continue to be important sites for the dead and they reveal the *longue durée* of Egyptian civilization and speak to the continuity of funeral practice. They also provide the material and daily reminder that death lies ahead.

A Meditation on Burials and Cemeteries: What Work Does Memory Do for Me? The Idiosyncrasies of Mass Burial

> "At any given time, the living see themselves in the midday of history. They are obliged to prepare a banquet for the past. The historian is the herald who invites the dead to the table."— Walter Benjamin[70]

Al-Jabartī's *ʿAjā'ib al-āthār* did not only eulogize the ulama, but the text also showed that epidemics were unbiased in who they could infect. One could not escape the wrath of virulent diseases irrespective of one's social status as was demonstrated by the passing of Ismail Bey. He outlined the ways that the disease waxed and waned during the spring. The description has less to do with the etiology in its clinical form but more with the impact that it had on the population. By describing how the disease was present among all layers of the population, al-Jabartī demonstrated the democratic nature of epidemics. If we are to believe his account, then it appears that the plague brought the urban poor, children, and women to the historical record. Nevertheless, al-Jabartī did not list their names or the conditions of their lives but the account paints a picture of the world that they inhabited.

At present, a mosque of Abū Hurairah continues to occupy a space in Giza and a visitor to the region would find little evidence to al-Jabartī's reference of the mass burial. This neighborhood is a working class community in its shape and composition; it has mosques, residential buildings, and schools. There are billboards, motorcycles, goods, and produce on the congested streets. The *mélange* of falafel aroma and exhaust fumes travels through various alleyways and pockets of this urban community. Further east, the pyramids tower over the community—in silence—along the hustle and bustle of prayer calls and urban life. Yet popular music overpowers the silence of these corpses. This is a neighborhood that no longer thinks of plague alongside death but of the political influx intermixed with a moribund revolution. And so for this reason I want to see how al-Jabartī's reference to the burial applies and explore what this means for an otherwise forgotten group.

70 Walter Benjamin, *The Arcades Project* (Cambridge, MA: Belknap Press, 2002), 481.

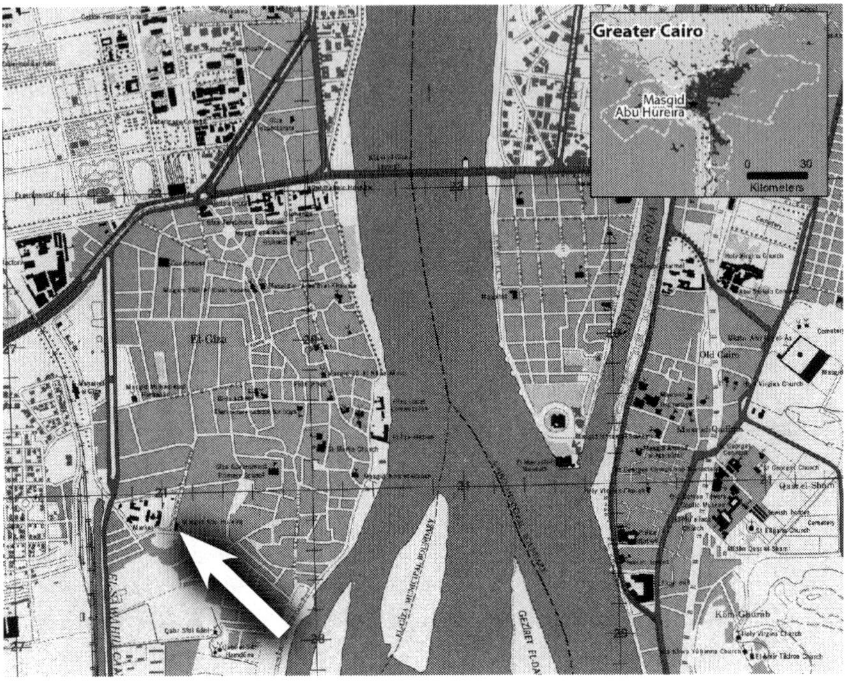

Map 1. A Contemporary Map of Old Cairo and Giza.
The arrow is pointing to the Mosque of Abū Hurairah.
The inner map shows the relative boundaries of the Greater Cairo area.

Geographically, Cairo is not strictly confined to current boundaries but the city is an ever-expanding metropole that has adjusted to an ever-expanding population. At the end of the eighteenth century, the population of Cairo was estimated to be 600,000 and currently, the population is over 18 million.[71] The reference to the mass burial was exceptional on many accounts and space was at the center of this. Since 1791, Cairo and its surrounding localities have significantly transformed. Yet a mosque bearing the name Abū Hurairah lays in Giza (Map 1). After acquiring a nearly complete list of registered mosques in Greater Cairo (over 5,100 in April 2014), I found two mosques that were called Abū Hurairah.[72] One mosque was

71 Estimates for the eighteenth-century populations were conducted by Daniel Panzac. See Panzac, *La peste*. According to UN statistics, Cairo's population in 2015 was 18,772,000. See: http://data.un.org/CountryProfile.aspx?crName=Egypt (accessed January 12, 2017).

72 The list was acquired by Princeton University Digital Map and Geospatial Information Center. The center purchased the list from Globe Technologies: http://www.gt-egypt.com/ (accessed January 12, 2017).

located on the right bank near the Muqattam hills and the other was located on the left bank in Giza. With further inquiry, I found that the coordinates of the Abū Hurairah mosque: 30°0'18" N 31°12'40" E. While there are flaws with maps and their boundaries, Map 1 is my rendition of the eighteenth century site interlaid with Cairo's twenty-first century expansion.[73]

There are many ways to document what this space looks like but I harp over mapping so that I can better understand the practicality of al-Jabartī's reference. The map allows one to decipher how the burial could have been carried out. It is in the context of having a non-memorial space that people can be "dumped" into a hole. At the same time, it is with their erasure from history and the rise of urbanization that those bodies are forgotten.

Death was imminent and rampant, but more importantly, there was a practical concern about the impact of the outbreak and what to do with the corpses. I believe that the plague, in eighteenth-century Egyptian and European discourse, generated a climate of fear amongst officials and commoners, and there were practical concerns about dealing with the less privileged dead. While al-Jabartī and his European contemporaries mentioned the death of Ismail Bey from the 1791 plague and the political matrix that overlaid his death, the only reference to the mass burial is by al-Jabartī. In the process of describing the development of a fervent disease to the broader population, the unmarked, in turn, became invisible. For non-elite persons in the historical record, invisibility is the default, yet plague overcomes the challenge of bringing out their experience in the historical record because of the scale of death. The mass burial near the mosque of Abū Hurairah—because it is unmarked—does not function as a site of memory for the contemporary residents of Giza because it is not currently recognized as a burial site. In contrast, cemeteries such as al-Qarafa are bounded and allow various people to enter and exit.

Since the nineteenth century, Egypt has had a special place in European and North American excavation projects, often for the sake of understanding ancient Egyptian culture and a persistence of burials. I consider my meditation on the

73 It bears noting that I do not consider my map a definitive and conclusive representation of Cairo and Giza. Instead, it stands as one of many layers that will mark the social and cultural space where my actors lived. While I do not consider myself a neo-imperialist, I am conscious that cartographers and those with access to tools for map making can inform historians about the power and capital associated with knowledge production. I make this statement with the following works in mind: Michel Foucault, *The Order of Things: An Archaeology of the Human Sciences* (New York: Vintage Books, 1973); D. Graham Burnett, *Masters of All They Surveyed: Exploration, Geography, and a British El Dorado* (Chicago: The University of Chicago Press, 2000).

burial site as less ambitious than a multi-team excavation project. Al-Jabartī's pit can be read as an "invisible" city of the dead that is buried beneath a visible city of the living. The composition and scale of this mass burial and the sort of labor needed to excavate these corpses would require a mass flow of human labor and financial capital. It could also entail displacing a large number of residents from this neighborhood to find these remains. As such, meditating on the site opens up other avenues for constructing memory. Because memory is often material and selective, theorizing around al-Jabartī's mass burial can provide alternative narratives for the plague of 1791.

A cemetery can be part of Cairene collective memory and an unmarked mass burial part of Cairene historical amnesia. The privileged dead can afford a tombstone or mausoleum and their structures still remind their descendants who they were, when they passed away, and their legacy. In contrast, the unmarked mass burial mutes the voices of the past. The late Haitian anthropologist Michel Trouillot wrote: "The bigger the material mass, the more easily it entraps us: mass graves and pyramids bring history closer while they make us feel small."[74] Giza is a complex site because it is a zone with some of the largest monuments (pyramids) and the least visible markers (al-Jabartī's pit). At the same time, the precarious life of the Cairene urban poor during the eighteenth century means their bodies were not only pushed aside but also forgotten.

Not all facts are created equal and I do not claim to be a fair arbiter of these events. Eighteenth-century Cairene residents were on equal footing for acquiring the plague, however, there were mass inequalities for how the rich and the poor were remembered. In this chapter, I argued that the epidemic crisis transforms conditions of possibility for burial and that the status of memory diminishes for commoners during a plague outbreak. The plague provides a unique opportunity to understand Egyptian medical history while also pointing to a range of burial practices. Upon occasion, al-Jabartī and his contemporaries referenced the various plague outbreaks and their impact on the city, commerce, and politics. There is also another layer that reveals the fortitude of death. Whether one was illiterate or literate, indigenous or denizens—anyone could be subject to death during an epidemic. What one finds from this whirlwind of accounts is that funeral rites were flexible during crisis. Thus, it appears that the plague put to rest the victims and their memory.

---

74 Michel-Rolph Trouillot, *Silencing the Past: Power and the Production of History* (Boston: Beacon Press, 1995), 29.

Edna Bonhomme (bonhomme@princeton.edu) is a history of science doctoral candidate at Princeton University who focuses on the history of epidemics and funeral rites in North Africa and the Middle East. She graduated from Reed College with a BA in Biology and from Columbia University with an MPH in Sociomedical Sciences. Before beginning her graduate work at Princeton, she worked as a research assistant in an immunology/genetics laboratory, coordinated with human rights groups in Haiti, and conducted public health research in New York City. Her dissertation examines plague, urbanization, and funeral rites in eighteenth-century Cairo and Tunis. Taking pre-colonial medical outbreaks as its point of departure, this project also sheds light on black slaves, public health, and quarantine measures. Additionally, this work entails conducting fieldwork in Cairene and Tunisian cemeteries for the purposes of understanding the relationship between eighteenth-century tombstones and twenty-first century cemeteries.

NOWHERE TO RUN TO, NOWHERE TO HIDE? SOCIETY, STATE, AND EPIDEMIC DISEASES IN THE EARLY NINETEENTH-CENTURY OTTOMAN BALKANS

ANDREW ROBARTS
Rhode Island School of Design

IN THE EARLY part of the eighteenth century, a Hungarian military commander in the service of the Ottoman army recounted in his memoirs the following story he heard while over-nighting in the Ottoman town of Karasu (Cherna Voda) in northeastern Bulgaria:

> Late at night four men with hoes and shovels came to the yard of an Orthodox priest and began to dig and throw earth as if they were making a grave. When he heard the noise at his door, the priest came outside and asked what these men were doing. They replied that they were burying a corpse. The priest asked that they dig the grave elsewhere, but the men kept on digging. The priest pondered the situation and asked if the corpse had died of the plague. Yes, the diggers replied, he died of the plague. Scared, the Priest offered the men three bottles of wine if they agreed to dig their grave elsewhere. They kept digging. The priest offered four jugs of wine then five. While this bargaining was taking place the Priest observed that the men had placed the corpse on a plank. Growing ever more scared, the Priest noticed that the digging of the grave had been completed. At this point the leader of the grave-diggers told the Priest that if he gave them five jugs of wine, they would bury the corpse somewhere else. The poor Priest, relieved and feeling saved, gave them the five jugs. The Priest secretly followed the men to see where they were carrying the corpse. With amazement, he saw that the corpse was no longer on the plank, had joined the men, and was drinking wine. The Priest did not know whether to laugh or cry. He had been swindled.[1]

1 This story can be found in the memoirs of Kelemen Mikesh, a long-time valet and advisor to the Hungarian prince Ferenc Rakoczi (1676–1735). Following a failed uprising against the Habsburg Empire, Rakoczi and his followers (including Mikesh) found refuge in the Ottoman Empire, first in Edirne, then in the environs of Istanbul (in Büyükdere and Yeniköy), and ultimately in Rodosto (Tekirdağ) where Mikesh died of plague in 1761. See *Madzharski Pŭtepisi za Balkanite, XVI–XIX v.* (Sofia: Izdatelstvo "Nauka i Izkustvo," 1976), 51–64.

As revealed in this vignette, the appearance and spread of epidemic diseases fostered an atmosphere of heightened anxiety among local populations in the Ottoman Balkans (Rumeli). For many Ottoman subjects in the Balkans flight (for safety and to escape social ostracism) was the common initial response to epidemic diseases. These disease-induced displacements disrupted the collection of taxes, hampered the recruitment of soldiers, and contributed to a breakdown in public order in the Empire's Balkan provinces.

This chapter will analyze the nexus between epidemic disease, human mobility, and the Ottoman state in the late eighteenth and early nineteenth centuries. Drawing upon Ottoman, Bulgarian, and Russian archival sources as well as Bulgarian, Russian and Western European travel accounts, it will argue that in the 1830s and 1840s, the Ottoman state—in the wake of a prolonged period of warfare and decentralization in Rumeli—expanded quarantine construction as a means to reassert central control over displaced and migratory populations in the Balkans.

The first section of this chapter will survey epidemic diseases in the Ottoman Balkans in the eighteenth and early nineteenth centuries. It will highlight how and in what ways disease-induced displacements resulted in the formation of new population settlements and alterations to the human geography of nineteenth-century Rumeli. Section two will explore the evolution of multi-confessional rituals and ceremonies staged to stave off death and disease and examine the development of "traditional" anti-disease and communal policing initiatives in the towns and villages of the Balkan countryside. The third section will analyze Ottoman initiatives to contain epidemics in the first half of the nineteenth century, focusing particularly on the role of lazarets and quarantine complexes as institutions of migration management and social control. Unlike the historical scholarship that has primarily approached quarantines as institutions constructed in an effort to combat the spread of disease, this chapter will argue that early-nineteenth century Ottoman quarantines rapidly evolved into all-purpose border posts where trade goods were inspected, customs collected, currency exchanged, criminals and fugitives surveilled, intelligence gathered, and migrants and refugees registered and provided with travel documents.

Overview of Epidemic Diseases in the Ottoman Balkans

In the eighteenth and early nineteenth centuries, few parts of Rumeli and the Danubian Principalities (Wallachia and Moldavia or, roughly, modern-day Romania) were spared the ravages of epidemic diseases.[2] It is important to note

---

2 For more on the history of epidemic diseases in the Ottoman Empire, see: Daniel Panzac, *La peste dans l'empire ottoman, 1700–1850* (Leuven: Éditions Peeters, 1985); Birsen

at the outset that when discussing outbreaks of epidemic diseases in the pre-modern period, the term "plague" has often been used as a catch-all term for a variety of diseases and ailments including typhus, malaria, and various viral infections.[3] My purpose here is not to wade too deeply into the historiographical discussion on the type and terminology surrounding the diseases prevalent in the Ottoman Balkans during the period under discussion, but rather to highlight the social and state responses to the appearance and spread of epidemic diseases (whether it be plague, cholera, or other diseases).

In the eighteenth and early nineteenth centuries outbreaks of what we believe to be plague lasted, on average, 1.5 years in the Balkans.[4] Depending upon various factors (including topography, settlement patterns, population density, and travel and transportation networks) plague spread outwards from Ottoman urban centers (principally Istanbul) at a rate of around one kilometer per day (or 200–400 kilometers per year).[5] At the start of the eighteenth century, an outbreak of infectious disease in Zağra-i Atik (Stara Zagora, in central Bulgaria) reduced the population of the town, through death and flight, by half.[6] Rusçuk (Ruse, in northern Bulgaria) was visited by the plague in 1703 as was Arbanasi (north of the Balkan

Bulmuş, *Plague, Quarantines and Geopolitics in the Ottoman Empire* (Edinburgh: University of Edinburgh Press, 2012); Yaron Ayalon, *Natural Disasters in the Ottoman Empire: Plague, Famine, and Other Misfortunes* (Cambridge: Cambridge University Press, 2014); Nükhet Varlık, *Plague and Empire in the Early Modern Mediterranean World: The Ottoman Experience, 1347–1600* (Cambridge: Cambridge University Press, 2015); Gülden Sarıyıldız, *Hicaz Karantina Teşkilatı* (Ankara: Türk Tarih Kurumu, 1996). See also Sam White's historiographical piece, "Rethinking Disease in Ottoman History" in *The International Journal of Middle East History* 42, no. 3 (2010): 549–67, for an excellent overview on the current state of the field in Ottoman disease studies.

3 In Ottoman sources, the terms *ṭāʿūn* and *vebā* are often used interchangeably to denote epidemic diseases. The term *ṭāʿūn*, however, tends to be specifically used to denote plague. I am following this convention here and when *ṭāʿūn* is used in the sources, I have translated it as "plague" and when *vebā* is used I have translated into the general term "epidemic disease." For more on the terminological issues surrounding the study of epidemic diseases in the Ottoman and Middle Eastern contexts, see Süheyl Ünver, "Taun Nedir? Veba Nedir?" *Dirim* 3–4 (1978): 363–66 and Tahsin Akpınar, "*Osmanlı Devleti'nde Karantina Usulünün Başlaması*," MA thesis, Marmara University, 1986, 4. As Sam White has noted, in reference to outbreaks of disease in early modern Ottoman cities, "bubonic plague was just one of many deadly pathogens in a complex disease environment." White, *The Climate of Rebellion in the Early Modern Ottoman Empire* (Cambridge: Cambridge University Press, 2011), 85–86.

4 Panzac, *La peste*, 208.

5 Nadia Manolova-Nikolova, *Chumavite Vremena (1700–1850)* (Sofia: "IF-94," 2004), 36–37.

6 Başbakanlık Osmanlı Arşivi/Prime Ministry's Ottoman Archives, Istanbul (BOA), İbnülemin Sıhhiye, 124/2, March 3, 1699.

Mountains near Turnovo) in 1729, Bender (astride the modern Moldovan-Ukrainian border) in 1737, Karasu in 1739, and Jassy (Iaşi, near the current Romanian-Moldovan border) in 1753.[7]

Generally temperate climate conditions, increased trade and migratory connections, regular outbreaks of Russo-Ottoman warfare, and a series of anomalous natural events (including a string of early and warm springs and high levels of seismological activity) made the Ottoman Balkans and Danubian Principalities a particularly active zone for the spread of diseases in the late eighteenth and early nineteenth centuries. Textiles, hides, and grains constituted a particularly conducive breeding environment for fleas and rats. The primary method for the long-range spread of plague between human populations was through trade in wool, silk, cotton, grains, and the personal effects (i.e., clothing) of merchants, migrants, and soldiers.[8] Dislocations and displacements caused by exogenous shocks to the normal patterns of life (i.e., earthquakes and floods) devastated already rudimentary levels of sanitation and—through reductions in food intake—severely compromised human immune systems.[9] These exogenous shocks extended the lifecycles of epidemic diseases and increased fatality rates.

From 1789 to 1795, a sustained plague epidemic in Filibe (Plovdiv, in Central Bulgaria) killed an estimated 10,000 people—or roughly thirty-three percent of the town's population.[10] In 1795, a Bulgarian émigré in Craiova (in modern-day Romania) wrote to a relative in Rumeli that a plague epidemic had struck the town,

---

7 *Madzharski Pŭtepisi za Balkanite, XVI–XIX v.,* 62; Manolova-Nikolova, *Chumavite Vremena,* 63–65.

8 Panzac, *Quarantaines et lazarets: l'Europe et la peste d'Orient, XVII*^{e}*–XX*^{e} *siècles* (Aix-en-Provence: Édisud, 1986), 21. While travelling by ship in the Black Sea region in the 1820s, the Englishman James Alexander observed that the clothes of Russian seamen who succumbed to plague were often appropriated by their fellow sailors, stored in rucksacks, and worn during subsequent voyages. *Angliski Pŭtepisi za Balkanite, XVI–XIX v.* (Sofia: Izdatelstvo "Nauka i Izkustvo," 1987), 699–700.

9 In 1821, an earthquake equivalent to a magnitude of 5 on the Richter scale occurred in northern Rumeli. Tremors and small earthquakes struck the Balkans annually from 1825–1830. On April 23, 1829 a massive earthquake (estimated to be between 8 and 9 on the Richter scale) ravaged southern Rumeli. In the same year, an unusually strong earthquake struck the Danubian Principalities. According to information gathered by the Russian Ministry of the Interior, during this earthquake tremors lasted 70 seconds in Jassy. Many of the buildings in this city were destroyed or heavily damaged. General data on climate and seismological conditions in early nineteenth-century Ottoman Empire can be found in Manolova-Nikolova, *Chumavite Vremena*, 48–53. Specific information on the November 1829 earthquake in the Danubian Principalities can be found in "O Zemletriasenii," *Zhurnal Ministerstva Vnutrennikh Del* (Kn. 1, 1829), 652–54.

10 Manolova-Nikolova, *Chumavite Vremena*, 90.

ten people were dying per day, and all economic activity had come to a standstill.[11] Outbreaks of epidemic disease in the years 1813–15—known in Bulgarian historiography as the time of the "*Purvata Chuma*" (first plague epidemic) or the period of the "*Goliamata Moria*" (great plague)—were particularly devastating. In the words of one individual who survived an outbreak of plague in Rumeli in 1814, "from east to west the plague killed half the world. The plague had come before, but never killed as it does now."[12] In September 1813, over 120 people died per day in the Ottoman Balkan town of Arbanasi. By the time the month was over, roughly thirty percent of the town's population had perished.[13] The majority of the population of the Dobrujan town of Vister (in northeastern Bulgaria) succumbed to plague in 1814—resulting, ultimately, in the disappearance of this town from later maps.[14] In the summer of 1814, roughly 50–60 people died per day in Stara Zagora. By September 1814, roughly 5,000 (around twenty-five percent) of the town's inhabitants had died of plague.[15] And in 1816, 5,000 inhabitants of Focşani (in Ottoman-controlled Moldavia) suffered the same fate (see maps 2 and 3).[16]

In the 1820s and 1830s, cholera and plague combined to produce a particularly powerful epidemiological threat to populations in the Ottoman Balkans.[17] From

11 *Bŭlgarski Istoricheski Arkhiv* (BIA), Fond 40 – Dimitraki Hadjitoshev Tsenovich (June 26, 1795).

12 Manolova-Nikolova, *Chumavite Vremena*, 76.

13 Ibid., 89.

14 *Fakiisko Predanie* (Sofia, 1985), 281, 349.

15 Manolova-Nikolova, *Chumavite Vremena*, 97.

16 William MacMichael, *Journey from Moscow to Istanbul in the Years 1817, 1818* (London: John Murray, 1819), 104.

17 Manolova-Nikolova, *Chumavite Vremena*, 77. Cholera is a highly infectious water-borne bacterial disease. Producing severe diarrhea, cholera manifests its symptoms within hours of contact and, if not treated, can be fatal within a 24-hour period. The appearance of the so-called Asiatic cholera (*cholera morbus*) in the Ganges plain in 1817 coupled with the increased use of steamship travel by Muslim pilgrims from the Indian Subcontinent, resulted in significant outbreaks of cholera in Mecca and Medina in the early part of the nineteenth century. Spread (via Astrakhan, on the north shore of the Caspian Sea, and Russian Black Sea ports) by Russian Muslim pilgrims returning from the Hijaz, the Russian Empire was the first European nation to suffer the ravages of the global cholera epidemic of the 1820s and 1830s. From 1823–31, over 250,000 Russians died of cholera. For more on cholera epidemics in the nineteenth century, see: David Arnold, *Colonizing the Body: State Medicine and Epidemic Disease in Nineteenth-Century India* (Berkeley: University of California Press, 1993); Michael Christopher Low, "Empire and the Hajj: Pilgrims, Plagues, and Pan-Islam under British Surveillance, 1865–1908," *International Journal of Middle East Studies* 40, no. 2 (2008): 269–90; Roderick McGrew, *Russia and the Cholera, 1823–1832* (Madison, WI: University of Wisconsin Press, 1965).

1828–29, plague and cholera epidemics struck the Black Sea and eastern Rumelian towns.[18] Victims of disease constituted the majority of the 17,000 inhabitants of Varna who died during the Russian siege of this key Black Sea port city in 1828. Overwhelmed grave-diggers in Varna hastily buried thousands of corpses in the early winter mud and snow, exposing—during the spring thaw in 1829—a landscape of protruding limbs and half-buried bodies in the fields around Varna.[19] In 1833, a cholera epidemic in the Macedonian town of Bitola killed over 400 people.[20] By the mid-1800s, a graveyard existed in Plovdiv (at the base of Cambaz Tepe) dedicated solely to the victims of early nineteenth-century plague epidemics.[21]

A bacterial disease, typhus flourished in the seventeenth and eighteenth centuries in crowded and unsanitary locales in the Ottoman Balkans such as towns and fortresses under siege, army bivouacs, and refugee camps.[22] Malaria, as well, ravaged populations in the Ottoman Balkans including those settled along the low-lying Black Sea coast (mainly in the area around Varna), in the marshy swampland of the Danubian estuary ("where ghastly mosquitoes—whose bite was capable of killing a man—bred and festered"), and in isolated pockets of the Rumelian interior and eastern Thrace ("where the air was bad").[23] Travelers in the Ottoman Balkans complained of aching fevers and the general malaise caused by breathing in "air full of noxious vapors."[24] And as Sam White has pointed out overcrowding, poor sanitation, and rudimentary water supply systems in Ottoman cities produced a cocktail of "ordinary" (but deadly) urban endemic diseases and infections such as anthrax, dysentery, fevers, gastro-intestinal disturbances, malaria, smallpox, and typhus.[25]

---

18 Varna, Sliven, Aytos, Karnobat, Ahyolu (Pomorie), Burgas, and Sizebolu (Sozopol) were affected. See Manolova-Nikolova, *Chumavite Vremena*, 73.

19 As reported by the English traveler James Alexander, *Angliski Pŭtepisi za Balkanite, XVI–XIX v*, 699.

20 BIA, Fond 27, Bratia Robevi.

21 "Unikalen Vŭzrozhdenski Rŭkopis: Konstantin D. Moravenov. Pametnik za Plovdivskoto Khristiiansko Naselenie v Grada i za Obshtite Zavedeniia po Proiznosno Predanie, Podaren na Bŭlgarskoto Chitalishte v Tsarigrad - do 1869," *Izvestia na Narodnata Biblioteka Kiril i Metodii* (Volume XIV, 1976), 511–631.

22 Bruce McGowan, *Economic Life in Ottoman Europe: Taxation, Trade and the Struggle for Land, 1600–1800* (Cambridge: Cambridge University Press, 1981), 86–87.

23 Helmuth von Moltke, *Unter dem Halbmond: Erlebnisse in der alten Türkei, 1835–1839* (Tübingen: Erdmann, 1979), 181.

24 "Vospominaniia Doktora Zeidlitsa o Turetskom Pokhod 1829 Goda," *Russkii Arkhiv* 1–4 (1878): 412–35; and "Tri Miesiatsa za Dunavaem," *Syn Otechetsva* 1, no. 5 (1833): 273–85.

25 White, *Climate of Rebellion*, 85–87, 153, 270–71.

Deaths from disease outnumbered combat fatalities in the Russo-Ottoman wars of the late eighteenth and early nineteenth century.[26] Reporting from Bucharest during the early stages of the Russo-Ottoman War of 1828–29, a Russian agent observed that "never in history have disease and warfare been as intertwined as they are at the present time."[27] Senior military officers lamented their inability to defend their soldiers from the depredations of the plague. To quote Feodor Tornay, the cousin and *aide-de-camp* of the Russian Field Marshal Dibich-Zabalkanski, "Generals and Commandants were at a loss to prevent deaths from plague among their officers and clerical staff. And on more than one occasion we encountered abandoned carts full of provisions and supplies surrounded by dead horses and merchants."[28] In 1828 and 1829, travelers and military servitors in the Danubian Principalities and Rumeli frequently remarked upon the large number of disease-related deaths in the Russian and Ottoman armies.[29]

In an effort to limit plague-related losses, soldiers—rather than billet in towns and villages suspected of being infected with disease—frequently bivouacked in open fields. For example, severe outbreaks of plague in the Wallachian capital of Bucharest in the summer of 1828 compelled Russian forces to camp at some distance from the city.[30] And, in the spring of 1829, repeated outbreaks of plague in eastern Rumeli prompted the Russian garrison in Aytos to relocate to an area several kilometers from the town center.[31] Additionally, as merchants trading in cloth, cotton, and woolen goods were often suspected of carrying disease into Russian military camps, Russian army regulations expressly forbid the sourcing of these kinds of goods from local populations.[32]

---

26 For example, during the Russian siege of Silistre in the summer of 1809 over half of General Bagration's army succumbed to illness and disease. L. A. Kasso, *Rossiia na Dunae i Obrazovanie Bessarabskoi Oblasti* (Moscow: [Pech. A. I. Snegirevoĭ], 1913), 73.

27 *Gosudarstvennyi Arkhiv Rossiiskoi Federatsii* (GARF), f. 109, op. 3a, d. 3195, l. 270 (May 2, 1828).

28 Manolova-Nikolova, *Chumavite Vremena*, 76–77. Due to severe outbreaks of plague in Russian military encampments, the summer fighting season was typically referred to as "*la mauvais saison*." GARF, f. 109, op. 3a, d. 3195, l. 76 and GARF, f. 109, op. 3a, d. 3195, l. 271.

29 See for example, "Zapisnaia Knizhka Grafa P. Kh. Grabbe," *Russkii Arkhiv* (Kn. 4, 1888), 33 and 44.

30 GARF, f. 109, op. 3a, d. 3195, l. 270.

31 Manolova-Nikolova, *Chumavite Vremena*, 206.

32 *Rossiiskii Gosudarstvennyi Voenno-Istoricheskii Arkhiv* (RGVIA), f. 14209, op. 3/163b, d. 19 (November 28, 1809).

Society's Response to the Spread of Epidemic Disease

"Chuesh li za chuma, Biagai v shuma"
("If you feel the plague coming, flee to the forest")[33]

Prior to the mounting of coordinated interventions by the Ottoman state to check the spread of epidemic diseases in the Balkans in the middle part of the nineteenth century, local communities implemented their own "traditional" measures. Developed over centuries, these mechanisms drew upon practical experience adopted in response to local environmental and social conditions rather than scientific or state-generated research. Balkan villagers heaped piles of dung in front of their homes and smeared their doors with tar as a preventative measure against the plague.[34] According to legend, Roma rarely contracted disease because they tended to live in smoky houses. The burning of rags and garbage became, therefore, a common response to the appearance of plague.[35]

These preventive measures sometimes included ritual offerings as plague was often depicted as a mythical personage (most often in the form of a female demon). As a defense against the plague Bulgarian women frequently placed offerings to "Old Woman Plague" (*Baba Chuma*) in their village's central square. A typical offering to *Baba Chuma* would include one roasted chicken, a bottle of wine, two shoes, and a cane. Other ritualistic defenses against the plague included sacrificing a bull, killing a blackbird, or walking over the roots of an old tree. The residents of the village of Gintsi (near Sofia) used herbs from the town of Izlas (at the confluence of the Danube and Olt rivers) as a fumigant against plague. The Olt-Danube confluence, it was believed, was the site (in biblical times) of an appeal made by the Angel Gabriel to the demon plague to spare humanity from the ravages of all diseases.[36]

Bulgarian subjects of the Ottoman Empire turned to prayer and religious devotion to ward off the contraction of disease. On February 10—a day otherwise known as the "Plague Day" (*Chumniden*) or the "Day of Good Health" (*Praznik za Zdrave*)—Balkan villagers would carry a special vessel filled with honey to the local church. Bread dipped into honey would be distributed to the children of the village to protect them from disease.[37] An active Christian devotional movement

33 Nineteenth-century Bulgarian proverb.

34 "Vospominaniia Doktora Zeidlitsa o Turetskom Pokhod 1829 Goda," 417.

35 Manolova-Nikolova, *Chumavite Vremena*, 190–92.

36 Ibid., 158–60, 190.

37 Ibid., 158–59.

dedicated to prayer and sacrifice as a defense against disease existed in early-modern Ottoman Rumeli. Adherents to this movement believed that the relics of Kharalambos (the patron saint and defender of plague victims) were capable of warding off disease.[38] One verse attributed to Kharalambos read in part "wherever one finds my relics and wherever people honor my memory there will be no hunger or plague or ruinous vapors. In these places there will be peace, health, and a feeling of security. In these places there will be an abundance of wheat and wine and a multitude of beasts of burden."[39]

In certain localities in Ottoman Rumeli multi-confessional rituals and ceremonies were performed to stave off death and disease. For example, in the mixed Christian-Muslim village of Trunchovitsa (near Pleven in north-central Bulgaria) anti-disease rituals involved an elaborate ceremony of sacrifice to the "Goddess of Plague" (*Boginiata Chuma*) performed to allay the Goddess's anger and to divert her attention away from the village. On the day of the ceremony, so-called "prophets of plague" advised the villagers of Trunchovitsa to fast and avoid the use of fire. Surrounded by all the villagers and inside of a space formed by the circling of wagons and carts, religious leaders from Trunchovitsa's three confessional communities (Muslims, Catholic, and Greek Orthodox) performed a common liturgy and read aloud a common prayer to protect the village from disease. Following the ceremony, the villagers would throw a specially-baked bread (unleavened and mixed with honey) from their carts into the center of the enclosure.[40]

Religious and societal authority figures appealed to the masses to attend to their personal cleanliness and touted the benefits of good personal hygiene as a preventative measure against disease. During the official opening of a new school in Plovdiv in 1834, the Greek Patriarch Kiril exhorted the students to clean themselves before coming to school in the morning and to strive, on a daily basis, to keep themselves, their clothes, and their books as clean as possible. And in the appendix of a Bulgarian phrasebook published in 1835, the publisher (Khristaki

38 The origins of Kharalambos and his devotional movement are somewhat shrouded. The basic theory is that an individual by the name of Kharalambos lived in Asia Minor sometime in the second or third century C.E. Kharalambos would often recite a prayer to God to save him from plague. While many of his fellow villagers died of plague, Kharalambos was repeatedly spared. Thus a belief developed that Kharalambos's prayers and his devotion to God were the route to salvation from epidemic diseases. See Manolova-Nikolova, *Chumavite Vremena*, 121–30.

39 In the 1830s and 1840s, compilations of these types of verses and prayers were some of the first books published in the Bulgarian language by Bulgarian-owned publishing houses. See ibid., 130–34.

40 Ibid., 183.

Pavloviç) opined that "for everyone health was the most important matter. Keep your hands, and face, and whole body clean. And for the best results, use running water instead of bathwater."[41]

Community policing measures were adopted to curb the spread of disease in Rumelian towns and villages. Houses deemed to be infected by plague were doused in vinegar, limed, or, in extreme cases, demolished.[42] Houses constructed out of straw and plaster were destroyed and stone houses built in their place. In the 1830s, entire neighborhoods in Turnovo (in north-central Bulgaria) were cordoned off and entry and exit to quarantined neighborhoods severely restricted. A red rag or fur hat flown from the roof of a house indicated to townspeople that an inhabitant had died of the plague. Town residents often appealed to local leaders to forcibly isolate neighbors suspected of being infected with plague.[43]

Plague-induced displacements resulted in the formation of new population settlements and significant alterations to the human geography of Rumeli. For example, on several occasions in the late eighteenth century, the town of Karnobat—upon the appearance of the plague—effectively dissolved and reformed several kilometers distant from the town's original site. Many residents of the town of Stara Zagora preferred to ride out plague epidemics in make-shift settlements in the Balkan Mountains. Here, caves, monasteries, and earthen dug-outs provided temporary refuge from plague-infested areas. Plague-free "quarantine villages" were established in the Rumelian countryside—usually in the environs of Bulgarian monasteries. For example, with the appearance of the plague in the early summer of 1837, frightened residents from the towns of Karlovo, Kazanlŭk, and Stara Zagora (all in central Bulgaria) erected a fortified camp in the environs of the Kalofer Monastery (located in central Bulgaria about 70 kilometers north of Plovdiv). No one was allowed to enter or leave the grounds of the camp and strict measures were adopted to disinfect imported food and supplies. In the fall, after the virulence of the plague had dissipated, the camp was dismantled and the inhabitants of the camp returned to their home towns.[44]

In response to the appearance of disease in 1837, Hoca Saroğlu and his three sons decided to flee from their home village of Iubelki. After wandering the countryside for about one month the Saroğlu family came upon the small settlement of Kemallar (located about 100 kilometers southwest of Silistre) where they settled

41 Ibid., 236–37.

42 Mark Mazower, *Salonica: City of Ghosts: Christians, Muslims, and Jews, 1430–1950* (New York: Alfred A. Knopf, 2005), 112.

43 Manolova-Nikolova, *Chumavite Vremena*, 186–90.

44 Ibid., 100–1.

permanently. In time neighborhoods grew up around these additional plague-induced settlements and today the town of Kemallar has a population of 13,000.[45]

The Ottoman State's Response to the Spread of Epidemic Disease

Prior to the 1830s, most of the quarantine-like structures in the Ottoman Empire existed along the empire's land frontiers or in the autonomous regions of the empire. A lazaret (pesthouse) existed in the Wallachian town of Izlas (at the confluence of the Olt and Danube Rivers) in 1740 and in the late eighteenth century three lazarets were erected around Bucharest.[46] Around the turn of the nineteenth century, a medical inspection post was established in the Wallachian town of Orşova, and small quarantine-like stations were operational on the Danube River at Kalaraşi and Zimnich.[47] All travelers crossing the Danube River from Silistre into Kalaraşi were obligated to undergo a seven-day period of medical observation. By 1813, several full-fledged medical inspection complexes lay astride all roads leading into Bucharest from the south.[48]

Wallachia and Moldavia were also the site of some of the more vigorous anti-disease measures undertaken in the Ottoman Empire in the early 1800s. These measures included the burning of infected houses in Bucharest, the increased surveillance of visitors to Bucharest, a prohibition against the import of clothing, the closing of coffee-houses and market stalls, the deportation of Roma, and the confinement of mendicants to monasteries.[49] During the Russo-Ottoman Wars of 1806–12 and 1828–29, lazarets were constructed around Bucharest and Jassy and quarantine posts established along the Danube River (in Braila, Galatz, and Giurgiu).[50]

In the early part of the nineteenth century, the Ottoman state increasingly viewed the implementation of anti-disease measures and the expansion of quarantine construction as a means to surveil and reassert central state control over displaced and migratory populations in the Balkans. In 1813, the provincial governor of Yanina (in northern Greece and southern Albania) Tepedelenli Ali Pasha ordered all postal stations in western Rumeli to be fumigated and disinfected.

---

45 Ibid., 184

46 Ibid., 200.

47 Panzac, *La peste,* 452–53; Manolova-Nikolova, *Chumavite Vremena*, 102.

48 Manolova-Nikolova, *Chumavite Vremena*, 205.

49 Panzac, *La peste*, 452–53; Manolova-Nikolova, 205.

50 RGVIA, f. 14209, op. 2/163a, d. 6, List 8 (February 17, 1808); RGVIA, f. 14209, op. 2/163a, d. 6, l. 35 (January–December 1808); RGVIA, f. 14209, op. 3/163b, d. 6, ch. 1, l. 46 (September 1810–January 1812); and *Rossiiskii Gosudarstvennyi Istoricheskii Arkhiv* (RGIA), f. 1263, op. 1, d. 602, ll. 50–63 (May 6–7, 1829).

Checkpoints were constructed to guard mountain passes leading into Yanina. Travelers crossing the Pindus Mountains from Thessaly (from the east) were detained at these new checkpoints and forced to undergo a period of medical observation. In Ohrid (in Macedonia), the local governor, Celaleddin Bey, had most of the monasteries around Lake Ohrid converted into lazarets.[51] By 1814, a medical complex existed in the important Danubian fortress-town of Vidin. This complex included facilities for the detention and observation of individuals afflicted with plague. The first military hospital constructed in Rumeli was included within this complex.[52] In the 1820s, travel restrictions were imposed on vessels crossing the Bosporus and the Dardanelles from the north and west.[53] A temporary lazaret was constructed in Edirne in the fall of 1829 and quarantine-like measures imposed on the town's population.[54] By the mid-1830s this temporary lazaret in Edirne had evolved into a full-scale quarantine station.[55]

Following the Russo-Ottoman War of 1828–29 a chain of quarantine stations was constructed along the northern shore of the Danube River and lazarets lay astride key interior commercial arteries in Wallachia.[56] This Danubian *cordon sanitaire* consisted of three main quarantine stations (in Braila, Galatz, and Giurgiu) and six secondary posts (in Kalaraşi, Pioa Pietri, Kalafat, Zimnich, Turnu Mugurele, and Severin). The largest quarantine station in Braila encompassed an area of 8,000 square meters and was composed of a mix of brick and wooden buildings. The complex was staffed by a doctor, a nurse practitioner, an interpreter, a secretary, two aides, and six guards. In 1831, the length of the quarantine at Braila fluctuated between four and sixteen days.[57]

To check clandestine cross-river movements, raised observation posts were erected along the northern shore of the Danube.[58] Military personnel were deployed to enforce quarantine regulations including the cleansing (in a mix of

---

51 Manolova-Nikolova, *Chumavite Vremena*, 204–5.

52 İsmail Eren, "Bulgaristan ve Romanya'daki Türk Sağlık Kuruluşları," *I. Türk Tıp Tarihi Kongresi: Kongreye Sunulan Bildiriler* (Ankara: Türk Tarih Kurumu, 1992), 75.

53 Manolova-Nikolova, *Chumavite Vremena*, 102.

54 Ibid., 207.

55 BOA, Hatt-ı Hümayun 737/34964–A (December 17, 1836).

56 The text of the article in the Treaty of Adrianople pertaining to quarantine construction on the Danube River can be found (in Russian) in *Dogovori Rossii s Vostokom* (Saint Petersburg: Tipografi O. I. Baksta, 1869), 82 and (in French) in Gabriel Noradounghian, *Recueil d'actes internationaux de l'empire ottoman, 1789–1856* (Paris: F. Pichon, 1900), 2: 175.

57 Panzac, *Quarantaines*, 156.

58 Panzac, "Politique sanitaire et fixation des frontières: l'exemple Ottoman (XVIIIe–XIXe siècles)," *Turcica* 31 (1999): 96–97.

chlorine and sulfur) of the personal effects of individual travelers and the merchandise of traders.[59] In his memoirs, the future Bulgarian Metropolitan Panaret Rashev described his experiences in the Giurgiu quarantine in 1829. Upon entering the complex, he was stripped naked and disinfected with lime. His coins were placed into pots of vinegar to be cleansed. While in quarantine, Rashev spent the night on the floor and used his own bedding.[60]

The promulgation of regulations governing the administration of this quarantine line and the adoption of any new measures in the Danubian Principalities required the approval of the Ottoman government.[61] Following the withdrawal of Russian occupation forces from the Danubian Principalities in the mid-1830s, control over the quarantine line reverted from Russian to Ottoman authority. The Ottoman state assumed supervision over the Danubian quarantine line, and senior-level quarantine officials were reassigned from Istanbul to the Danubian Principalities.[62]

Following the conclusion of the Russo-Ottoman War of 1828–29, the retreating Russian army abandoned and left behind a significant amount of anti-disease infrastructure. For example Russian military engineers had constructed temporary (or mobile) quarantine stations (*quarantines volantes*) in occupied Ottoman territory to shield soldiers from infected civilian populations.[63] Sited around the Wallachian capital of Bucharest, in key Danubian fortress towns (such as Ismail, Kilia, and Hirsova), and at important fortified transportation hubs (such as Novipazar in northeastern Bulgaria and Nova Zagora in eastern Rumeli), many of these temporary quarantine stations were eventually expanded by the Ottomans into full-scale and permanent quarantine stations.[64]

---

59 Panzac, *Quarantaines*, 96.

60 BIA, Fond 8, Panaret Rashev. For each of these sanitation procedures he was charged ten rubles. Upon completing his quarantine obligations, Rashev was asked to pay an additional 20 rubles as a "departure" fee. Memoirs penned by migrants on the move across the Ottoman-Russian Black Sea frontier in the early part of the nineteenth century indicate that bribery was rife along Russian-controlled quarantine lines. See for example, "Vospominaniia Doktora Zeidlitsa o Turetskom Pokhod 1829 Goda," 423, 426.

61 A.P. Zablotskii-Desiatovskii, *Graf P.D. Kiselev i ego Vremia* (Saint Petersburg: Tip. M. M. Stasiulevicha, 1882), 360–63.

62 On Ottoman quarantine administration in the Danubian Principalities, see BOA, Hatt-ı Hümayun 1144/45467–B (August 14, 1835); BOA, Hatt-ı Hümayun 1144/45467–G (August 14, 1835); BOA, Cevdet Sıhhiye 15/717 (1837–1838); BOA, Cevdet Sıhhiye 27/1343 (April 22, 1841).

63 GARF, f. 109, op. 4a, d. 7, l. 74.

64 RGIA, f. 1263, op. 1, d. 602, ll. 50–63; RGVIA, f. 14209, op. 2/163a, d. 11, l. 32 (May 6–7, 1829); and "Vospominaniia Doktora Zeidlitsa o Turetskom Pokhod 1829 Goda," 423, 426.

Following a successful Russian siege in the summer and fall of 1828, the Russian army immediately established a *cordon sanitaire* around the Black Sea port-city of Varna, closed the gates of the city to all commercial traffic, and constructed several quarantine stations in the port area. In the city center, Russian military hospitals treated civilian victims of the plague. Further down the Black Sea coast in Burgas, abandoned houses along the city's bay were converted into temporary quarantine stations and in Pomorie the Russian army established quarantines and military hospitals to intern and treat civilians suspected of carrying the plague.[65]

The implementation of state-initiated public health and migration management measures in Ottoman Rumeli established the groundwork for the formation of a comprehensive quarantine system in the Balkans in the 1830s. These measures included the prohibition of all population movements in and out of the towns of Sofia and Plovdiv, the quarantining of villages around Turnovo, and the severing of transportation links between the towns of Pirot and Nish (along today's Bulgarian-Serbian border). In 1836, two lazarets were constructed on the southern shore of the Danube River in Ruse and Silistre. Merchants and migrants passing through these two important transportation hubs were obliged to undergo a twelve-day period of medical observation.[66] With the reopening of the Pirot-Nish road in 1837, soldiers were posted to control travel between these two towns and all travelers arriving from Pirot were placed into quarantine in Nish.[67] By the mid-1840s, of the total 81 quarantines operational in the Ottoman Empire outside of Istanbul, 25 were located in Rumeli and along the western Black Sea coast.[68]

Smyrna (İzmir): An Example of an Ottoman Quarantine Complex

My purpose here in including a brief discussion of the regulations in place at the Ottoman Quarantine complex in Smyrna (İzmir) is threefold. First, I would like to highlight the ways in which Ottoman quarantine stations served as surveillance

---

65 Manolova-Nikolova, *Chumavite Vremena*, 26–27.

66 Ibid., 209.

67 Panzac, *La peste*, 477–78.

68 In the late 1830s and early 1840s, quarantine stations were constructed in the following Dobrujan and Rumelian towns: Maçin, Tulça, Constanţa, Galatz, Balçık, Babadağ, Silistre, Ruse, Sviştov, Nikopol, Vidin, Varna, Burgas, Sozopol, Edirne, Plovdiv, Şipka, Ahyolu (Pomorie), Shumen, Kazanlŭk, Turnovo, Sofia, Aytos, Sliven, and Dimetoka. BOA, Cevdet Sıhhiye 8/371 (undated, probably 1841 or 1842); Gülden Sarıyıldız, "Karantina Teşkilatının Kuruluşu ve Faaliyetleri, 1838–1876," MA thesis, Istanbul University, 1986, 76–84; Süheyl Ünver, "Les épidémies de choléra dans les terres balkaniques aux XVIIIe et XIXe siècles," *Etudes Balkaniques* 4 (1973), 96.

posts and sites for information-gathering on merchants, migrants, diplomats, and travelers entering and moving through the Ottoman Empire in the 1840s. Second, given the centralized, comprehensive and empire-wide nature of Ottoman quarantine administration in the middle part of the nineteenth century, it is reasonable to assume that the procedures in place in İzmir closely resembled those in place in other Ottoman quarantine stations, including those recently constructed in the Balkans. And third, the full report upon which this brief account is taken provides us with the most detailed description we have of a mid-nineteenth Ottoman quarantine complex.

In 1844, the Russian Ministry of Interior published a report on the Ottoman quarantine complex in İzmir (Smyrna).[69] The author of the report (identified only as A. Y.) noted that the İzmir quarantine complex formed an important hub in what he referred to as the "Turkish quarantine system." According to A. Y., quarantine guards were responsible for supervising the movements of all travelers arriving at the port of İzmir, for overseeing intake and processing procedures at the main quarantine building, and for providing security in both the main quarantine building and in the lazaret. Every ship entering the port was met by a quarantine guard. The passengers and goods on the ship were inspected and the ship's *patente* handed over from the captain to the quarantine guard. Carried in a tin box, this *patente* contained information on the overall health of the passengers, the home port of the vessel, and the ports through which it had passed while *en route* to İzmir. Those with a clean *patente* were authorized to fly a yellow flag indicating that the vessel had been permitted to dock in the main harbor and allowed to engage in direct contact with merchant houses and residents in İzmir. Ships suspected of carrying plague-ridden cargo or transporting individuals suspected of being afflicted with infectious diseases were towed to a long wooden pier leading directly into the courtyard of the main quarantine building. In this building the passengers were registered and inspected by the quarantine's medical officer. These intake and processing procedures were overseen by armed guards.

---

69 "Karantin i Gospitali v Smirn," *Zhurnal Ministerstva Vnutrennikh Del* 8 (1844), 295–312. As I have argued elsewhere, in the late eighteenth and early nineteenth centuries, the Ottoman and Russian states (at both the imperial and local levels) undertook joint initiatives to police their mutual Black Sea borderland. This entailed exchanging information and coordinating activities concerning population movements and the spread of disease between the two empires. This visit to the Ottoman quarantine in İzmir by a Russian Ministry of Interior official should be understood in this context. See my "Imperial Confrontation or Regional Cooperation?: Bulgarian Migration and Ottoman-Russian Relations in the Black Sea Region, 1768–1830s," *Turkish Historical Review* 3, no. 2 (2012), 149–67.

The Secretary of the Chancellery of the İzmir quarantine acted as the main registrar for the complex. In this capacity he recorded information on all arrivals in the quarantine complex including their overall health status and determinations made regarding the amount of time they were required to remain in quarantine.[70] As part of his record-keeping requirements, the Secretary of the Chancellery maintained three separate registers. The first register contained information on all arriving ships in İzmir including their port of origin, the name of their captain, the number of sailors and passengers on each ship, the types of goods carried, and the name of the merchant house or shops in İzmir where the goods were to be delivered. The second register recorded health and disease-related information, such as the name of each ship arriving in İzmir from places known to have been infected with plague, the required quarantine period for passengers on infected ships, the date on which the passengers had completed their quarantine period, and the date on which the passengers were discharged from the complex. The third register contained annual mortality statistics for the city of İzmir, including the number of deaths in any given year, the name, gender, age, and occupation of the dead, and the cause of death. On a bi-weekly basis, the director of the İzmir quarantine was required to submit a statistical report to Istanbul with information on plague-related deaths.[71] According to A. Y.'s report, it is clear that the İzmir quarantine served not only as the main repository for information on disease and public health in İzmir but also as the clearinghouse for intelligence gathered on merchants and travelers arriving in the city's harbor.

Quarantines as Multi-Purpose State Institutions

As was the case in İzmir, lazarets and quarantine stations in the Ottoman Balkans served as comprehensive Ottoman customs and surveillance posts. In Rumeli, however, quarantine stations also demarcated land borders and served as the primary land-based border crossing posts into the Ottoman Empire from the north

70 The Secretary of the Chancellery assigned to the İzmir quarantine complex in 1844 had previously served as a scribe at a Greek quarantine station located on the island of Siros (in the Cyclades about 150 kilometers southeast of Athens)—an indication, perhaps, of the career trajectory and upward mobility available to experienced quarantine officials in the Eastern Mediterranean. In the 1830s, the three largest and most important Greek quarantine facilities in the Aegean were located in Piraeus, Siros, and Santorini. See Manolova-Nikolova, *Chumavite Vremena*, 211–12.

71 Translated from Russian, the name of the Istanbul-based bureaucratic entity, which received and processed the health-related statistics forwarded from the İzmir quarantine was "The Ottoman Board of Public Health."

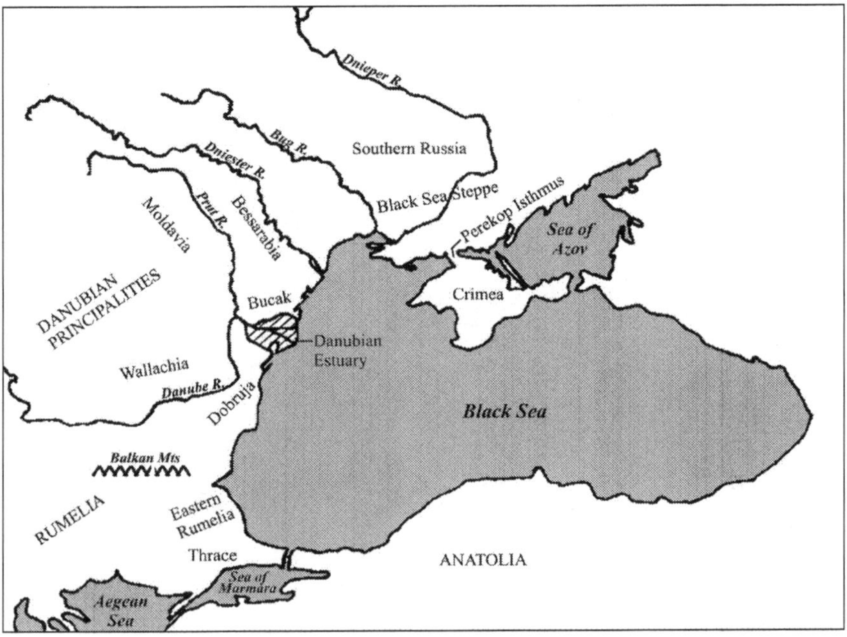

Map 2. The Black Sea Region.

and west. In the 1830s, newly-constructed lazarets lined the recently-established Ottoman-Serbian and Ottoman-Greek borders. Along the Ottoman-Serbian border, a series of guard stations (manned by militia drawn from the local populace) and makeshift barriers (constructed out of thickets and straw) radiated outward from a central headquarters lazaret. By 1837, a large five-lazaret border and surveillance complex operated in Aleksinac (just north of Nish along the Ottoman-Serbian border). Surrounded by a wooden fence, the interior courtyard of this complex was, at any given time, capable of holding over 1,200 people. In Thessaly—along the new Ottoman-Greek border—all travelers entering and exiting the Ottoman Empire were required to undergo an extended period of quarantine (nine days for ordinary travelers and fifteen days for merchants). Upon the appearance of plague, lazaret posts were militarized and regular army units were dispatched to bolster border-control, surveillance, and disease-monitoring efforts.[72]

As mentioned above, the staffing list and spatial distribution of buildings in the Ottoman quarantine complex in İzmir indicate that the lazaret function was only one of many parts of a full-scale quarantine operation. Non-medical interro-

72 Manolova-Nikolova, *Chumavite Vremena*, 211–12.

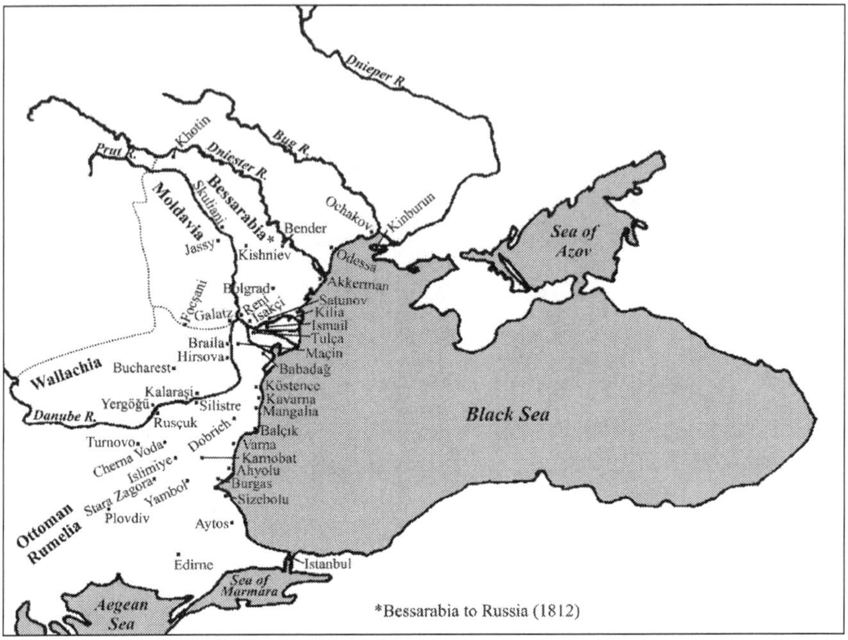

Map 3. Cities, Towns, and Political Divisions in the Black Sea Region (Late Eighteenth and Early Nineteenth Centuries).

gation units operated within quarantine complexes in Istanbul and, in addition to medical personnel, many Ottoman quarantine facilities employed a staff of multilingual officials specifically assigned to issue health certificates (*sıhhiye tezkiresi* or *karantina tezkiresi*) to individual travelers.[73] In the Balkans and Danubian Principalities, customs houses were commandeered and converted into quarantine stations and customs collectors were reappointed as quarantine officials.[74] In this manner, the normal functions of Ottoman customs houses were subsumed within the overall operation of quarantine complexes. For example, in the 1830s, Bulgarian merchants paid customs duties upon entering into quarantine stations along the Danube River.[75]

In response to severe outbreaks of cholera in the 1830s, a provisional Quarantine Council was formed in Istanbul to oversee the implementation of previously *ad-hoc* quarantine, disease control, and sanitation measures in the Ottoman

73 Sarıyıldız, "Karantina Teşkilatı," 84–92.

74 BOA, Hatt-ı Hümayun 523/25542 (1839).

75 Manolova-Nikolova, *Chumavite Vremena*, 103.

Empire.[76] The maintenance of public order and the provision of security were among the core competencies of the Council.[77] Military officials worked with members of the Council on the development and implementation of the *cordons sanitaires* and oversaw the establishment of security perimeters around Ottoman quarantine complexes.[78] Retired soldiers were employed to help staff newly established quarantine stations in Rumeli. At the municipal level, the Ottoman gendarmerie (*zaptiye*) was often charged with implementing local anti-disease and sanitation measures.[79] Officials were dispatched by the Council in Istanbul to assist provincial authorities in the Balkans in suppressing the spread of disease. Typically seconded from the large Kuleli quarantine station in Istanbul, these officials were charged with reporting on any irregularities in the administration of provincial quarantines and gathering information on the quality and effectiveness of Ottoman quarantine lines.[80] By the 1840s, the Council was operating a training academy within the Kuleli complex. In time, the graduates of this academy rose to leadership positions in various quarantine posts in the empire and eventually replaced the medical professionals who, in the 1830s, had formed the initial leadership *cadre* in Ottoman quarantines.[81]

As indicated in the above-described operations in place at the Ottoman complex in İzmir, quarantine officials were required to compile registration lists with the full names, family composition, current and previous places of residence, and occupation of all individuals and families entering and exiting Ottoman quarantine stations.[82] In a similar vein, quarantine directors and *qadis* were directed to

76 The overall competency of the Ottoman Quarantine Council was threefold: to establish quarantines in important border, coastal, and interior cities throughout the Empire; to eliminate internal outbreaks of epidemic diseases; and to dispatch doctors and officials in a timely manner to places where they were needed. The Quarantine Council was subordinate to the Ottoman Foreign Ministry. BOA, Hatt-ı Hümayun 524/25572-B (1839); Ünver, "Les épidémies de choléra," 96; Sarıyıldız, "Karantina Teşkilatı," 48.

77 Sarıyıldız, "Karantina Teşkilatı," 46–47. For an in-depth discussion on Mahmud II (r. 1808–39)'s efforts to improve safety and security on Ottoman roads, see Yusuf Halaçoğlu, "Osmanlı İmparatorluğu'nda Menzil Teşkilatı Hakkında Bazı Mülahazalar," *Osmanlı Araştırmaları* 2 (1981), 123–32.

78 BOA, Hatt-ı Hümayun 523/25542 (1839).

79 Sarıyıldız, "Karantina Teşkilatı," 32–36.

80 BOA, Cevdet Sıhhiye 13/625 (September 23, 1839); BOA, Cevdet Sıhhiye 22/1063 (September 26, 1840); BOA, Cevdet Sıhhiye 27/1325 (1839–40).

81 Ünver, "Les épidémies de choléra," 97.

82 Ufuk Gülsoy, "1828 Yılında İstanbul'a Getirilen Varnalı Muhacirler," *Tarih İncelemeleri Dergisi* 7 (1992): 252–70. An example of a Galata *defter* with registration lists of arrivals in

gather basic health statistics on populations. This information was forwarded to the Council and compiled into a monthly report for the Grand Vizier.[83] As part of an empire-wide information-gathering network, quarantine directors in the Balkans communicated on a regular basis with members of the Council in Istanbul.[84]

Conclusion

In the late eighteenth and early nineteenth centuries, epidemic diseases (plague, cholera, typhus, malaria or other unidentified pathogens) ravaged the populations of Rumeli and the Ottoman-controlled Danubian Principalities of Moldavia and Wallachia. In response, the townspeople and villagers of the Ottoman Balkans implemented time-honored measures such as fumigation, ritual offerings to mythical personages, and the sacrifice of animals, and engaged in multi-confessional ceremonies and rituals such as the performance of common liturgies and the reading aloud of common prayers. Many also opted to flee from their homes in search of safety from disease. These disease-induced displacements and socio-economic disruptions contributed to lawlessness and a breakdown in public order in the Ottoman Balkans, severely hampered Ottoman tax-collection efforts, reduced Ottoman military preparedness, and limited the Ottoman state's overall war-making capabilities.[85]

Istanbul can be found in BOA, Hatt-ı Hümayun 1021/42649 (November 19, 1829).

83 The holdings of the BOA contain numerous examples of these reports and statistical tabulations. See, for example, BOA, Hatt-ı Hümayun 523/25564–C (January 15, 1839); BOA, Hatt-ı Hümayun 524/25567–C (April 15, 1839); BOA, Hatt-ı Hümayun 524/25571–B (December 17, 1838); BOA, Hatt-ı Hümayun 524/25571–C (December 17, 1838); BOA, İrade Dahiliye 17/782 (July 7, 1840).

84 BOA, Cevdet Sıhhiye 27/1330 (1840s); Ünver, "Les épidémies de choléra," 91.

85 Ottoman tax collectors in İpsala province (south of Edirne) reported that they were unable to perform their duties because of the disruptions caused by a plague epidemic. See BOA, İbnülemin Sıhhiye 107/1–2 (June 7, 1699). In 1814, a Bulgarian inhabitant of Stara Zagora noted that Ottoman tax collection efforts were severely hampered by the death and displacement caused by an outbreak of a severe plague epidemic. See Manolova-Nikolova, *Chumavite Vremena*, 75. During the Russo-Ottoman War of 1768–1774, large-scale desertions among soldiers stationed in the strategic Danubian estuary fortress-town of Isakçı were, in large measure, the direct consequence of a plague epidemic. See Coşkun Yılmaz and Necdet Yılmaz, eds., *Osmanlılarda Sağlık* (Istanbul: Biofarma, 2006), 2: 355. Following the Russo-Ottoman War of 1806–1812, the inability to collect revenue in northern Rumeli impeded the Ottoman ability to repair fortresses along the Danube River. See BOA, Cevdet Askeriye 1177/52473 (February 20, 1814). In 1814, the displacement of many of the skilled factory workers employed at an important Ottoman weapons manufacturing facility in Sliven resulted in a shortfall in the plant's monthly output of armaments. See BOA, Cevdet Askeriye 600/25315 (July 9, 1814).

In the 1830s, following a prolonged period of Russo-Ottoman warfare and administrative decentralization in the Balkans, the Ottoman state moved to regain control over the economy and society of its Balkan possessions. The centralizing and post-war reconstruction initiatives undertaken by the Ottoman state included the implementation and strengthening of anti-disease and public health measures as well as the extension and institutionalization of a previously *ad-hoc* quarantine regime. In time, Ottoman quarantines evolved into all-purpose border posts and served as multi-purpose state institutions in Rumeli. The implementation of enhanced social control measures and the evolving role of quarantine stations highlights the general connection between disease suppression, migration management, and border control in the early nineteenth-century Ottoman Balkans.

Andrew Robarts (arobarts@risd.edu) is Assistant Professor of History at the Rhode Island School of Design where he teaches courses on Middle Eastern, Ottoman, and Russian History. He is the author of *Migration and Disease in the Black Sea Region: Ottoman-Russian Relations in the Late Eighteenth and Early Nineteenth Centuries* (Bloomsbury Academic Press), *Black Sea Regionalism: A Case Study* (Oxford University Press), and "Reconstruction, Resettlement, and Economic Revitalization in pre-Tanzimat Ottoman Bulgaria," in *Wealth in the Ottoman and Post-Ottoman Balkans: A Socio-Economic History*, ed. Evguenia Davidova (I. B. Tauris).

CHOLERA, PILGRIMAGE, AND INTERNATIONAL POLITICS OF SANITATION: THE QUARANTINE STATION ON THE ISLAND OF KAMARAN*

GÜLDEN SARIYILDIZ
Istanbul University

OYA DAĞLAR MACAR
Istanbul Commerce University

THIS CHAPTER WILL focus on Kamaran quarantine station in the context of the late nineteenth- and early twentieth-century international sanitary politics. Located on Kamaran Island on the southern tip of the Red Sea, this was one of the largest quarantine facilities in the world at the time of its establishment in 1882. It was built primarily for the purpose of blocking the spread of cholera, which, in the nineteenth century was believed to come from the east, in particular South Asia. Given its strategic location and the competing international interest to claim jurisdiction over it, the Kamaran quarantine offers a unique lens to study international politics of sanitation in the late nineteenth century. What was the reason for the establishment of a quarantine station on Kamaran Island? What were the characteristics of the Kamaran station? What were the British sanitary policies in the Red Sea in the nineteenth century, with respect to the Kamaran station? And what were the political and economic expectations that informed these policies? Using a wealth of archival documents, this chapter will survey the international debates and controveries behind the establishment of the quarantine, its construction, organization, and function.

Following the devastating cholera pandemic of 1865, an International Sanitary Conference was held in Istanbul in 1866, in which India was accepted as the origin of the pandemic.[1] In the same meeting, it was decided that a quarantine station

---

* This essay, originally written in Turkish, has been translated and revised for publication by Nükhet Varlık.

1 Bedi N. Şehsuvaroğlu, "Türkiye Karantina Tarihine Giriş I: Dünya Karantina Teşkilatı," *İstanbul Tıp Fakültesi Mecmuası* 20, no. 3 (1957): 15; Valeska Huber, "The Unification of the Globe by Disease? The International Sanitary Conferences on Cholera, 1851–1894," *The Historical Journal* 49, no. 2 (2006): 462; Sheldon Watts, "Cholera Politics in Britain in 1879: John Netten Radcliffe's Confidential Memo on 'Qurantine in the Red Sea'," *The Journal of the Historical Society* 7, no. 3 (2007), 331; Handan Kılınç, "Isolating the Subject: Cholera,

needed to be established at the entry point to the Red Sea in order to monitor Muslim pilgrims coming from the Indian Ocean. As per the decision of the conference, the Ottoman Empire was entrusted with this responsibility.[2] Hence, the Ottoman administration sent a commission to the region to explore where the quarantine station could be built. As a result of investigations, it was decided that the island of Kamaran would be ideal for this purpose. The geographic location would make possible to monitor the movement of ships coming to the Red Sea through the Bab-el-Mandeb Straits, which connected it to the Gulf of Aden. Moreover, the terrain of the island was found to be suitable for holding quarantine procedures.[3]

After its inauguration in 1882, the quarantine quickly became an important point in the service of international sanitary efforts, in additon to its critical role in controling health conditions locally. For the Muslim world, its significance was especially prominent during the pilgrimage season. Every year, tens of thousands of Muslims went to the Holy Cities in the Hijaz region for pilgrimage. According to the agreements drawn at the International Sanitary Conference, all pilgrims-to-be who entered the Red Sea from the south had to go through mandatory health screening.[4] Among those were Muslims from mainly India, Java, and the Persian Gulf, as well as those coming from Afghanistan and Central Asia.[5] Only after an

Control, and Sanitary Discourse in the Istanbul International Sanitary Conference of 1866," MA thesis, Boğaziçi University, 2005, 57.

2 Başbakanlık Osmanlı Arşivi (Prime Ministry's Ottoman Archives), Istanbul [hereafter BOA], İrade Meclis-i Mahsus, 1387: Report of the Commission dated Feb. 2, 1867; "Kamaran'da Müessesat-ı Sıhhiye-yi Osmaniye: Tahaffuzhane ve Memurin," *Servet-i Fünun* 24, no. 604 (1902): 86; Gülden Sarıyıldız, *Hicaz Karantina Teşkilatı* (Ankara: Türk Tarih Kurumu, 1996), 26; The British Delegate on the Constantinople Board of Health, "Some Turkish Lazarets and Other Sanitary Institutions in the Near East, I," *The Lancet* 169, no. 4365 (Apr. 27, 1907): 1188.

3 BOA, İrade Sıhhiye, 4058.

4 For the International Sanitary Conferences, see Norman Howard-Jones, *The Scientific Backround of International Sanitary Conferences, 1851–1938* (Geneva: World Health Organization, 1975); Arne Barkhuus, "The Sanitary Conferences," *Ciba Symposium* 5, no. 7 (1943): 1563–79; William F. Bynum, "Policing Hearts of Darkness: Aspects of the International Sanitary Conferences," *History and Philosophy of the Life Sciences* 15 (1993): 421–34; Emine Melek Atabek, *1851'de Paris'te Toplanan I. Milletlerarası Sağlık Konferansı ve Türkler* (Istanbul: Cerrahpaşa Tıp Fakültesi Yayınları, 1974); Kılınç, "Isolating the Subject." For the International Sanitary Convention of Paris, 1894, see BOA, İrade Sıhhiye, 2 (Şevval 1314 / March-April 1897); The British Delegate on the Constantinople Board of Health "Some Turkish Lazarets I," 1188; Huber, "Unification," 469.

5 Between 1887 and 1902, 42 percent of the pilgims screened at Kamaran were from Malay, 40.8 percent from India, and 17.2 percent from South Asia, Iran, and Mesopotamia.

initial screening at the quarantine station on Kamaran Island were they allowed to proceed to the port of Jidda.[6] The quarantine also served for the screening of those who traveled to the Mediterranean via the Suez Canal, after pilgrimage.[7] In brief, this quarantine station was of key importance for Muslims who wanted to go on pilgrimage.

For Europe, Kamaran was a point of confluence where intertwined interests and expectations converged. The island already had considerable strategic and commercial influence over maritime traffic in the Red Sea. For European ships that carried Muslim pilgrims, this was a promising business. The advent of steamships in the nineteenth century and the opening of the Suez Canal in 1869 contributed to an increased pilgrimage traffic in the Red Sea—so much so that shipping companies started to offer scheduled pilgrimage voyages. At this time, the overland caravan routes started to lose their primacy for pilgrimage. Pilgrims now preferred sea travel, which was faster, safer, and more comfortable. While British and Dutch ships carried pilgrims from their colonies in India, Java, and Indonesia, French and Austrian maritime companies served the Muslims of the Ottoman Empire, North Africa, and Europe. Tens of thousands of Muslim pilgrims every year yielded considerable profits to European carriers.[8]

European carriers were aware of the sanitary implications of this business: carrying large groups of pilgrims from South and Southeastern Asia—where epidemic diseases were thought to have originated—could facilitate the spread of disease. Controling the spread of epidemic diseases was especially challenging

---

See Kuneralp, "Osmanlı Yönetimindeki (1831–1911) Hicaz'da Hac ve Kolera," trans. Münir Atalar, *Osmanlı Tarihi Araştırma ve Uygulama Merkezi Dergisi (OTAM)* 7 (1996): 510.

6 Léonard Fischer, *Pèlerinage de la Mecque* ([Strasbourg: Imprimerie de Hauss, 1908]), India Office Library and Records [hereafter IOL], T 13328 (d), 10.

7 BOA, Eyalet-i Mümtaze (05) Mısır, 5-C/187.

8 Adrien Proust, *Sıhhiye Politikasında Yeni Bir Cevelan Yani Sıhhiye Mesele-i Siyasiyesinin Hal ve Tesviyesi Cihetini Tayin: Hicaz Hacları*, trans. Ahmed Nermi, Istanbul University Rare Books Collection, ms. TY 4631, 17; Jonathan Miran, "Space, Mobility, and Translocal Connections Across the Red Sea Area since 1500," *Northeast African Studies*, 12, no. 1 (2012): xix; William Facey, "The Red Sea: The Wind Regime and Location of Ports," in *Trade and Travel in the Red Sea Region: Proceedings of Red Sea Project I Held in the British Museum, October 2002*, eds. Paul Lunde and Alexandra Porter, 7–17 (Oxford: Archaeopress, 2004); Kirti N. Chaudhuri, *Trade and Civilisation in the Indian Ocean: History from the Rise of Islam to 1750* (Cambridge: Cambridge University Press, 1985); Colette Dubois, "The Red Sea Ports during the Revolution in Transportation, 1800–1914," in *Modernity and Culture from the Mediterranean to the Indian Ocean*, eds. Leila Tarazi Fawaz and C. A. Bayly (New York: Columbia University Press, 2002); Ashin Das Gupta, *Merchants of Maritime India, 1500–1800* (Aldershot: Ashgate/Variorum, 1994).

during pilgrimage season owing to increased mobility involving the sustenance and accommodation of large numbers of pilgrims, as well as the practice of ritual animal sacrifice. In addition, maintaining hygiene was burdensome on account of excessive heat and water scarcity in the region. The multiple sanitary challenges of keeping mass mobilities in check made it imperative to screen the health of travelers before they arrived at Mecca. Kamaran was a perfect site to serve that purpose. The island could stop the spread of disease believed to be arriving from South Asia, and its further dissemination to the Hijaz region, and eventually to Europe. For this reason, European states regarded the quarantine station on the island as a sanitary barrier. At the intersection of international political and sanitary interests, Kamaran was a top agenda item for discussion in the international sanitary conferences held in Paris (1894) and Venice (1897).[9]

Kamaran Quarantine and Its Significance

Research suggests that the Kamaran quarantine was one of the world's largest quarantine complexes at the turn of the twentieth century. In 1893, the number of pilgrims that went through Kamaran was 31,673.[10] In 1907, this number further increased to 36,363.[11] According to the report issued by the Ottoman Sanitary Council (*Meclis-i Umur-ı Sıhhiye*) in June 1899, the site was organized as a quarantine complex.[12] In addition to the buildings that served for isolation of travelers, there were designated areas for meeting the needs of pilgrims on the island, such as hospitals and restaurants. With the addition of new buildings, the complex continued to grow and change over time. Sustained efforts of the Ottoman administration to maintain and improve the complex turned it into a key transit point, not only for the pilgrims coming from South and Southeast Asia but also for European colonial agents.

What further contributed to the prominence of the quarantine at Kamaran was the British political and commerical interests in the region. Britain had growing aspirations to control the Red Sea to secure the trade routes leading to India and to command over trade. At times, Britain's commercial interests were prioritized over medical concerns in the application of quarantine procedures. It is quite

---

9 Watts, "Cholera Politics in Britain," 328, 338.

10 BOA, Meclis-i Umur-u Sıhhiye (meeting minutes of the Ottoman Sanitary Council) [hereafter MUSM], session held on June 13, 1893.

11 Kuneralp, "Osmanlı Yönetimindeki (1831–1911)," 510.

12 For the report, see Administration sanitaire de l'empire Ottoman, *Rapport sur les travaux du lazaret de Camaran par la commission envoyée sur les lieux, en Juin 1899* (Constantinople: Imp. A. Zellich Fils, 1899).

interesting to trace such conflicting concerns raised during discussions about quarantine procedures in the international sanitary conferences and the changes adopted to modify them.

Despite its obvious importance in the late nineteenth and early twentieth centuries, the Kamaran quarantine remained hitherto unexplored in the historical scholarship. Even though there are several studies about the region's political and economic importance, the issue of sanitation and quarantine has not received thorough scholarly attention. Studies on the Ottoman quarantines are limited for the most part. Despite its significance for the Ottoman system of quarantines, the Kamaran station has been only the subject of a handful of studies. This lack of interest may have resulted from the location of the Red Sea that situated it at the periphery of Ottomanist historiography. Recently, historians of the Ottoman Empire have started paying more attention to questions of health and sanitation. An early study on Kamaran quarantine was John Baldry's 1978 article.[13] Gülden Sarıyıldız's 1996 study on the Hijaz quarantines also discusses the Kamaran station.[14] There are scattered references to the Kamaran quarantine in the secondary literature.[15] Beyond this, all research on the Kamaran quarantine needs to be based on primary sources. British archival collections contain important information on the quarantine. For example, there is discussion on the Kamaran quarantine in a nineteen-page report.[16] Another report presents information regarding the establishment and characteristics of the Kamaran quarantine, as well as the procedures applied during the pilgrimage of 1885.[17] A third report by Léonard Fischer, *Pèlerinage de la Mecque*, gives an account of the pilgrimage in 1906–7, including a

13 John Baldry, "The Ottoman Quarantine Station on Kamaran Island, 1882–1914," *Studies in History of Medicine* 11, nos. 1–2 (1978): 3–137.

14 Sarıyıldız, *Hicaz Karantina Teşkilatı*, 54–59. Also see idem, "Osmanlı Sıhhiye Rüsum Tarifesi ve Muhtelit Sıhhiye Rüsum Tarifesi Komisyonları: Kapitülasyona Giden Bir Süreç," in *"Osmanlıdan Cumhuriyete" Sosyo-Kültürel Siyasi Yansımalar: Prof. Dr. Ali İhsan Gencer anısına*, Sarıyıldız et al., eds. (Istanbul: Derin Yayınları, 2015), 273-318.

15 J. E. Peterson, "The Islands of Arabia: Their Recent History and Strategic Importance," *Arabian Studies* 7 (1985): 23–35; Nigel Groom, "The Island of Two Moons: Kamaran 1954," The British-Yemeni Society, July 2002. http://al-bab.com/albab-orig/albab/bys/articles/groom02.htm (accessed January 13, 2015).

16 The report that discusses pilgrimage voyages between the Hijaz and the ports of British India also touches upon the Kamaran quarantine. See: *The Mecca Pilgrimage: Appointment By The Government Of India Thos. Cook And Son as Agents for the Control of the Movements of Mahomedan Pilgrims from All Parts of India to Jeddah for Mecca, Medina, etc., and Back* (London: n.p., 1886), IOL, V 8644 (a).

17 Dr. Duca, *Le pèlerinage de 1885 et la quarantaine de Camaran: rapport au Conseil supérieur de santé* (Constantinople, 1885), IOL, 8644 (c).

brief dicussion of the Kamaran quarantine.[18] More important, the Ottoman archival records can offer a wealth of information on Kamaran. Hundreds of documents kept at the Prime Ministry's Ottoman Archives in Istanbul, currently awaiting the attention of scholars, contain invaluable details on the history of the Kamaran quarantine. The present essay has benefited from documents kept at collections such as Yıldız, Office of the Grand Vizier (*Sadaret*), Ministry of Health (*Sıhhiye Nezareti*), and Chamber of Documents (*Bab-ı Ali Evrak Odası*). In addition, we have examined the relevant minutes of the meetings of the Ottoman Sanitary Council. Maps of the Kamaran quarantine and photographs of the quarantine complex kept at Istanbul University's Rare Books Collection have also been utilized in this study.

The Establishment of the Quarantine Station

In the year 1882, before the beginning of the pilgrimage season, construction work continued apace in the small Red Sea island of Kamaran. Administratively speaking, the island was part of the Ottoman province of Yemen. Traditionally, the population of the island made a living by fishing and harvesting oysters and corals. However, with the establishment of the quarantine, the island would quickly become a harbor for a massive number of ships and pilgrims. Upon the completion of the construction, all ships coming from south of the Bab-el-Mandeb Straits would stop here for the health screening of pilgrims.

As mentioned above, the idea of building a quarantine station in southern Red Sea was first proposed in the International Sanitary Conference of 1866. The conference met to discuss the cholera pandemic of 1865, which had swept across Europe before it was transported to North America. The pandemic caused high mortality everywhere it spread—15,000 died in the Hijaz alone.[19] The punishing effects of the pandemic were further aggravated by the special circumstances of that year's pilgrimage. On years when pilgrims' gathering in Mount Arafat (east of Mecca) fell on a Friday, pilgrimage was considered as "Greater Pilgrimage" (*hacc-ı ekber*) and attracted a greater number of Muslims. The pilgrimage of 1865 was one such year that was attended by a greater number of pilgrims than usual.[20] Two British ships (*Persia* and *North-Wind*) coming from India were believed to have brought the infection to the Hijaz, as cholera broke out shortly after their arrival.[21]

---

18 IOL, T 13028 (d).

19 Michael Christopher Low, "Empire and the Hajj: Pilgrims, Plagues, and Pan-Islam Under British Surveillance, 1865–1908," *International Journal Middle East Studies* 40 (2008), 270.

20 Dr. Duca, *Le pèlerinage de 1885*; Sarıyıldız, *Hicaz Karantina Teşkilatı*, 14.

21 Kuneralp, "Osmanlı Yönetimindeki (1831–1911)," 503–4.

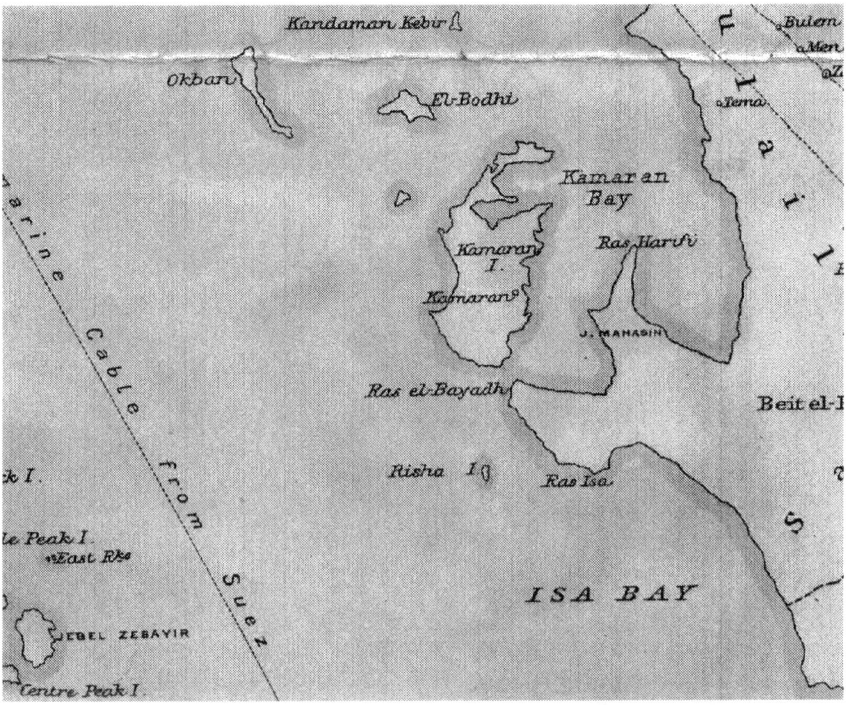

Map 4. Kamaran Island and the Red Sea (Source: Prime Ministry's Ottoman Archives, Istanbul, Maps Catalog, HRT_h_1723).

When the international conference met in Istanbul the next year, there was consensus on not only that India was the source of the pandemic but also that the Muslim pilgrimage was of critical importance in facilitating its spread.[22] It was proposed that a quarantine station be built at an entry point to the Red Sea to screen incoming ships and passengers. In addition, proposals were made for improving the overall conditions of health and hygiene in the Hijaz with the ultimate goal of curbing the spread of cholera.[23]

After the conference, the Ottoman administration sent three different commissions to the area to investigate the spread of the pandemic. These commissions started to explore the Red Sea coast with the purpose of establishing a sanitary

22 Kılınç, "Isolating the Subject," 60; Kuneralp, "Osmanlı Yönetimindeki (1831–1911)," 505.

23 IOL, T 13328 (d), 67; The British Delegate on the Constantinople Board of Health, "Some Turkish Lazarets I," 1188; Kılınç, "Isolating the Subject," 63; Kuneralp, "Osmanlı Yönetimindeki (1831–1911)," 505.

organization.[24] This was also the beginning of the Ottoman initiative for promoting public health and sanitation in the Muslim Holy Cities—something the empire's administration did not undertake before that time. Commissions sent from Istanbul during pilgrimage season inspected health conditions in the Hijaz and proposed measures to improve them.[25] Egypt also decided to establish surveillance against epidemics in the Red Sea, sent its own sanitary commission to the Hijaz, and planned a sanitary organization in the region to start with the pilgrimage of 1867. Quite displeased by Egypt's acting as an independent state, the Ottoman administration responded by emphasizing its own efforts, and appointing physicians and other health personnel to serve in the Hijaz and Yemen. At the same time, it moved toward taking the necessary steps leading to the establishment of quarantines.[26] The first task was to determine the location of the quarantine.

Kamaran, a small coral island at the southern tip of the Red Sea, north of Yemen, would make a good fit for building a quarantine station. Both the location of the island and its physical characteristics were suitable for this purpose. On the east coast of the island lay a large bay that was naturally protected from winds. It could safely harbor twenty large ships.[27] The island had five villages as settled areas.[28] One of the villages, Kamaran, was located at the southern tip of the bay and suitable for building a quarantine station on many acccounts. It was large. Its climatic and topographic conditions were moderate. Most importantly, it had wells supplying clean drinking water.[29] This was especially fortunate, given the demand for water by pilgrims in the hot climate of the region.

24 Kasım İzzeddin, *Mekke-i Mükerremede Kolera ve Hıfzıssıhha* (Istanbul: Mahmud Bey Matbaası, 1911), 32.

25 Sarıyıldız, *Hicaz Karantina Teşkilatı*, 15–19.

26 Following the 1831 cholera pandemic, the Ottoman administration decided to establish quarantines across the empire. In 1838, Sultan Mahmud II (r. 1808–39) ordered the inauguration of the Ottoman Sanitary Council to oversee and administer quarantines. In 1872, there were a total of 148 quarantine stations serving the empire (30 in the Black Sea, 28 in Marmara Sea, 65 in the Aegean, 13 in the Adriatic, 9 in Syria, and 3 on the African coast). In addition, there were check points in Soulina, Trabzon, Batumi, Çanakkale, İzmir, Beirut, and Istanbul (Kavak, Büyükdere, Salacak, and Yenikapı) increasing the total number of facilities up to 159. See BOA, Bâbıâli Evrak Odası, 4314/323540. Also see Andrew Robarts, "Nowhere to Run to, Nowhere to Hide? Society, State, and Epidemic Diseases in the Early Nineteenth-Century Ottoman Balkans," (221–41).

27 Baldry, "Ottoman Quarantine Station," 22.

28 The five villages on the island were Kamaran, Yemen, Furra (Fourre), Mekrem (Makram) and Zeyla (Seila). See BOA, Sadaret Mektubi Mühimme Kalemi Evrakı, 570/17; The British Delegate on the Constantinople Board of Health "Some Turkish Lazarets I," 1189.

29 BOA, Şura-yı Devlet, 2255/12; "Kamaranda Müessesat-ı Sıhhiye-i Osmaniye," *Servet-i*

Even though the plans to build a quarantine station were active since 1866, the actual construction did not take place immediately. During the pilgrimages of 1866 and 1867, Ottoman sanitary commissions of Muslim physicians were sent to serve in the Hijaz. After three years' experience in the Hijaz, a permanent sanitary administration was established. Physicians and sanitary officials were appointed to serve in Mecca, Medina, and Jidda. Temporary quarantines were set up on the coast of Jidda, Lit, and Yanbu.[30] A new cholera outbreak that started to spread in the Hijaz and that was particularly punishing in Mecca in 1881 prompted building a simple and temporary quarantine station to isolate Yemeni pilgrims, both on their way to pilgrimage and on their return journey.[31]

These steps to establish sanitation undertaken by the Ottoman administration were highly costly. Moreover, the Ottoman finances were exhausted by the Russo-Turkish war of 1877–78. Given the financial hardships of the Ottoman administration at the time and the great distance of Kamaran to Istanbul, the quarantine did not start until 1882. Dr. Duca, inspector general of the Ottoman Sanitary Council between 1902 and 1907, supervised the construction of the new quarantine complex.[32] This was a facility that could serve six thousand people at once.[33] The first year it was opened, it processed eight thousand pilgrims.[34] Kamaran was the largest of the Red Sea quarantines, both in size and the number of people it served.

As mentioned above, the island was initially part of the province of Yemen's *Luhayya* district.[35] After the establishment of the quarantine complex, however, its administrative status was changed. In 1884, the island was converted into a sub-

---

Fünun 24, no. 603 (1902): 71.

30 Kasım İzzeddin, *Hicaz Sıhhiye İdaresi Senevi Raporu, Hicaz'da Teşkilat ve Islahat-ı Sıhhiye* (Istanbul: Matbaa-yı Amire, 1328 [1912 or 1913]), 4–7.

31 IOL, V. 8644

32 As the inspector general for the Ottoman Sanitary Council, Dr. Duca (Pasha) represented the empire at the 11th International Sanitary Conference in Paris (1903) and at the 5th Sanitary Dues Tariff Commission (1904). He retired from his post in 1908. See BOA, Sadaret Mektubi Mühimme Kalemi Evrakı, 586/23, 599/24; BOA, Sadaret Mümtaze Kalemi, Mısır (05), 15-B/93; BOA, İrade Sıhhiye, 4/3; BOA, MUSM 1902–1903, 1903–1904, 1904–1905, 1905–1906, and 1906–1907.

33 BOA, İrade-Şura-yı Devlet, 4058; Bedi N. Şehsuvaroğlu, "Türkiye Karantina Tarihine Giriş: Türkiye'de Karantina Tesis ve Teşkilleri," *İstanbul Tıp Fakültesi Mecmuası* 3 (1957): 319–39; The British Delegate on the Constantinople Board of Health, "Some Turkish Lazarets I," 1188.

34 At this time, in addition to Kamaran, other Red Sea quarantines (al-Hudaydah, Abou Saad, and Vasta) also served the region. See Sarıyıldız, *Hicaz Karantina Teşkilatı,* 55.

35 BOA, Şura-yı Devlet, 2255/2.

Table 2. Number of Pilgrims Quarantined at the Kamaran Station (1882–1906). Source: "Some Turkish Lazarets and Other Sanitary Institutions in the Near East, I," *The Lancet* 169, no. 4365 (Apr. 27, 1907): 1189.

Year / H.	Year / C.E.	Pilgrims
1299	1882	9,067
1300	1883	20,016
1301	1884	12,746
1302	1885	17,303
1303	1886	15,031
1304	1887	13,707
1305	1888	20,932
1306	1889	18,723
1307	1890	20,184
1308	1891	23,464
1309	1892	24,032
1310	1893	31,907
1311	1894	22,417

Year / H.	Year / C.E.	Pilgrims
1312	1895	23,378
1313	1895–1896	30,448
1314	1896–1897	14,210
1315	1897–1898	15,229
1316	1898–1899	14,075
1317	1899–1900	11,155
1318	1900–1901	18,336
1319	1901–1902	17,729
1320	1902–1903	15,822
1321	1903–1904	32,452
1322	1904–1905	22,349
1323	1905–1906	32,116

district (*nahiye*) by bringing a nearby village (*Salif*) under its control.[36] Then, it was declared to be part of al-Hudaydah.[37] With the order of the sultan, the Istanbul Sanitary Council appointed an administrator to the island to oversee all affairs of the quarantine. Two units of troops were sent to the island to guarantee the safety of the pilgrims and the quarantine.[38] The Porte was hoping to assert greater control over the island as a result of these administrative changes.

During the construction of the quarantine, there were discussions about evacuating the residents of the village. It was proposed that only the quarantine personnel remained on site, as a precautionary measure. In some years, as it would be the case in 1893, some thirty thousand pilgrims were quarantined on the island.[39] According to the decision of the Istanbul Sanitary Council, no individuals were to reside on the island other than quarantine officials. As it were, the island previ-

36 BOA, Şura-yı Devlet, 2255/10 and 2484/41.

37 BOA, Şura-yı Devlet, 2255/21.

38 BOA, Şura-yı Devlet, 586/21.

39 BOA, Dahiliye Mektubî Kalemi, 1607/17.

ously served as a site for keeping exiled individuals. Even though the Ministry of Health suggested that the exiles were transferred to the island of Farasan (north of Kamaran; off the western coast of Yemen), these individuals were allowed to stay on Kamaran Island on the condition that they were strictly isolated from quarantined individuals.[40] Initially, the quarantine complex was fully functional only for six months during the pilgrimage season (between May and October).[41] At other times, it was only staffed by watchmen in charge of safety and maintenance of the buildings.[42] In later years, the complex was kept open year around.

The Structure of the Quarantine Complex

At the time of its establishment, pilgrims were housed in simple bungalow-like structures (*ariş*). These were wooden huts covered with bamboo on the interior and exterior surfaces. The roof was covered with a thin layer of date palm leaves. The interior was divided with straw panels made of palm leaves. Pilgrims would spread straw or a rug to sit on the desert sand ground.[43] In addition to the bungalows, temporary tents were set up to house the pilgrims when necessary.

Given the tropical climate of the region, these simple structures offered some advantages. For example, they were inexpensive to build and could be easily replaced, if necessary. Although they could offer some protection from sunlight and heat, the porous material used for the walls and the roof could let in air, rainwater, and dust, as well as such pests as insects and mice. Moreover, they were difficult to disinfect. Open to damage, they required frequent repairs or rebuilding, which could be considerably costly, given the increased cost of labor, greater demand by increased number of pilgrims, demand for new personnel, and the like.[44] Neither the bungalows nor the tents offered adequate protection from

40 BOA, Şura-yı Devlet, 2566/8. In January 1889, the number of individuals exiled to Kamaran from the Yemen province was about 20. See BOA, Dahiliye Nezareti Mektubi Kalemi, 1627/97. During discussions in the International Conference of 1894 in Paris, the question of evacuating the island's population was brought up again.

41 BOA, Bâbıâli Evrak Odası, 146/10881; Kaymakam Dr. Mehmed Şakir, *Hindistan Kolerası ve Irak'ın Islahatı*, Istanbul University, Rare Books Collection, ms. TY 5071 (Istanbul, 1895), 663.

42 The British Delegate on the Constantinople Board of Health, "Some Turkish Lazarets I," 1189.

43 IOL, V. 8644(c); The British Delegate on the Constantinople Board of Health, "Some Turkish Lazarets and Other Sanitary Institutions in the Near East, III," *The Lancet* 169, no. 4367 (May 11, 1907): 1319–20.

44 BOA, Sadaret Mektubi Mühimme Kalemi, 570/17.

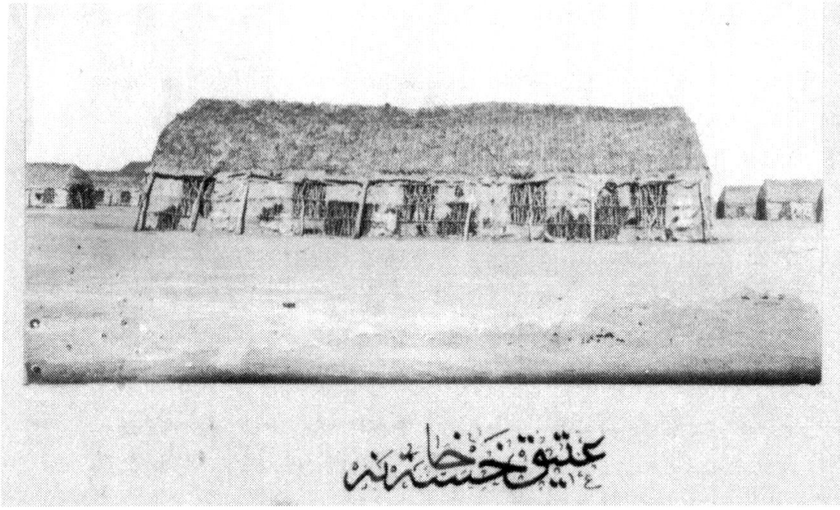

Figure 3. Old Hospital, Kamaran Island. Source: Istanbul University, Rare Books Collection; courtesy of Gülden Sarıyıldız.

tropical heat and rain.[45] Damage caused by fires and rain quickly deteriorated the huts, which had to be rebuilt in 1887.[46] Eventually, these structures were gradually replaced by more comfortable masonry buildings.

Renovation of the Quarantine Complex

According to official statistics of 1895, the quarantine complex processed about 24,000 pilgrims every year, on average.[47] The increasing number of pilgrims called for renovation of existing facilities. The extensive maintenance and repair held in 1887 did not meet the need. The repeated cholera outbreaks of 1890, 1891, and 1893 caused terrible damage in the Hijaz. The international conference that

45 The British Delegate on the Constantinople Board of Health, "Some Turkish Lazarets III," 1320.

46 Damage owing to the environment was greater in the sea-level bungalows that were on the outer circles. For example, the bungalows on rows 1, 3, and 6 were destroyed by water at times of heavy rain. Even though the island did not receive much rainfall around the year, heavy rains could occur a few times during the winter. Taking this into account, sea-level bungalows were built in a manner to withstand heavy rainfall. Newer bungalows were larger, much sturdier, and had porches. For the report of the administrator of al-Hudaydah dated August 19, 1884, see BOA, Şura-yı Devlet, 2255/12; The British Delegate on the Constantinople Board of Health, "Some Turkish Lazarets III," 1319.

47 BOA, Sadaret Hususi Maruzat Evrakı, 336/60.

met in Venice in 1892 emphasized the importance of securing sanitary control over the Suez Canal, Egypt, and the Red Sea for protecting Europe from infections coming from Asia. Improving the Sanitary Council of Alexandria and establishing a sanitary control center, a disinfection unit, and a hospital in the Suez Canal, as well as monitoring the ships that crossed the canal were among the proposals discussed and agreed upon in the Venice meeting. The new measures were implemented in November 1893, after the approval of the Khedivate of Egypt.[48] It should be pointed out that behind the adoption of these new sanitary regulations was the desire of European states to assert control over the maritimate traffic of the Red Sea, as much from north of it, as from the south.

In 1893, one of the deadliest cholera outbreaks killed between thirty to fourty thousand pilgrims in the Hijaz.[49] The dreadfully high number of fatalities was mostly caused by that year's being a Greater Pilgrimage—just was the case in 1865. Rumor had it that cholera first broke out among the Indian pilgrims in the quarantine of Kamaran, which was then carried to Mecca by Yemeni pilgrims.[50] In the conference held in Paris the next year, pilgrimage and the Red Sea quarantines were once again under scrutiny. But this time, there was also discussion about taking precautions in the Persian Gulf.[51]

The nature of Ottoman quarantines and the procedures followed in them also stirred discussion in the international meetings.[52] A major source of concern was that they followed older methods of disinfection. In Europe, the use of new machinery eased such procedures, whereas the Ottoman quarantines still used older equipment.[53] Being fully aware of the need for modernization, the Porte spent ten to twenty thousand *liras* every year to modernize the equipment and to renovate facilities. Yet a substantial modernization effort required as much as 100,000 *liras*.[54]

Sultan Abdulhamid II (r. 1876–1909) ordered comprehensive sanitary reforms. To that end, Cozzonis Efendi, the inspector general of Ottoman quarantines, was sent to Europe to examine the methods of quarantine and disinfection

48 Şehsuvaroğlu, "Türkiye Karantina Tarihine Giriş," 16.

49 Kasım İzzeddin, *Mekke-i Mükerremede Kolera,* 67; Proust, *Sıhhiye Politikasında Yeni Bir Cevelan Yani Sıhhiye Mesele-i Siyasiyesinin Hal ve Tesviyesi-Hicaz Hacları,* trans. Ahmed Nermi, Istanbul University, Rare Books Collection, ms. TY 4199, 111.

50 Sarıyıldız, *Hicaz Karantina Teşkilatı,* 66.

51 BOA, MUSM, session dated June 13, 1893.

52 BOA, MUSM, session dated February 23, 1893.

53 BOA, MUSM, session dated January 17, 1892.

54 BOA, İrade Dahiliye, 96943.

practiced there.[55] A special commission was formed to assess the reform of quarantines. The commission prepared a report about reforming the quarantines at Kamaran, Abou Saad, and Vasta in the Red Sea, as elsewhere. It was submitted to the Council and approved in 1894.[56] However, the reform package could not be implemented immediately. In 1895, the Ministry of Health petitioned the Porte emphasizing the critical importance of the Kamaran quarantine and requested the implementation as soon as possible.[57] The next year, it was decided that the older bungalow-like structures on Kamaran Island be replaced by new masonry buildings, with the addition of shops, a warehouse, and a restaurant.[58] Toward the end of the construction work, a scientific sub-committee was to be sent to the island. The Porte appointed A. Rivet, the chief inspector of the Ministry of Trade and Public Works and the engineer of the sanitary reform project, along with Robet Land, a German engineer elected by European embassies, to serve in the committee. The committee was in charge of inspecting the facilities, auditing the funds used for reforms, verifying that the buildings were constructed according to plans, and preparing a report. Both Rivet and Land went to the island in June 1899, yet the latter died before constructions were completed. Rivet prepared the report himself and submitted it to the Council upon his return.[59]

In November 1902, the Ottoman newspaper *Servet-i Fünun* described the Kamaran quarantine station as follows: "The quarantine station was divided into four sections, which were apart from each other of about 200–250 meters. In addition, there were two spearate wards reserved for patients suffering from cholera, plague, and typhoid fever. Built on the sea shore, these facilities were situated at a distance of about 500–600 meters from each other and from other buildings, so as to minimize contacts between them. In the first section, there was a mosque and twenty brick-iron units, with domes that allowed adequate air flow inside. In addition, there was a unit reserved for elite pilgrims, as well as residences of physicians and the head guardian. Overall, the first section could house up to 1,000 pil-

---

55 Cozzonis Efendi, an Ottoman doctor of Italian origin, served as a sanitary inspector at the quarantine of İzmir between 1885 and 1887, and as inspector general of Ottoman quarantines between 1888 and 1902. See Pelin Böke, "İzmir Karantina Meclisi'nin Kuruluşu ve Faaliyetleri (1840–1900)," *Çağdaş Türkiye Tarihi Araştırmaları Dergisi* 8, nos. 18–19 (2009): 137–59; BOA, Yıldız Resmi Maruzat Evrakı, 56/10.

56 On January 2, 1894. See BOA, Sadaret Mektubi Mühimme Kalemi Evrakı, 570/12 and BOA, Sadaret Mektubi Mühimme Kalemi Evrakı, 570/17.

57 BOA, Sadaret Mektubi Mühimme Kalemi Evrakı, 570/12.

58 BOA, Şura-yı Devlet, 586/21.

59 BOA, Sadaret Mektubi Mühimme Kalemi Evrakı, 578/2.

grims. The second section had ten units that could house up to 600 pilgrims. The fifth and sixth sections, both reserved for infected patients, were different than others. Five to six times larger than the other sections, they comprised eight sub-sections, each built about eighty meters away from the others. In each sub-section, there were three units that could house up to fifty pilgrims each. Each section was surrounded by a fence separating it from the others."[60]

Along with renovations in the facilities, disinfection machinery was also renewed. Three units were reserved for large and stationary disinfection machines.[61] Bought from Europe, this new machinery could disinfect up to one hundred people in fifteen minutes. In addition to clothing and other personal items, the steam machinery could disinfect such larger pieces as carpets, bedding, and straw chairs.[62] In the event of a failure in the units supplying water to disinfection equipment, water could be acquired from the wells of Kamaran, through the newly built channels.

A unit was reserved as the residence of the sanitary inspector. Another two-storied brick-and-iron building housed offices for sanitary secretaries, a pharmacy, and a large warehouse on the lower floor, and residences for officials and physicians on the upper. A coal storage of 700 tons was built further away from smaller residences reserved for the head guardians. Telephone lines were set up between the residences of sanitary inspectors and physicians in order to facilitate communication. A narrow tram line of eleven kilometers encircled the entire complex, transporting pilgrims as well as cargo.[63] In addition to this, a brick factory was built to supply new constructions and reduce building costs.[64]

Access to water was an important issue on the island. As a result, a number of precautions were taken. In order to supply distilled water to the pilgrims free of charge, a large distillation unit was built. The equipment could process up to sixty tons of water a day. It was supported by an additional water storage unit of 160-ton capacity and machines supplying up to five tons of ice per day.[65] Other hygienic

---

60 "Kamaran'da Müessesât-ı Sıhhiye-i Osmaniye: Üçüncü Makale Tahaffuzhane ve Aksamı," *Servet-i Fünun* 24, no. 605 (1902): 103.

61 The British Delegate on the Constantinople Board of Health, "Some Turkish Lazarets III," 1318–19.

62 BOA, Sadaret Mektubi Mühimme Kalemi Evrakı, 570/17.

63 BOA, Sadaret Mektubi Mühimme Kalemi Evrakı, 570/17; "Kamaran'da Müessesât-ı Sıhhiye-i Osmaniye," 106.

64 "Kamaran'da Müessesat-ı Sıhhiye-yi Osmaniye: Tahaffuzhâne ve Memurin," *Servet-i Fünun* 24, no. 604 (1902), 87.

65 "Kamaran'da Müessesat-ı Sıhhiye-yi Osmaniye: Tahaffuzhâne ve Memurin," 85–87;

measures were implemented as well. For example, flushable toilets were installed. Similar to Paris and other European cities, odor-free barrels were used for cleaning privy vaults, which were then disposed of in a distant bay.[66]

Quarantine Procedures at Kamaran

There were different quarantine procedures in place depending on where pilgrims were coming from. For example, pilgrims who came from India were quarantined up to ten days. In the event of a new outbreak of disease, the observation time could be extended. Those who came from Dutch India, Ceylon, and the Persian Gulf were kept under isolation for five days.[67]

Once arrived at the facilities, all pilgrims were to take showers, and their clothes and belongings to be disinfected, while the ships and their crew cleaned and disinfected. Pilgrims were kept in sections reserved for them, undergoing medical screening twice daily. Those suspected of being infected with plague or cholera were kept isolated from other pilgrims. If the infection was confirmed, they were sent to the hospital to receive treatment. The section where disease broke out was to be quarantined for twelve days for the first case and for ten days each time afterwards. After completing the isolation period and receiving approval from a physician, pilgrims were allowed to continue to the Hijaz. Before departing, they were disinfected once again.[68]

Pilgrims were required to pay a fee to the quarantine complex. They were also responsible for paying for their own sustenance during their stay. Those with the means, could eat at the restaurant or buy their needs from shops.[69] The island had a factory producing canned food, established by the initiative of French engineer Émile Roullet.[70] Pilgrims could cook their own food, granted they brought along rice and flour. Water was offered to all free of charge.[71]

Pilgrims undertaking the journey had to consider quarantine expenses. Thomas Cook and Son, a British transportation company that carried pilgrims between India and Mecca calculated the total cost for an Indian pilgrim as 300

Kasım İzzeddin, *Mekke-i Mükerremede Kolera*, 57.

66 "Kamaran'da Müessesât-ı Sıhhiye-i Osmaniye," 103.

67 Watts, "Cholera Politics in Britain," 331.

68 The British Delegate on the Constantinople Board of Health, "Some Turkish Lazarets I," 1188–89.

69 BOA, Şura-yı Devlet, 586/21.

70 Kuneralp, "Osmanlı Yönetimindeki (1831–1911)," 510.

71 BOA, Sadaret Hususi Maruzat Evrakı, 336/60.

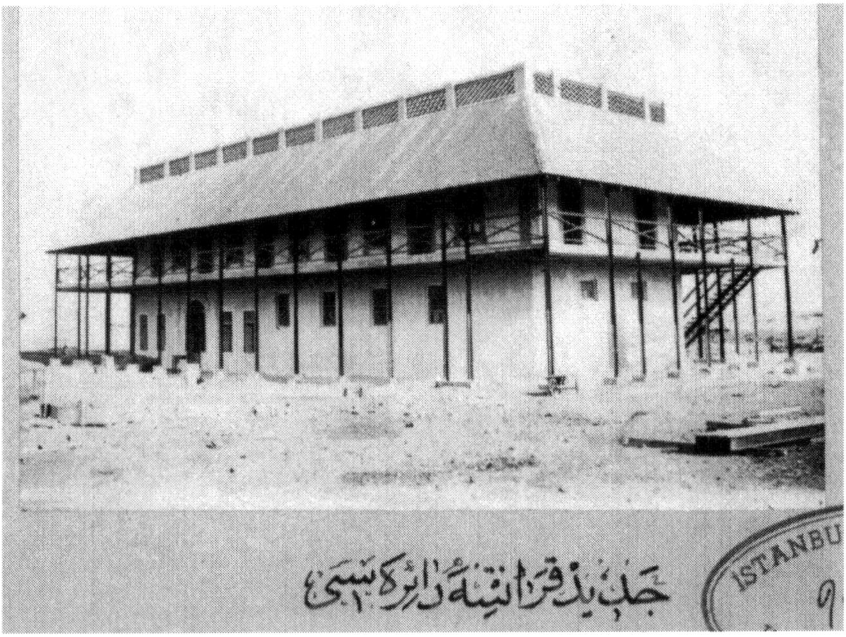

Figure 4. New Quarantine Unit, Kamaran Island. Source: Istanbul University, Rare Books Collection; courtesy of Gülden Sarıyıldız.

Indian rupees.[72] However, not all pilgrims could meet these expenses. For those who did not have the means, all expenses were met by the quarantine authority. The majority of "pauper pilgrims" from British India only paid small freight fees for their voyage and arrived at the Red Sea quarantines penniless. Regardless, the quarantine authority had to accept poor pilgrims and meet their expenses for sustenance while keeping them in isolation. Unable to pay necessary fees, destitute pilgrims inflicted large losses to sanitation revenues.[73] In 1893, the quarantine administration was authorized for an allowance of 20,000 *kuruş* to meet the sustenance of poor pilgrims returning from the Hijaz.[74] About one thousand destitute pilgrims from Yemen, Iran, and Iraq were offered help that year.[75]

---

72 "The Mecca Pilgrimage: Appointment by the Government of India Thos. Cook and Son Agents for the Control of the Movements of Mahomedan Pilgrems from All Parts of India to Jeddah for Mecca, Medina etc., and Back," IOL, V 8644 (a).

73 BOA, Şura-yı Devlet, 2674/3.

74 BOA, MUSM, session held on August 1, 1893.

75 BOA, Dahiliye Mektubî Kalemi, 180/43.

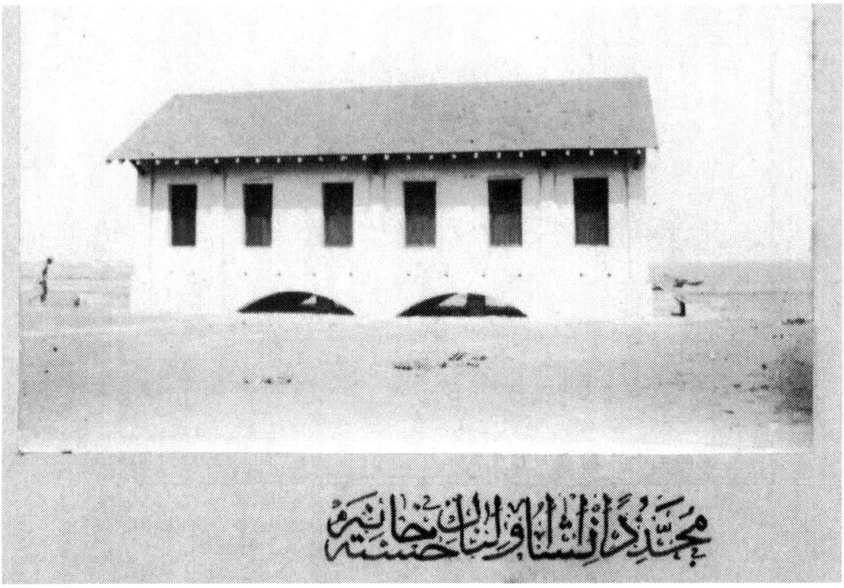

Figure 5. Rebuilt Hospital, Kamaran Island. Source: Istanbul University Rare Books Collection; courtesy of Gülden Sarıyıldız.

It is clear that these expenses were beyond what many pilgrims could afford. At times, pilgrims complained about excess sanitary fees charged and overpriced food sold at the quarantine.[76] The Ottoman documents suggest that such complaints were taken seriously and followed up in order to circumvent the abuse of the system.

Criticism of the Kamaran Quarantine

Since the time of its inauguration, there were ongoing criticisms about the Kamaran quarantine, primarily raised by Britain and India. The criticism pointed at inadequate medical conditions, insufficient and salty water, expensive food, short supply of gas and kitchen utensils, poor accommodation conditions, and the abusive attitudes of guards to the pilgrims. When Kamaran first opened, the Mohammedan Association, an influential Muslim organization in India, petitioned the government in Bombay to push against the mandatory quarantine at Kamaran. According to the Indian government, quarantine procedures at Kamaran were cruel and aimed at nothing more than raising revenue for the Ottoman administra-

76 BOA, Sadaret Hususi Maruzat Evrakı, 336/60.

tion. Moreover, it was claimed that the quarantine had no visible medical benefits. The Indian government took its allegations so far as to claim that "the conditions at Kamaran are so terrible that the chances of cholera spreading out of Kamaran is greater than those of Indian ports."[77]

In 1895, the Indian government conducted an inquiry about Kamaran. According to the government's statements, the regulations at Kamaran were found less than satisfactory. Arthur Alban, the British ambassador to the Porte, claimed that pilgrims faced pressure, overcrowdedness, and other problems at Kamaran and demanded that conditions be reformed. Moreover, the Ottoman pilgrim vessels were also criticized by the British for being crowded, unhygienic, and medically inadequate.[78] All of these criticisms called for the Ottoman government's investigation of the conditions on site and if allegations were indeed true, the problems had to be addressed.

It appears that the criticism raised by the British and Indian governments was highly inaccurate as it was clearly motivated by political and commercial interests. This was primarily owing to the financial burden caused by the Kamaran quarantine for shipping companies that did business in the Red Sea. The companies complained that the bill of health was too high and that their cargo were stolen during quarantine. The same year, Britain had to give in to international pressures and require new quarantine regulations on all ships leaving Indian ports, which caused considerable delays in commerce and travel. In particular, India suffered heavily from economic complications, as more than half of its imports were from Britain. The groups that suffered from the effects of the quarantine raised their frustration against those measures in the Anglo-Indian press outlets. *The Gazette* and the Indian government declared that quarantine had no medical basis but that it only was a result of Europe's jealousy for Britain's colonial trade.[79]

It was clear to the Ottoman administration that the Kamaran quarantine had significant shortcomings, which was the reason behind repeated efforts to reform it. Nevertheless, it appears that quarantine procedures were carefully followed on site. Archival records suggest that many Indian ships, both commercial and carrying the pilgrims, tried to avoid the quarantine by following alternative itineraries, sometimes illegally.[80] Dr. Spiridion C. Zavitziano, United States Sanitary Commis-

---

77 Mark Harrison, "Quarantine, Pilgrimage, and Colonial Trade: India 1866–1900," *The Indian Economic and Social History Review* 29, no. 2 (1992), 124–25.

78 Harrison, "Quarantine, Pilgrimage, and Colonial Trade," 136.

79 Harrison, "Quarantine, Pilgrimage, and Colonial Trade," 126.

80 For sanitary fugitives, see BOA, MUSM, session held on July 31, 1890; BOA, Sadaret Mektubi Mühimme Kalemi Evrakı, 575/14; BOA, Dahiliye Mektubî Kalemi, 2151/19.

sioner, observed that many Indian Muslims circumvented strict quarantine procedures at Kamaran by going to Muscat first, and then to Jidda with other ships, thus avoiding quarantine altogether. All of these efforts to avoid Kamaran can be taken as evidence that quarantine procedures were in fact being followed closely. It seems very likely that it was the strict quarantine administration that caused the resentment among its critics.

A report prepared by the Russian military engineer and geographer Leonid Artamonov, who was appointed by the Ethiopian emperor Menelik II to investigate a plague outbreak in 1899, discussed the Kamaran quarantine along with other Red Sea quarantines. Artamonov compared the Red Sea quarantines to those of the Indian Ocean. Although critical of the quarantine at Aden, he praised Kamaran by saying that sanitary controls were done properly and that the quarantine was reliable.[81] He wrote, "Camaran, with its magnificent quarantine structures and its complete disinfection plant, is unique as a Red Sea station, and constitutes the best and only real defence against the introduction of plague and cholera."[82]

Occasionally, there were warnings about the conditions of the quarantine. One of these was the observation about the presence of large numbers of rats on the island and the danger they posed in spreading disease. This observation by Dr. Creudiropoulos, a physician of the Ottoman sanitary service at Kamaran was included in a report prepared in 1899.[83] Another major shortcoming of the quarantine station was the lack of a bacteriological laboratory. This issue was brought up by quarantine physicians during meetings held for discussing how to reform Kamaran. In a meeting held in 1898, The British delegate E. D. Dickson objected to the proposal on account of the high cost of building such a laboratory and for potential conflicts with quarantine procedures already in place.[84] According to the testimony of Dr. Zavitziano, the British sanitary commissioner was opposed to the purchase and installation of disinfecting furnaces and the establishment of a bacteriology laboratory.[85]

---

81 Spiridion C. Zavitziano, "Turkey: Sanitary report from Constantinople," *Public Health Reports (1896–1970)* 14, no. 16 (1899), 573.

82 Zavitziano, "Turkey: Sanitary report from Constantinople," *Public Health Reports (1896–1970)* 14, no. 18 (1899), 668.

83 In the same report, it is also stated that the Ottoman administration did not attempt to poison the rats and that the residents of the island had to be evacuated. See "Plague cases at the lazaretto of Camaran," *Public Health Reports (1896–1970)* 14, no. 23 (1899), 888–89.

84 "Current Quarantine measures," *Public Health Reports (1896–1970)* 13, no. 43 (1898), 1220.

85 Spiridion C. Zavitziano and Cozzonis, "Turkey: Drought in the Hedjaz," *Public Health Reports (1896–1970)* 15, no. 4 (1900), 198.

A laboratory, however, was sorely needed at Kamaran. In a report dated May 25, 1899, the Ottoman sanitary inspector Dr. Creudiropoulos wrote, "a fully-equipped bacteriological laboratory in Camaran is indispensable."[86] He stated that it would be nearly impossible to identify epidemic diseases like plague and cholera without a microscope. He also emphasized the importance of making the right diagnosis in a timely manner for preventing the spread of epidemics. For him, Kamaran had a critical role to play in the larger sanitary effort. He wrote, "Camaran is an exceptional place," and continued, "unique for the scientific problems to be solved. Science will profit very much from the bacteriological experience at Camaran, which must not be fitted only for epidemiological, but for hygienic work also."[87]

Britain often opposed the diagnosis of epidemics at quarantine stations, including at Kamaran. While discussing the diagnosis decisions of quarantine physicians at the latest meeting of the Superior Sanitary Council, Dr. Zavitziano noted the attitude of the British delegates. In a report dated September 15, 1899, it was stated that Dr. Creudiropoulos made a diagnosis of plague at Kamaran and warned that the disease was going to continue. But the British sanitary representative disagreed with that diagnosis. The latter believed that this was not plague since no previous epidemics of plague had been observed in the city of Chittagong where pilgrims-to-be had come from. In a similar case, a British delegate opposed the diagnosis of Dr. Moschides, the quarantine physician at Basra, about the disease seen at the ship named *Haydari* being plague, whereupon he forced the commission members to vote against that diagnosis. Critical of the commission's decision being manipulated by the British delegate's opinion, Dr. Zivitziano wrote, "By said decision the superior sanitary commission shows that the sanitary physicians in the Ottoman service are not able to make a diagnosis, which diagnosis can only be made by the members of the superior sanitary commission," and warned against future embarrassment, as long as the commission continued making decisions in like manner.[88]

It seems unreasonable to argue that the British attitude was motivated by medical reasons. It had become customary in British politics to criticize and complain about the Ottomans internationally, in a manner to call for sustained European pressure over it.[89] At the same time, Britain tried to discredit the reputation

86 Zavitziano, "Turkey: Sanitary report from Constantinople, Plague in Jiddah," *Public Health Reports (1896–1970)* 14, no. 35 (1899), 1446.

87 Zavitziano, "Turkey: Sanitary report from Constantinople, Plague in Jiddah," *Public Health Reports (1896–1970)* 14, no. 35 (1899), 1447.

88 Zavitziano, "Turkey: Sanitary report from Constantinople, Sanitary condition of Constantinople," *Public Health Reports (1896–1970)* 14, no. 37 (1899), 1542.

89 Harrison, "Quarantine, Pilgrimage, and Colonial Trade," 136.

of the Ottoman caliph over Muslims, by criticizing that the Ottoman sanitation regulations in Jidda and Mecca were inadequate and by claiming that the Ottoman quarantine officials treated pilgrims badly and abused them.[90]

British Politics in the Red Sea and on the Island of Kamaran

Despite being a small island, Kamaran had been subjected to Mamluk, Portuguese, and Egyptian invasions in its history, largely owing to its strategic location. In the nineteenth century, it was Britain, France, and Italy that were politically active in the region.[91] By this time, the Red Sea had become the site of conflicting interests of European states. Britain, in particular, had interests in the region not only to secure the trade routes leading to India but also to control the Indian Ocean trade via the Red Sea. The British were involved in profitable arms trade on the coast of Yemen and Ethiopia. In addition, British ships transported coffee from Yemen to England.

Since the early nineteenth century, the British interest in southern Arabian Peninsula was expanding. Napoleon's invasion of Egypt facilitated Britain's pursuit of power in the area. It first established power in the Gulf of Aden and on the coast of Somalia. In the 1830s, it sought to control islands, such as Socotra (east of the Horn of Africa), Perim (in the Bab-el-Mandeb Straits), and Kamaran, as well as ports like Mocha (on the Red Sea coast of Yemen). In 1839, the acquisition of a small but strategically important base in Aden afforded Britain to expand its power in the area. From there, it could exert control over the Bab-el-Mandeb Straits and the Red Sea. Aden was indeed an important addition to the British possessions. As a natural port, it was an important stop for merchant vessels and a trading *entrepôt*. For the British ships coming from India, this was an ideal stop to replenish supplies. To that end, a coal station was built there. Aden also became an important hub for postal services. Mail sent from cities like Bombay or Calcutta was first brought here and sorted before being forwarded to their final destination.[92]

The advent of the steamship and the opening of the Suez Canal in 1869 contributed to the rising commercial potential of the region. In addition to trading goods, British, Egyptian, and Dutch vessels also carried large numbers of Muslim pilgrims. Every year, about twenty to twenty-five thousand pilgrims were ferried from India to Jidda and the other ports of the Hijaz. The demand for travel was so

---

90 For further details, see Harrison, "Quarantine, Pilgrimage, and Colonial Trade."

91 J. E. Peterson, "The Islands of Arabia," 24.

92 Sarah Searight, "A Waghorn Letter Book for 1840," *Journal of the Royal Asiatic Society* 7, no. 2 (1997): 240.

high that steamship companies started to offer scheduled pilgrimage voyages for the Muslims of South and Southeast Asia. The opening of the Suez Canal almost entirely replaced the already declining traditional caravan routes. While in 1865, the number of pilgrims that traveled over land was about 50,000, there was a steep decline after that.[93] Ferrying pilgrims had become a profitable business in the last decades of the nineteenth century. Yet this was not the only reason for the European interest in the region. Mecca and Medina were great markets for selling European goods because of an increasing number of pilgrims who went there every year. During pilgrimage season, products from Britain and the Low Countries were highly sought by the pilgrims. The commercial vitality of the region attracted to the area, not only the British but also other European merchants, including the French, Italian, and the Dutch—all seeking to receive a better share from this market.[94]

Fully cognizant of these changes, the Ottoman Empire pursued an active policy to strengthen its military and administrative presence in the region. The proposal made during the International Sanitary Conference in Istanbul for building a quarantine station at the entrance of the Red Sea was perfectly compatible with Ottoman interests. It was understood that this strategically important quarantine station could promote the Ottoman political and administrative power in the region. This was also an opportunity to curb possible military interventions of European powers, especially that of Britain. Hence the Porte recognized the establishment of the quarantine station as a critical enterprise for preserving its interests in the area.

Several years before the quarantine was built, Britain had tried to acquire the island in order to use it as a coaling station. When the establishment of a new quarantine in southern Red Sea was proposed at the 1866 conference in Istanbul, Britain was displeased. During the conference, the British delegates firmly denied that cholera spread from India, as they saw this claim conflicting with their commercial interests.[95] If the origin of cholera pandemics were to be acknowlegded as India, Britain would have to be most adversely affected. Any disease known to have originated in and spread from India would have been regarded as Britain's responsibility. This could involve establishing quarantines and imposing sanitary surveillance procedures to companies. From an economic point of view, this could be a major drawback for the British shipping companies that ferried tens of thousands of passengers every year without taking any sanitary precautions. Quaran-

93 Kuneralp, "Osmanlı Yönetimindeki (1831–1911)," 499, 504.

94 Miran, "Space, Mobility, and Translocal Connections," xix.

95 Foreign Office Records [hereafter FO], 195/864, session held on February 22, 1866, 2; FO, 78/2006, 1. Also see FO, 78/2008; Kılınç, "Isolating the Subject," 44, 57–60.

tines could interfere with the business. The long wait during quarantines could cause major loss of revenue for companies. Moreover, quarantines could disrupt the trade between India and Europe. From a political point of view, Britian was concerned that Muslims in India would find quarantine restrictions to pilgrimage offensive and that this would create widespread resentment, which would pose a challenge for the British rule in India.[96] Given the calculated outcomes of the position, the British denied that cholera spread from India but instead argued that it was a problem endemic to the region. Nevertheless, this position was not accepted at the international conference.[97]

Notwithstanding, Britain was not alone in defending its own interests in the region. Throughout the conference, European states used cholera as a political tool to negotiate their ambitions to control Egypt and the Hijaz. Several European states used medical concerns in a manner to mask their political interests. This was especially transparent in the case of discussions on cholera's spread. The emerging consensus among the delegates was that cholera spread to Europe via the pilgrimage route. Hence, it was decided that the Porte would meet this challenge by implementing rigorous sanitary control in the region. This way, they could continue to exert pressure, if indirectly, on Egypt and the Hijaz where only Muslims were allowed to enter.[98]

For the Ottoman administration, the decisions reached at the Istanbul conference were mixed. On the one hand, the establishment of quarantine stations in the Red Sea and instituting sanitary regulations in the Hijaz would be a heavy blow to the already frail Ottoman economy. Such an effort would require careful financial planning. Moreover, there was increasing international pressure about a timely and resolute response. On the other hand, the Ottoman administration could acquire great political advantages from this venture. The quarantine and other sanitary regulations could promote Ottoman presence and power in the Red Sea and the Arabian Peninsula. In particular, sanitary success in the Hijaz could increase the Ottoman prestige in the Holy Cities and along pilgrimage routes.[99] The Ottoman administrators seized this opportunity to use sanitary efforts for political ends. Starting in 1870s, they actively used the ideology of pan-Islamism, by using the press to reach out to Muslims. Sultan Abdulhamid II pursued this ideology more adamantly, adopting it as the ideology of the state and reenacting

96 Low, "Empire and the Hajj," 271.

97 FO, 78/2006, 1; FO, 78/2008, 18; Harrison, "Quarantine, Pilgrimage, and Colonial Trade."

98 Kılınç, "Isolating the Subject," 85–88.

99 Low, "Empire and the Hajj," 280.

the power of the caliphate among the Muslims of the world. In doing so, he greatly benefitted from quarantines and politics of sanitation. The Ottoman efforts to impose quarantines and maintain sanitation in the Red Sea and the Hijaz to check the spread of epidemics, turned Abdulhamid into a "protector" and "patron" of all Muslims.

In order to improve the monitoring and record-keeping of Indian pilgrims, the Porte issued a new regulation in 1880 that required all passengers arriving to Jidda to possess a passport. Those without a passport were to be denied admission at the port. It was also announced that all pilgrims-to-be had to have sufficient funds to cover their return journey. From now on, pilgrims-to-be were required to present at Jidda the passport they had acquired from their country of departure and the funds for their return trip. The purpose of this new regulation was to solve the problem of the pauper pilgrims and the burden they brought to the Ottoman economy. The Porte also announced that very strict procedures were to be followed for screening pilgrims' sanitary conditions.

These changes forced the hand of British India to reform its procedures. Starting in 1874, the British Consul at Jidda was to oversee the movement of all pilgrims ferried on British-flagged vessels.[100] The new regulation about requiring the pilgrims to secure funds for return trips was difficult to impose. The Indian administration was unwilling to enforce it, fearing the reaction of the Muslims. However, it had to endorse the passport requirement for the pilgrims, owing to international pressures.[101] On July 12, 1882, the Indian Ministry of the Interior announced that all Indian pilgrims were to be issued passports. This service was going to be limited to Indian citizens only. The Indian government declared that all other pilgrims who wished to travel from Indian ports were responsible for securing their own travel documents. In order to regulate the pilgrimage traffic, changes were made in 1883 to the the Native Passenger Ships Act of 1876, reforming the equipment, acquisition of victuals, and sanitary conditions of vessels ferrying Indian pilgrims. It became mandatory to have a health official on board, for vessels carrying over hundred pilgrims. The Indian authorities also printed pamphlets, such as *A Manual for the Guidance of Officers and Others Concerned in the Red Sea Pilgrim Traffic* and distributed to all units. A new vice consul was appointed to Jidda to facilitate the accommodation and other needs of Indian pilgrims in the Hijaz. A Muslim consul was appointed to al-Hudaydah to assist their problems while undergoing quarantine procedures. In addition, manuals were prepared in English, Hindi, and Persian for distribution to the pilgrims, informing them about the cost of the pil-

100 Baldry, "The Ottoman Quarantine Station," 29.

101 Harrison, "Quarantine, Pilgrimage, and Colonial Trade," 124.

grimage journey, the difficulties of travel, the mandatory ten-day quarantine on Kamaran Island, and the expenses related to it.[102]

All these regulations focused on improving the travel of pilgrims on vessels and railways. The British envisioned consolidating pilgrimage business, which would then be contracted to a British company. The sanitary conferences of Istanbul (1866) and Vienna (1874) had underscored the necessity of regulating the ferrying of pilgrims and called for a reform package, based on the British model. Responding to this call, the Ottoman Sanitary Council prepared a new statute in 1879 that limited the authority of consuls. According to the new statute, the consuls were not allowed to interfere in the execution of the provisions; they were only to assist the sanitary officials.[103] The statute also mandated that the 24-hour precautionary quarantine (practiced since 1866 to vessels pronounced to be healthy) be increased after the inauguration of the Kamaran complex, to five and at times to ten days (depending on circumstances).[104]

In response to this new statute implemented by the Porte, the British sought to promote their consul in Kamaran to an official position.[105] Also, they reviewed the privileges of shipping companies in order to create a monopoly in the business of ferrying pilgrims. Until that time, no hygienic regulations were followed on British vessels, not least against the spread of cholera.[106] For this reason, cases of cholera, dysentery, tuberculosis, and bronchitis were commonly seen in the vessels. Pilgrims suffered from the poor hygiene of the vessels, which they often complained about.[107] The Indian government was subjected to endless complaints from the Muslims. The terrible conditions of pilgrimage journeys were being criticized internationally. As an attempt to stop widespread criticism and to gain the support of Muslim leaders in the country, Indian autorities passed the Bombay Pilgrims Bill in 1886. The new law aimed to regulate pilgrimage to stop overcrowded, uncontrolled, and overpriced journeys. This reorganization was also expected to suppress unlicensed pilgrimage business and fraud. In the framework of this new law, British India granted the monopoly of pilgrimage to the British shipping com-

102 IOL, V 8644 (a).

103 BOA, İrade Meclis-i Mahsus, 3071. Also see Sarıyıldız, *Hicaz Karantina Teşkilatı*, 50.

104 BOA, MUSM, session held on April 3, 1895.

105 In January 1903, two British ships sailed to Kamaran after taking the British consul in al-Hudaydah and attempted to raise the British flag in the building where the consul resided. The Ottoman administration contested this attempt and sent Captain Veli Bey to oversee the crisis. See BOA, Bâbıâli Evrak Odası, 1969/147649.

106 Kuneralp, "Osmanlı Yönetimindeki (1831–1911)," 506–7.

107 IOL, V. 8644 (c).

pany Thomas Cook and Sons. The company was expected to offer transportation for pilgrims, reorganize the administration of pilgrimage, provide sustenance, and improve sanitary conditions with the support and guidance of the government. The government relied on the company's prestige to overcome these problems.[108]

The agreement signed with Thomas Cook and Sons was published as an ordinance in the *Gazette of India* and in other local newspapers. It was claimed that the agreement was expected to reform the current conditions radically. According to the agreement signed with Thomas Cook and Sons, the company was granted the right to manage pilgrimage trips and fares both on steamships and on railways. The passports prepared and authorized by Indian authorities would be then forwarded to local company officials. The company was to keep records of the pilgrims' identity information. In this effort, local authorities in India were tasked to assist company officials. The extensive consessions granted to Thomas Cook and Sons testify to the British scheme for exercising greater control over pilgrimage traffic through British companies.

Soon after the agreement, Thomas Cook and Sons opened new offices in Bombay and Jidda. The company promised to offer a safer, more comfortable, and affordable pilgrimage journey. Yet it took some time for the company to launch its pilgrimage trips in compliance with new procedures. In a letter sent to A. McKenzie, the Secretary to the Government, John Mason Cook, the owner of the company, stated that the company was working hard to have the vessels and trains ready for the 1887 pilgrimage season. Cook also mentioned that he had been in touch with local officials, observed the difficulties faced by pilgrims during their journeys, and that he had plans to remedy the problems.[109]

In 1887, a revised Native Passenger Ships Act was passed. This new law required improved sanitary conditions on vessels and imposed heavier penalties for failure to execute them. Nevertheless, the anticipated improvements did not seem to occur. Depsite all the regulations, pilgrimage trips suffered from overcrowdedness, unsatisfactory sanitation, and other problems. A testimony to the miserable conditions of the journey comes from Muhammad Yakub Alikhan, a retired hospital inspector, who in 1889 observed the terrible conditions of the pilgrimage vessel named *Tanjore*. The disclosure of his testimony was scandalous for Thomas Cook and Sons that admitted overselling pilrimage trips to maximize profit. Similar scandals followed suit. The company officials indirectly accepted the allegations by stating that the business was not as profitable as had been expected, they were carrying pilgrims at a loss, and they did not receive the antici-

108 Harrison, "Quarantine, Pilgrimage, and Colonial Trade," 132.

109 IOL, V 8644 (a).

pated support from the Muslim community. Despite the company's declaration, the Indian government continued to defend it and pay for its losses. When cholera broke out on a ship named *S. S. Deccan* in the year 1891, it became clear that this arrangement could not be maintained for much longer.[110] The company declared the business unprofitable and quit in 1893.[111]

In July 1915, British war ships bombarded and invaded the island. This meant the acquisition of the island which they saw as strategically important. During the invasion of Kamaran, the British forces captured recalcitrant Ottoman officials and exiled them to Hyderabad. According to the information supplied by the guardians of Medina, the sanitary physician and engineer of the Hijaz, as well as the inspector and chest-keeper of Jidda were taken as war captives and sent to Aden.[112] This, however, was against international conventions.[113] In retaliation, the Ottomans captured British civilians and treated them as prisoners of war. Eight British civilians from Istanbul were sent to exile in Afyonkarahisar.[114] Before a mutual agreement could be reached between Britain and the Porte, two of the eight Ottoman sanitary officials captured at Kamaran had died in exile in Aden and the remaining six were sent to Thayetmyo in Burma. In December 1915, the two states agreed to exchange their prisoners of war.[115] On August 12, 1916, when Britain informed the Porte that the captives in Thayetmyo were being shipped from Egypt to Athens, the Ottoman authorities decided to send five of the eight British prisoners to Istanbul.[116]

For the Ottomans, the British occupation of the island was not only a political exploit. It also had a religious implication. A correspondence dated July 17, 1915 between the Ottoman Ministry of the Interior and the Ministry of Foreign Affairs states that the reason behind the British occupation of the island was to disturb the pilgrims and obstruct their religious duty. For Ottoman officials, this meant defiance of Islamic law.[117] A telegram dated August 1, 1915 sent from Istanbul to the embassy in Tehran voiced criticism about the British occupation as an

110 Harrison, "Quarantine, Pilgrimage, and Colonial Trade," 133.

111 Low, "Empire and the Hajj," 271.

112 BOA, Hariciye Nezareti Siyasi, 2187/9, inset 7.

113 This was contrary to the principles of the Geneva Convention of 1906, which offered protection to military health personnel and civilians that provide medical assistance to military personnel. See Atalay Kocatepe, *Silahlı Çatışma Hukuku Açısından Cenevre Sözleşmeleri ve Ek Protokolleri El Kitabı* (Istanbul, 2006), 13.

114 BOA, Dahiliye Nezareti Emniyet-i Umumiye, 5. şube, 81/53, inset 1.

115 BOA, Hariciye Nezareti Siyasi, 2187/9, inset 27.

116 BOA, Hariciye Nezareti Siyasi, 2187/5, inset 29.

117 BOA, Hariciye Nezareti Siyasi, 2187/4, inset 9.

act targeting Muslim pilgrims and interfering with the performance of their religious duty. The telegram called for spreading the word as much as possible in Iran and in other Muslim countries.[118] The Ottoman response to the British occupation of the island can be better understood in the political context of the time. Too exhausted for military response to the occupation, the Ottomans were seeking support from other Muslim countries. For their part, the British were fully aware of the possible consequences of occupying the island, close to the pilgrimage season. It was clear that this would interfere with quarantine procedures and cause health problems locally as well as internationally. Yet Britain's political interests outweighed its concern for sanitation.

Conclusion

The Kamaran quarantine station was established by the Ottoman Empire in 1882 following the agreement reached at the International Sanitary Conference in Istanbul (1866). All Muslims coming for pilgrimage to the Hijaz from South and Southeast Asia, as well as those coming from eastern Africa, the Persian Gulf, and the Yemen were quarantined at Kamaran. Quarantine was not only for pilgrim vessels; all ships coming from south of the Red Sea had to stop at Kamaran Island for sanitary inspection. To meet the high volume of traffic, Kamaran was built as a large quarantine complex. The physical structures and the disinfection plant were renovated and upgraded twice to meet the growing needs and techological changes of its time, making Kamaran the largest and most advanced quarantine station in the world.

Kamaran was seen as a *cordon sanitaire* that could stop cholera from spreading to Europe, which made it the focus of attention for European states. The quarantine procedures and renovation works often became the subject of discussion in international sanitary conferences, which turned Kamaran into a political site. The Red Sea trade had become increasingly important in the nineteenth century, especially after the advent of the steamships and the opening of the Suez Canal. The Red Sea basin was critical for the British and Dutch empires, in particular, for political and commercial reasons. In addition to transporting raw materials and commodities to Europe, they also made large profits ferrying tens of thousands of Muslim pilgrims every year. Moreover, British and Dutch products were in high demand in the markets of Mecca and Medina during pilgrimage season. This demand made this area gradually more attractive to European merchants and entrepreneurs, as the Red Sea trade continued to grow throughout the nineteenth century. In conjunction with this, the region grew in political importance,

118 BOA, Hariciye Nezareti Siyasi, 2187/9, inset 7.

becoming a site of conflicting political interests of European states. The Ottoman Empire observed the increasing importance of the region and used this opportunity to build a presence for itself in the region in a manner to protect its own political interests against those of the European powers.

In this context, the decision of the International Sanitary Conference held in Istanbul was very important. In 1865, one year before the conference, cholera had brought devastating results globally. Research suggested that the source of the pandemic was India. It was critical to develop adequate preventive measures against a new cholera pandemic that could arrive from this region. Hence the discussions at the conference largely reflected sanitary anxieties of Europe. However, it was clear that European powers tried to use the threat of cholera to serve their own political interests. Even though the Kamaran quarantine was established by the Ottoman Empire as a result of pressures coming from European states, the Ottomans would not be allowed to govern it alone, given the island's strategic importance. European states in general, and Britain, in particular, tried to have a say over quarantine procedures, renovations, and even the administration of the quarantine station. To this end, Britain tried to promote the British consul at Kamaran to an official rank. At the same time, it pursued an active policy to bring the Red Sea pilgrimage trips under its control. One significant step in this direction was to entrust a British shipping company with the transportation of pilgrims between British India and the Hijaz.

Kamaran quarantine was a strategic point for the political interests of the Ottoman Empire in the region. Not unlike European states, the Ottomans also saw Kamaran as a critical institution for asserting political power. It carried out quarantine procedures and preventive health measures with great care in order to protect Kamaran from external interventions. Even though this was a time when the Ottoman state was financially bankrupt, it allocated the necessary budgetary resources to support Kamaran's renovations. At international sanitary conferences, it maintained an uncompromising attitude toward attempts for intervention from European states. Moreover, to protect the island from a possible British invasion, the Porte supplied Kamaran with military support and sent the navy to the island, using the excuse of securing the quarantine. However, these efforts of the Ottoman Empire failed with the onset of World War I. In 1915, Britain invaded Kamaran Island and hence its quarantine. Given its circumstances, the Ottoman state did not entertain any hopes of getting Kamaran back from Britain. Instead, it protested the invasion of the island, not by political means but by way of religious propaganda. In letters sent to Muslim countries, the Ottoman state proclaimed that the British invaded the island to stop Muslim pilgrimage and that this was a major attack on Islamic law. Curiously, neither the Ottomans nor the British made any explanations to address medical and sanitary concerns.

Gülden Sarıyıldız (guldensariyildiz@yahoo.com) is Professor in the Department of Information and Document Management at Istanbul University, where she has been teaching since 2000. Previously, she taught at Trakya University. Prof. Sarıyıldız is interested in the history of Ottoman bureaucracy, state organization, and medicine. She has published widely on epidemics, sanitary policies, and quarantine in the nineteenth century, especially in the Hijaz region. In addition to numerous articles and book chapters, she is the author of *Hicaz Karantina Teşkilatı (1865-1914)* (Quarantine Organization in the Hijaz (1865–1914)) (1996), *Sicill-i Ahval Komisyonunun Kuruluşu ve Faaliyetleri (1879–1909)* (2004), *Sokak Yazıcıları: Osmanlılarda Arzuhal ve Arzuhalciler* (2010), and editor of *Nezihi Aykut Armağanı* (Festschrift to Nezihi Aykut) (2011), *Prof. Dr. Ali İhsan Gencer Anısına Osmanlıdan Cumhuriyete Sosyo-Kültürel Siyasi Yansımalar* (2015). She holds a PhD from Istanbul University.

Oya Dağlar Macar (oyadr@ticaret.edu.tr) is Associate Professor of History in the Department of Political Science and International Relations at Istanbul Commerce University, where she currently teaches. Previously, she was a post-doctoral fellow at Fort Hays State University (Hays, KS) and visiting scholar at Hellenic College Holy Cross Greek Orthodox School of Theology (Brookline, MA). Her research focuses on twentieth-century Ottoman political and medical history. Along with several articles and book chapters, she is the author of *War, Epidemics, and Medicine in the Ottoman Empire: From the Balkan Wars through the Great War (1912-1918)* (2008) and *Balkan Savaşları'nda Salgın Hastalıklar ve Sağlık Hizmetleri* (Epidemic Diseases and Health Services during the Balkan Wars (1912-1918)) (2009), as well as co-author of *Rus Ordusu Türkiye'de* (Russian Army in Turkey) (2010). She holds a PhD from Boğazici University.

BIBLIOGRAPHY

Select Published Works

ʿAbd al-Karīm, Aḥmad ʿIzzat. *Tārīkh al-Taʿlīm fī ʿAṣr Muḥammad ʿAlī*. Cairo: Maktabat al-Nahḍa al-Miṣriyya, 1938.

Abu El-Haj, Nadia. *Facts on the Ground: Archaeological Practice and Territorial Self-Fashioning in Israeli Society*. Chicago: The University of Chicago Press, 2001.

Abu-Lughod, Lila. "Islam and the Gendered Discourses of Death." *International Journal of Middle East Studies* 25, no. 2 (1993): 187–205.

Abul-Magd, Zeinab. "A Crisis of Images: The French, Jihad, and the Plague in Upper Egypt, 1798–1801." *Journal of World History* 23 (2012): 315–43.

——. *Imagined Empires: A History of Revolt in Egypt*. Berkeley: University of California Press, 2013.

Adıvar, Adnan. *Osmanlı Türklerinde İlim*. Istanbul: Remzi Kitabevi, 1970.

Afkhami, Amir Arsalan. "Defending the Guarded Domain: Epidemics and the Emergence of an International Sanitary Policy in Iran." *Comparative Studies of South Asia, Africa and the Middle East* 19 (1999): 122–36.

Ágoston, Gábor. *Guns for the Sultan: Technology, Industry, and Military Power in the Ottoman Empire*. Cambridge: Cambridge University Press, 2004.

Agrawal, C. M. *Natural Calamities and the Great Mughals*. Bodh Gaya, India: Kanchan Publications, 1983.

Ahmed, Moinuddin et al. "Continental-Scale Temperature Variability During the Past Two Millennia." *Nature Geoscience* 6 (2013): 339–46.

Akasoy, Anna. "Islamic Attitudes to Disasters in the Middle Ages: A Comparison of Earthquakes and Plagues." *The Medieval History Journal* 10, nos. 1–2 (2007): 397–410.

Akdağ, Mustafa. *Celâlî İsyanları, 1550–1603*. Ankara: Ankara University Press, 1963.

——. *Türkiye'nin İktisadi ve İçtimai Tarihi*. Ankara: Türk Tarih Kurumu, 1971.

——. *Türk Halkının Dirlik ve Düzenlik Kavgası*. Ankara: Bilgi, 1975.

Akhisarlı Şeyh İsa Menakıbnamesi (XVI. Yüzyıl), İlyas İbn-i Isa Akhisari Saruhani (ö. 967/1559), edited by Sezai Küçük and Ramazan Muslu. Istanbul: Aşiyan Yayınları, 2003.

Albert, Jeff, Magnus Bernhardsson, and Roger Kenna (eds). *Transformations of Middle Eastern Natural Environments: Legacies and Lessons*. New Haven, CT: Yale School of Forestry and Environmental Studies, 1998.

Alderson, Anthony D. *The Structure of the Ottoman Dynasty*. Oxford: Oxford University Press, 1956.

Alexander, John T. *Bubonic Plague in Early Modern Russia: Public Health and Urban Disaster*. Baltimore: Johns Hopkins University Press, 1980.

ʿAlī ibn Rabbān al-Ṭabarī. *Firdaws al-ḥikmah fī al-ṭibb*, edited by M. Z. Siddiqi. Berlin, 1928.

Altizer, Sonia, Rebecca Bartel, and Barbara A. Han. "Animal Migration and Infectious Disease Risk." *Science* 331 (2011): 296–302.

Angliski Pŭtepisi za Balkanite, XVI–XIX v. Sofia: Izdatelstvo "Nauka i Izkustvo," 1987.

ʿAntebi, Avraham. *Sefer yoshev ohalim*. Jerusalem: Mekhon ha-Ktav, 1981.

Antes, John. *Observations on the Manners and Customs of the Egyptians, the Overflowing of the Nile and Its Effects; with Remarks on the Plague, and Other Subjects*. London: J. Stockdale, 1800.

Appel, Toby A. *The Cuvier-Geoffroy Debate: French Biology in the Decades before Darwin*. New York: Oxford University Press, 1987.

Appuhn, Karl. "Ecologies of Beef: Eighteenth-Century Epizootics and the Environmental History of Early Modern Europe." *Environmental History* 15 (2010): 268–87.

Arnold, David. *Colonizing the Body: State Medicine and Epidemic Disease in Nineteenth-Century India*. Berkeley: University of California Press, 1993.

d'Arvieux, Laurent. *Mémoires du chevalier d'Arvieux*. Paris: C. J. B. Delespine, 1735.

ʿAtāʾī, Nevʿizade. *Hadāʿikü'l-hakāʿik fī tekmileti'ş-şekā'ik: Zeyl-i şekāʿik*. Istanbul, [1852].

Atabek, Emine Melek. *1851'de Paris'te Toplanan I. Milletlerarası Sağlık Konferansı ve Türkler*. Istanbul: Cerrahpaşa Tıp Fakültesi Yayınları, 1974.

Ayalon (Neustadt), David. "The Historian Al-Jabartī and His Background." *Bulletin of the School of Oriental and African Studies* 23, no. 2 (1960): 217–49.

——. "The Plague and Its Effects upon the Mamluk Army." *Journal of the Royal Asiatic Society* 66 (1946): 67–73.

——. "Regarding Population Estimates in the Countries of Medieval Islam." *Journal of the Economic and Social History of the Orient* 28 (1985): 1–19.

Ayalon, Yaron. *Natural Disasters in the Ottoman Empire: Plague, Famine, and Other Misfortunes*. Cambridge: Cambridge University Press, 2015.

——. "Ottoman Urban Privacy in Light of Disaster Recovery." *International Journal of Middle East Studies* 43, no. 3 (2011): 513–28.

Aykut, Nezihi, ed. *Hasan Bey-zâde Târîhi*, 3 vols. Ankara: Türk Tarih Kurumu, 2004.

Baer, Marc. "The Great Fire of 1660 and the Islamization of Christian and Jewish Space in Istanbul." *International Journal of Middle East Studies* 36, no. 2 (2004): 159–81.

Bahrani, Zainab, Zeynep Çelik, and Edhem Eldem, eds. *Scramble for the Past: A Story of Archaeology in the Ottoman Empire, 1753–1914*. Istanbul: SALT, 2011.

Baldry, John. "The Ottoman Quarantine Station on Kamaran Island: 1882–1914." *Studies in History of Medicine* 11, nos. 1–2 (1978): 3–137.

Bankoff, Greg. "A Question of Breeding: Zootechny and Colonial Attitudes toward the Tropical Environment in the Late Nineteenth-Century Philippines." *Journal of Asian Studies* 60 (2001): 413–37.

Baptista, Johanne and Antonio Loick. *Historia Pestis quae ab Anno 1708 ad 1713 Transylvaniam, Hungariam, Austriam, Pragam & Ratisbonam, Aliasque Conterminas Provincias Depopulabatur [etc.]*. Styria: Joseph Grünewald, 1715.

Barenstein, Jennifer Duyne and Esther Leemann. *Post-Disaster Reconstruction and Change: Communities' Perspectives*. Boca Raton, FL: CRC Press, 2013.

Barker, John. *An Account of the Present Epidemical Distemper Amongst the Black Cattle*. London: A. Millar, 1745.

Bautista R. E. "Racial Differences in Coping Strategies Among Individuals with Epilepsy." *Epilepsy and Behavior* 29 (2013): 67–71.

Bayram, Mikâil, ed. *Şeyh Evhadü'd-din Hamid el-Kırmânî ve Menâkıb-nâmesi*. Istanbul: Kardelen Yayınları, 2005.

Beinart, William, and Peter Coates. *Environment and History: The Taming of Nature in the USA and South Africa*. London: Routledge, 1995.

Benedict, Carol Ann. *Bubonic Plague in Nineteenth-Century China*. Stanford: Stanford University Press, 1996.

Benedictow, Ole Jørgen. *The Black Death, 1346–1353: The Complete History*. Woodbridge, UK: Boydell Press, 2004.

Bent, J. Theodore. *Early Voyages and Travels in the Levant*. London: Hakluyt Society, 1893.

Bertelli, Pietro. *Vite Degl'imperatori de Turchi*. (n.p., [1596]).

Beyhan, Mehmet Ali. "1811–1812 İstanbul Veba Salgını, Etkileri ve Alınan Tedbirler." In *1. Uluslararası Türk Tıp Tarihi Kongresi / 10. Ulusal Türk Tıp Tarihi Kongresi Bildiri Kitabı (20–24 May 2008)*, edited by Ayşegül Demirhan Erdemir et al., 2: 1029–36. Konya: Türk Tıp Tarihi Kurumu, 2008.

Biraben, Jean-Noël. *Les hommes et la peste en France et dans les pays européens et méditerranéens*, 2 vols. Paris: Mouton, 1975.

Bjørneboe, Lars. *In Search of the True Political Position of the 'Ulama: An Analysis of the Aims and Perspectives of the Chronicles of Abd al-Rahman al-Jabartī (1753–1825)*. Aarhus: Aarhus University Press, 2007.

Blanchard, Ian. "The Continental European Cattle Trades, 1400–1600." *Economic History Review* 39 (1986): 427–60.

Blancou, Jean. *History of the Surveillance and Control of Transmissible Animal Diseases*. Paris: Office International des Épizooties, 2003.

Blažina-Tomić, Zlata, and Vesna Blažina. *Expelling the Plague: The Health Office and the Implementation of Quarantine in Dubrovnik, 1377–1533*. Montreal: McGill-Queen's University Press, 2015.

Boeckl, Christine M. *Images of Plague and Pestilence: Iconography and Iconology*. Kirksville, MO: Truman State University Press, 2000.

Börekçi, Günhan. "İnkırâzın Eşiğinde Bir Hanedan: III. Mehmed, I. Ahmed, I. Mustafa ve 17. Yüzyıl Osmanlı Siyasî Krizi." *Dîvân Disiplinlerarası Çalışmalar Dergisi* 26 (2009): 45–96.

Borisenkov, Ye. P. "Documentary Evidence from the U.S.S.R.." in *Climate Since A.D. 1500*, edited by R. S. Bradley and P. D. Jones, 171–83. London: Routledge, 1995.

Borromeo, Elisabetta. *Voyageurs occidentaux dans l'empire ottoman, 1600–1644: inventaire des récits et études sur les itinéraires, les monuments remarqués et les populations rencontrées (Roumélie, Cyclades, Crimée)*. Paris: Maisonneuve & Larose, 2007.

Borsch, Stuart J. *The Black Death in Egypt and England: A Comparative Analysis*. Austin, TX: University of Texas Press, 2005.

———. "Plague Depopulation and Irrigation Decay in Medieval Egypt." *The Medieval Globe* 1 (2014): 125–56.

Bowers, Kristy Wilson. *Plague and Public Health in Early Modern Seville*. Rochester: University of Rochester Press, 2013.

Boyar, Ebru. "British Archeological Travellers in Nineteenth-Century Anatolia: Anatolia 'Without' Turks." *Eurasian Studies* 1, no. 1 (2002): 97–113.

———. "'An Inconsequential Boil' or a 'Terrible Disease'? Social Perceptions of and State Responses to Syphilis in the Late Ottoman Empire." *Turkish Historical Review* 2 (2011): 101–24.

Brantz, Dorothee. "'Risky Business': Disease, Disaster and the Unintended Consequences of Epizootics in Eighteenth- and Nineteenth-Century France and Germany." *Environment and History* 17 (2011): 35–51.

Brentjes, Sonja. *Travellers from Europe in the Ottoman and Safavid Empires, 16th-17th Centuries: Seeking, Transforming, Discarding Knowledge*. Farnham: Ashgate, 2010.

———. "The Interests of the Republic of Letters in the Middle East, 1550–1700." *Science in Context* 12, no. 3 (1999): 435–68.

Broad, J. "Cattle Plague in Eighteenth-Century England." *Agricultural History Review* 31 (1983): 104–15.

Broughton, John Cam Hobhouse. *A Journey Through Albania: And Other Provinces of Turkey in Europe and Asia, to Constantinople, During the Years 1809–1810*. London: James Cawthorn, 1813.

Brown, Edward. *The Travels and Adventures of Edward Brown, Esq.* London: J. Applebee, 1739.

Brown, Karen and Daniel Gilfoyle, eds. *Healing the Herds: Disease, Livestock Economies, and the Globalization of Veterinary Medicine*. Athens: Ohio University Press, 2010.

Brummett, Palmira. "Dogs, Women, Cholera, and Other Menaces in the Streets: Cartoon Satire in the Ottoman Revolutionary Press, 1908–11." *International Journal of Middle East Studies* 2 (1995): 433–60.

Brumont, Francis. "Les Moutons de la grange de Quintanajuar en vieille-Castille (1623–1834)." In *Les animaux malades en Europe occidentale (VIe–XIXe siècle)*, 117–24. Toulouse: Presses universitaires du Mirail, 2005.

Brunsma, David et al., eds. *The Sociology of Katrina: Perspectives on a Modern Catastrophe*. Lanham: Rowman and Littlefield, 2007.

al-Budayri, Aḥmad. *Ḥawādith dimashq al-yawmiyya*. Cairo: al-Jamʿiyya al-Miṣriyya, 1959.

Buell, Paul D. "Qubilai and the Rats." *Sudhoffs Archiv* 96, no. 2 (2012): 127–44.

Bulliet, Richard W. "The Camel and the Watermill." *International Journal of Middle East Studies* 42, no. 4 (2010): 666–68.

——. *Cotton, Climate, and Camels in Early Islamic Iran: A Moment in World History*. New York: Columbia University Press, 2009.

Bulmuş, Birsen. *Plague, Quarantines and Geopolitics in the Ottoman Empire*. Edinburgh: Edinburgh University Press, 2012.

Büntgen, Ulf et al. "Filling the Eastern European Gap in Millennium-Long Temperature Reconstructions." *Proceedings of the National Academy of Sciences* 110 (2013): 1773–78.

Burak, Guy. *The Second Formation of Islamic Law: The Hanafī School in the Early Modern Ottoman Empire*. Cambridge: Cambridge University Press, 2015.

Burke, Edmund III. "Pastoralism and the Mediterranean Environment." *International Journal of Middle East Studies* 42, no. 4 (2010): 663–65.

——. and David Prochaska. *Genealogies of Orientalism: History, Theory, Politics*. Lincoln: University of Nebraska Press, 2008.

Burleigh, Nina. *Mirage: Napoleon's Scientists and the Unveiling of Egypt*. New York: HarperCollins, 2007.

Burnett, D. Graham. *Masters of All They Surveyed: Exploration, Geography, and a British El Dorado*. Chicago: The University of Chicago Press, 2000.

Burrell, R. M. "The 1904 Epidemic of Cholera in Persia: Some Aspects of Qājār Society." *Bulletin of the School of Oriental and African Studies* 51 (1988): 258–70.

de Busbecq, Ogier Ghiselin. *The Turkish Letters of Ogier Ghiselin de Busbecq, Imperial Ambassador at Constantinople, 1554–1562: Translated from the Latin of the Elzevir Edition of 1663*. Baton Rouge: Louisiana State University Press, 2005.

Bynum, William F. "Policing Hearts of Darkness: Aspects of the International Sanitary Conferences." *History and Philosophy of the Life Sciences* 15 (1993): 421–34.

Cahn, Théophile. *La vie et l'oeuvre d'Étienne Geoffroy Saint-Hilaire*. Paris: Presses universitaires de France, 1962.

Campbell, Bruce M. S. *The Great Transition: Climate, Disease and Society in the Late-Medieval World*. Cambridge: Cambridge University Press, 2016.

——. "Nature as Historical Protagonist: Environment and Society in Pre-Industrial England." *The Economic History Review* 63 (2010): 281–314.

——. "Physical Shocks, Biological Hazards, and Human Impacts: The Crisis of the Fourteenth Century Revisited." In *Le interazioni fra economia e ambiente biologico nell'Europa preindustriale secc. XIII–XVIII*, edited by Simonetta Cavaciocchi, 13–32. Florence: Firenze University Press, 2010.

Campbell, Gwyn. "Disease, Cattle, and Slaves: The Development of Trade between Natal and Madagascar, 1875–1904." *African Economic History* 19 (1990): 105–33.

Carmichael, Ann G. *Plague and the Poor in Renaissance Florence*. Cambridge: Cambridge University Press, 1986.

——. and Arthur M. Silverstein. "Smallpox in Europe before the Seventeenth Century: Virulent Killer or Benign Disease." *Journal of the History of Medicine and Allied Sciences* 42, no. 2 (1987): 147-68.

Carrière, Charles, Marcel Courdurié, and Ferréol Rebuffat. *Marseille ville morte: la peste de 1720*. Marseille: M. Garçon, 1968.

Çavusoğlu, Semiramis. "The Kadızadeli Movement: An Attempt of Şerîʿat-Minded Reform in the Ottoman Empire." Unpublished PhD dissertation, Princeton University, 1990.

Celalüddin Hızır (Hacı Paşa). *Müntahab-ı Şifâ*, edited by Zafer Önler. Ankara: Türk Dil Kurumu, 1990.

Chareyron, Nicole. *Pilgrims to Jerusalem in the Middle Ages*. Translated by Donald Wilson. New York: Columbia University Press, 2005.

Chaudhuri, Kirti N. *Trade and Civilisation in the Indian Ocean: History from the Rise of Islam to 1750*. Cambridge: Cambridge University Press, 1985.

Chiffoleau, Sylvia. *Genèse de la santé publique internationale: de la peste d'Orient à l'OMS*. Rennes: Presses universitaires de Rennes, 2012.

Çırakman, Aslı. *From the "Terror of the World" to the "Sick Man of Europe": European Images of Ottoman Empire and Society from the Sixteenth Century to the Nineteenth*. New York: Peter Lang, 2002.

Clemow, F. G. "The Constantinople Board of Health, A Brief Historical Survey." *Reprinted From the Lancet* 201, no. 5204 (1923): 1074–76.

Clot-Bey, Antoine Barthélemy. *Aperçu general sur l'Égypte*, 2 vols. Bruxelles: Meline, Cans, 1840.

Coates, Peter. "Emerging from the Wilderness (or, from Redwoods to Bananas): Recent Environmental History in the United States and the Rest of the Americas." *Environment and History* 10, no. 4 (2004): 407–38.

Cogrossi, Carlo Francesco. *Nuova Idea del Male Contagioso de' Buoi* [1714]. Rome: Società Italiana di Microbiologia, 1953.

Cole, Juan. *Napoleon's Egypt: Invading the Middle East.* New York: Palgrave Macmillan, 2007.

Collins, Billie Jean, ed. *A History of the Animal World in the Ancient Near East.* Leiden: Brill, 2002.

Conrad, Lawrence I. "Arabic Plague Chronologies and Treatises: Social and Historical Factors in the Formation of a Literary Genre." *Studia Islamica* 54 (1981): 51–93.

——. "Epidemic Disease in Central Syria in the Late Sixth Century: Some New Insights from the Verse of Ḥassān ibn Thābit." *Byzantine and Modern Greek Studies* 18 (1994): 12–58.

——. "Epidemic Disease in Formal and Popular Thought in Early Islamic Society." In *Epidemics and Ideas: Essays on the Historical Perception of Pestilence,* edited by Terence Ranger and Paul Slack, 77–99. Cambridge: Cambridge University Press, 1992.

——. "A Ninth-Century Muslim Scholar's Discussion of Contagion." In *Contagion: Perspectives from Pre-modern Societies,* edited by Lawrence I. Conrad and Dominik Wujastyk, 163–77. Aldershot: Ashgate, 2000.

——. "The Plague in the Early Medieval Near East." Unpublished PhD dissertation, Princeton University, 1981.

——. "Scholarship and Social Context in the Near East." In *Knowledge and the Scholarly Medical Traditions,* edited by Don Bates, 81–101. Cambridge: Cambridge University Press, 1995.

——. "*Ṭāʿūn* and *Wabāʾ*: Conceptions of Plague and Pestilence in Early Islam." *Journal of the Economic and Social History of the Orient* 25 (1982): 268–307.

——. Michael Neve, Vivian Nutton, Roy Porter, and Andrew Wear, *The Western Medical Tradition: 800 B.C.–1800 A.D.* Cambridge: Cambridge University Press, 1995.

Coste, Joël. *Représentations et comportements en temps d'épidémie dans la littérature imprimée de peste (1490–1725): contribution à l'histoire culturelle de la peste en France à l'époque moderne.* Paris: Honoré Champion, 2007.

Crawshaw, Jane L. Stevens. *Plague Hospitals: Public Health for the City in Early Modern Venice.* Farnham: Ashgate, 2012.

Crecelius, Daniel. "The Importance of Qusayr in the Late Eighteenth Century." *Journal of the American Research Center in Egypt* 24 (1987): 53–60.

——. *The Roots of Modern Egypt: A Study of the Regimes of Ali Bey al-Kabir and Muhammad Bey Abu al-Dhahab, 1760–1775.* Minneapolis: Bibliotheca Islamica, 1981.

Cronon, William. "The Trouble with Wilderness; Or, Getting Back to the Wrong Nature." *Environmental History* 1, no. 1 (1996): 7–28.

Crosby, Alfred W. *The Columbian Exchange: Biological and Cultural Consequences of 1492.* Westport, CT: Greenwood Press, 1972.

——. *Ecological Imperialism: The Biological Expansion of Europe, 900–1900*. Cambridge: Cambridge University Press, 1986.

——. "Smallpox." In *The Cambridge World History of Human Disease*, edited by Kenneth F. Kiple, 1008–13. Cambridge: Cambridge University Press, 1993.

Cunningham, Andrew and Perry Williams, eds. *The Laboratory Revolution in Medicine*. Cambridge: Cambridge University Press, 1992.

Curry, John J. "The Growth of a Turkish-Language Hagiographical Literature Within the Halveti Order of the 16th and 17th Centuries." *The Turks*, edited by Hasan Celal Güzel et al., 3: 912–20. Ankara: Yeni Türkiye Press, 2002.

——. "The Intersection of Past and Present in the Genesis of an Ottoman Sufi Order: The Life of Cemâl el-Halveti (d. 900/1494 or 905/1499) and the Origins of the Halveti *Tarîqa*." *Journal of Turkish Studies (In Memoriam Şinasi Tekin III)* 32 (2008): 121–41.

——. *The Transformation of Muslim Mystical Thought in the Ottoman Empire: The Rise of the Halveti Order 1350–1650*. Edinburgh: Edinburgh University Press, 2010.

——. and Erik S. Ohlander, eds. *Sufism and Society: Arrangements of the Mystical in the Muslim World, 1200–1800*. London: Routledge, 2012.

Curth, Louise Hill. *The Care of Brute Beasts: A Social and Cultural Study of Veterinary Medicine in Early Modern England*. Leiden: Brill, 2010.

Cutler, Sally J., Anthony R. Fooks, and Wim H. M. van der Poel. "Public Health Threat of New, Reemerging, and Neglected Zoonoses in the Industrialized World." *Emerging Infectious Diseases* 16 (2010): 1–7.

Cvetkova, Bistra A. "Le service des celeps et le ravitaillement en bétail dans l'Empire ottoman (XVe–XVIIIe siècles)." *Études Historiques* 3 (1966): 145–72.

Dağlar, Oya. *War, Epidemics, and Medicine in the Late Ottoman Empire (1912–1918)*. Haarlem: Sota, 2008.

al-Damurdashi's Chronicle of Egypt, 1688–1755: Al-Durra al-Musana fi Akhbar al-Kinana. Translated and annotated by Daniel Crecelius and ʿAbd al-Wahhab Bakr. Leiden: Brill, 1991.

Daniels, Ronald et al., eds. *On Risk and Disaster: Lessons from Hurricane Katrina*. Philadelphia: University of Pennsylvania Press, 2006.

Darwin, Charles. *On the Origin of Species by Means of Natural Selection, or the Preservation of Favoured Races in the Struggle for Life*. London: John Murray, 1859.

Davis, Diana K. "Brutes, Beasts, and Empire: Veterinary Medicine and Environmental Policy in French North Africa and British India." *Journal of Historical Geography* 34 (2008): 242–67.

——. "Introduction: Imperialism, Orientalism, and the Environment in the Middle East." In *Environmental Imaginaries of the Middle East and North Africa*, edited by Diana K. Davis and Edmund Burke III, 1–22. Athens: Ohio University Press, 2011.

——. "Prescribing Progress: French Veterinary Medicine in the Service of Empire." *Veterinary Heritage* 29 (2006): 1–7.

——. and Edmund Burke III, eds. *Environmental Imaginaries of the Middle East and North Africa*. Athens: Ohio University Press, 2011.

Davis, James Cushman. *Pursuit of Power: Venetian Ambassador's Reports on Spain, Turkey and France in the Age of Phillip II: 1560–1600*. New York: Harper and Row, 1970.

Demirsoy, Vildan Taşkıran. "Analysis of a Manuscript: *Risāla-i Tibbi't-Turkî*: Treatment of Head Diseases in Ottoman Medicine." *Journal of the International Society for the History of Islamic Medicine* 12–13, nos. 23–26 (2013–14): 8–20.

Derham, William. "The History of the Great Frost in the Last Winter, 1708 and 1708/9." *Philosophical Transactions of the Royal Society* 26 (September 1708): 454–78.

Derry, Margaret E. *Bred for Perfection: Shorthorn Cattle, Collies, and Arabian Horses since 1800*. Baltimore: Johns Hopkins University Press, 2003.

Devinsky, Orrin and George Lai. "Spirituality and Religion in Epilepsy." *Epilepsy and Behavior* 12, no. 4 (2008): 636–43.

Diamond, Jared M. *Collapse: How Societies Choose to Fail or Succeed*. New York, 2005.

——. *Guns, Germs, and Steel: The Fates of Human Societies*. London: W. W. Norton, 1998.

Dieckerhoff, W. *Geschichte der Rinderpest und ihrer Literatur*. Berlin: T. C. F. Enslin, 1890.

Dolev, Eran. "'I Am Campaigning Against Mosquitoes': General Allenby's Campaign against Malaria, Palestine 1918." *Korot* 21 (2011): 75–88.

Dols, Michael W. *The Black Death in the Middle East*. Princeton, NJ: Princeton University Press, 1977.

——. *Majnūn: The Madman in Medieval Islamic Society*, edited by Diana E. Immisch. Oxford: Clarendon Press, 1992.

——. "Al-Manbiji's *Report of the Plague*: A Treatise on the Plague of 764–5/1362–4 in the Middle East." In *The Black Death: The Impact of the Fourteenth-Century Plague*, edited by Daniel Williman, 65–76. Binghamton, NY: Medieval and Renaissance Texts and Studies, 1982.

——. "The Second Plague Pandemic and Its Recurrences in the Middle East: 1347–1894." *Journal of the Economic and Social History of the Orient* 22 (1979): 162–89.

——. "The Theory of Magic in Healing." In *Magic and Divination in Early Islam*, edited by Emilie Savage-Smith, 87–101. Aldershot: Ashgate, 2004.

Donner, Fred McGraw. *Narratives of Islamic Origins: The Beginnings of Islamic Historical Writing*. Princeton: Darwin Press, 1998.

Dorwart, Reinhold. "Cattle Disease (Rinderpest?): Prevention and Cure in Brandenburg, 1665–1732." *Agricultural History* 33 (1959): 79–85.

Dossie, Robert. *Memoirs of Agriculture and Other Oeconomical Arts*. London: J. Nourse, 1771.

Dubois, Colette. "The Red Sea Ports during the Revolution in Transportation, 1800–1914." In *Modernity and Culture from the Mediterranean to the Indian Ocean*, edited by Leila Tarazi Fawaz and Christopher A. Bayly, 58–74. New York: Columbia University Press, 2002.

Duggan, Ana et al. "17th century *Variola* Virus Reveals the Recent History of Smallpox." *Current Biology* 26 (2016): 1-6.

du Mont, Jean. *A New Voyage to the Levant Containing an Account of the Most Remarkable Curiosities in Germany, France, Italy, Malta, and Turkey*. London: M. Gillyflower, 1696.

Dunlop, Robert H. and David J. Williams. *Veterinary Medicine: An Illustrated History*. St. Louis: Mosby, 1996.

Dwight, H. G. O. *Memoir of Mrs. Elizabeth B. Dwight Including an Account of the Plague of 1837*. New York: M. W. Dodd, 1840.

Ebrahimnejad, Hormoz. "Introduction: For a History of Modern Medicine in Non-Western Countries." In *The Development of Modern Medicine in Non-Western Countries: Historical Perspectives*, edited Hormoz Ebrahimnejad, 1–22. London: Routledge, 2009.

Echenberg, Myron J. *Plague Ports: The Global Urban Impact of Bubonic Plague, 1894–1901*. New York: New York University Press, 2007.

Eisenstein, Herbert. *Einführung in die arabische Zoographie: Das tierkundliche Wissen in der arabisch-islamischen Literatur*. Berlin: Dietrich Reimer, 1990.

Eldem, Edhem. *Death in Istanbul: Death and its Rituals in Ottoman-Islamic Culture*. Istanbul: Ottoman Bank Archives and Research Centre, 2005.

——. "Death and Funerary Culture." In *Encyclopedia of the Ottoman Empire*, edited by Gábor Ágoston and Bruce Alan Masters, 177–80. New York: Facts on File, 2009.

Ellenbaum, Ronnie. *The Collapse of the Eastern Mediterranean: Climate Change and the Decline of the East, 950–1072*. Cambridge: Cambridge University Press, 2012.

Enenkel, Karl A. E. and Paul J. Smith, eds. *Early Modern Zoology: The Construction of Animals in Science, Literature and the Visual Arts*, 2 vols. Leiden: Brill, 2007.

Engler, S. et al. "The Irish Famine of 1740–1741: Famine Vulnerability and 'Climate Migration'." *Climate of the Past* 9 (2013): 1161–79.

Erder, Leila. "Population Rise and Fall in Anatolia, 1550–1620." *Middle East Studies* 15 (1979): 322–45.

Erler, Mehmet. *Osmanlı Devleti'nde Kuraklık ve Kıtlık Olayları (1800–1880)*. Istanbul: Libra Yayınevi, 2010.

Essner, Cornelia. "Cholera der Mekkapilger und Internationale Sanitätspolitik in Ägypten (1866–1938)." *Die Welt des Islams* 32 (1992): 41–82.

Evered, Emine Ö. and Kyle T. Evered. "Sex and the Capital City: The Political Framing of Syphilis and Prostitution in Early Republican Ankara." *Journal of the History of Medicine and Allied Sciences* 68, no. 2 (2013): 266–99.

Evered, Kyle T. and Emine Ö. Evered. "Governing Population, Public Health, and Malaria in the Early Turkish Republic." *Journal of Historical Geography* 37, no. 4 (2011): 470–82.

——. "Syphilis and Prostitution in the Socio-Medical Geographies of Turkey's Early Republican Provinces." *Health and Place* 18, no. 3 (2012): 528–35.

——. "State, Peasant, Mosquito: The Biopolitics of Public Health Education and Malaria in Early Republican Turkey." *Political Geography* 31, no. 5 (2012): 311–23.

Evliyâ Çelebi, *Evliyâ Çelebi Seyahatnâmesi*. Istanbul: Yapı Kredi Yayınları, 1994–2007.

Faber, J. A. "Cattle-Plague in the Netherlands During the Eighteenth Century." *Medelingen van de Lanbouwhogeschool Te Wageningen* 62 (1962): 1–7.

Facey, William. "The Red Sea: The Wind Regime and Location of Ports." In *Trade and Travel in the Red Sea Region: Proceedings of Red Sea Project I Held in the British Museum, October 2002*, edited by Paul Lunde and Alexandra Porter, 7–17. Oxford: Archaeopress, 2004.

Fahmy, Khaled. *All the Pasha's Men: Mehmed Ali, His Army and the Making of Modern Egypt*. Cambridge: Cambridge University Press, 1997.

——. "Women, Medicine, and Power in Nineteenth-Century Egypt." In *Remaking Women: Feminism and Modernity in the Middle East*, edited by Lila Abu-Lughod, 35–72. Princeton, NJ: Princeton University Press, 1998.

Fairhead, James, and Melissa Leach. *Misreading the African Landscape: Society and Ecology in a Forest-Savanna Mosaic*. Cambridge: Cambridge University Press, 1996.

The Famine in Asia-Minor: Its History, Compiled from the Pages of the "Levant Herald." Istanbul: Isis Press, 1989.

Fancy, Nahyan. *Science and Religion in Mamluk Egypt: Ibn al-Nafis, Pulmonary Transit and Bodily Resurrection*. London: Routledge, 2013.

Faroqhi, Suraiya. "Seeking Wisdom in China: An Attempt to Make Sense of the Celâli Rebellions." In *Zafar-nama: Memorial Volume to Felix Tauer*, edited by Rudolf Vesely and Eduard Gombar, 101–24. Prague: Enigma, 1996.

——. *Towns and Townsmen of Ottoman Anatolia*. Cambridge: Cambridge University Press, 1984.

——. ed. *Animals and People in the Ottoman Empire*. Istanbul: Eren, 2010.

Ferrières, Madeleine. *Sacred Cow, Mad Cow: A History of Food Fears*. Translated by Jody Gladding. New York: Columbia University Press, 2006.

Finkel, Caroline. *Osman's Dream: The Story of the Ottoman Empire, 1300–1922*. London: John Murray, 2005.

Firpo, Luigi, ed. *Relazioni di ambasciatori veneti al senato, tratte dalle migliori edizioni disponibili e ordinate cronologicamente*, 13: *Costantinopoli (1590–1793)*. Torino: Bottega d'Erasmo, 1984.

Fleischer, Cornell H. *Bureaucrat and Intellectual in the Ottoman Empire: The Historian Mustafa Ali: 1541–1600*. Princeton: Princeton University Press, 1986.

Fleming, George. *Animal Plagues: Their History, Nature, and Prevention*. London: Champman and Hall, 1871.

Fletcher, Joseph. "Turco-Mongolian Monarchic Tradition in the Ottoman Empire." *Harvard Ukranian Studies* 3–4 (1979–80): 236–51.

Foucault, Michel. *The Order of Things: An Archaeology of the Human Sciences*. New York: Vintage Books, 1973.

Frandsen, Karl-Erik. *The Last Plague in the Baltic Region, 1709–1713*. Copenhagen: Museum Tusculanum Press, 2010.

Friedman, Donald Flanell. *The Symbolist Dead City: A Landscape of Poesis*. New York: Garland, 1990.

Frost, Robert. *The Northern Wars*. New York: Longman, 2000.

Gage, Kenneth L. et al. "Climate and Vectorborne Diseases." *American Journal of Preventive Medicine* 35 (2008): 436–50.

Gallagher, Nancy. *Medicine and Power in Tunisia, 1780–1900*. Cambridge: Cambridge University Press, 1983.

——. *Egypt's Other Wars: Epidemics and the Politics of Public Health*. Syracuse, NY: Syracuse University Press, 1990.

Geoffroy Saint-Hilaire, Isidore. *Vie, travaux et doctrine scientifique d'Étienne Geoffroy Saint-Hilaire*. Paris: P. Bertrand, 1847.

Gerlach, Stephan. *Türkiye Günlüğü: 1573–1576*. 2 vols. Istanbul: Kitap Yayınevi, 2007.

Getz, Faye Marie."Black Death and the Silver Lining: Meaning, Continuity, and Revolutionary Change in Histories of Medieval Plague." *Journal of the History of Biology* 24, no. 2 (1991): 265–89.

al-Ghazzī, Kāmil bin Ḥusayn. *Kitāb nahr al-dhahab fī taʾrīkh ḥalab*. Aleppo: Dār al-Qalam al-ʿArabī, 1992.

Gijsbers, Wilhelmina Maria and Peter A. Koolmees, "Food on Foot: Long-Distance Trade in Slaughter Oxen Between Denmark and the Netherlands (14th-18th Century)." *Historia Medicinae Veterinariae* 26 (2001): 115–27.

Giladi, Avner. "Concepts of Childhood and Attitudes towards Children in Medieval Islam." *Journal of the Economic and Social History of the Orient* 32 (1989): 121–52.

Gladitz, Charles. *Horse Breeding in the Medieval World.* Dublin: Four Courts Press, 1997.

Grabar, Oleg. "The Earliest Islamic Commemorative Structures, Notes and Documents." *Ars Orientalis* 6 (1966): 7–46.

Grajera, Alfonso Rodríguez and Mireille Mousnier. "Les maladies et l'état sanitaire des animaux dans la couronne de Castille à l'époque moderne." In *Les animaux malades en Europe occidentale (VIe–XIXe siècle)*, 153–78. Toulouse: Presses universitaires du Mirail, 2005.

Green, Monica H. "Editor's Introduction to *Pandemic Disease in the Medieval World: Rethinking the Black Death*." *The Medieval Globe* 1 (2014): 9–25.

——. "Taking 'Pandemic' Seriously: Making the Black Death Global." *The Medieval Globe* 1 (2014): 27–61.

——. ed. *Pandemic Disease in the Medieval World: Rethinking the Black Death. The Medieval Globe* 1 (2014).

Greenwood, Anthony. "Meat Provisioning and Ottoman Economic Administration." In *Abdullah Kuran İçin Yazılar*, edited by Çiğdem Kafesçioğlu and Lucienne Thys-Şenocak, 191–210. Istanbul: Yapı Kredi Yayınları, 1999.

Griffiths, John. *Travels in Europe, Asia Minor and Arabia.* London: T. Cadell and W. Davies, 1805.

Griswold, William. *The Great Anatolian Rebellion, 1591–1611.* Berlin: Klaus Schwarz, 1983.

Grove, Jean and A. Battagel. "Tax Records from Western Norway as an Index of the Little Ice Age Environmental and Economic Deterioration." *Climatic Change* 3 (1983): 265–82.

Güçer, Lütfi. *Osmanlı İmparatorluğunda Hububat Meselesi ve Hububattan Alınan Vergiler.* Istanbul: Istanbul University Press, 1964.

Gupta, Ashin Das. *Merchants of Maritime India, 1500–1800.* Aldershot: Ashgate, 1994.

Guy, William A. *Public Health: A Popular Introduction to Sanitary Science.* London: Renshaw, 1870.

Habesci, Elias. *The Present State of the Ottoman Empire.* London: R. Baldwin, 1784.

Halevi, Leor. *Muhammad's Grave: Death Rites and the Making of Islamic Society.* New York: Columbia University Press, 2007.

Hamont, Pierre Nicolas. *L'Egypt sous Méhémet-Ali*, 2 vols. Paris: Léautey et Lecointe, 1843.

Hamza, Hani. *The North Cemetery of Cairo.* Cairo: The American University in Cairo Press, 2001.

Hanioğlu, M. Şükrü. *A Brief History of the Late Ottoman Empire.* Princeton: Princeton University Press, 2008.

Hanna, Nelly, ed. *Money, Land and Trade: An Economic History of the Muslim Mediterranean.* London: I. B. Tauris, 2002.

——. and Raouf Abbas, eds. *Society and Economy in Egypt and the Eastern Mediterranean, 1600–1900*. Cairo: The American University in Cairo Press, 2005.

Harper, James G. *The Turk and Islam in the Western Eye, 1450–1750: Visual Imagery Before Orientalism*. Aldershot: Ashgate, 2011.

Harrison, Mark. "Quarantine, Pilgrimage, and Colonial Trade: India 1866–1900." *The Indian Economic and Social History Review* 29, no. 2 (1992): 117–44.

Hathaway, Jane. *Al-Jabarti's History of Egypt*. Princeton: Markus Wiener Publishers, 2009.

Hatina, Meir. *ʿUlamaʾ Politics and the Public Sphere: An Egyptian Perspective*. Salt Lake City: University of Utah Press, 2010.

Heberer, Johann Michael. *Aegyptiaca servitus*. Graz: Akademische Druck und Verlagsanstalt, 1967.

Hecker, J. F. C. *Der schwarze Tod im vierzehnten Jahrhundert*. Berlin: F. A. Herbig, 1832.

——. *The Epidemics of the Middle Ages*. Translated by B. G. Babington. London: Trübner, 1859.

Heinrich, Ingo et al. "Winter-to-Spring Temperature Dynamics in Turkey Derived from Tree Rings since AD 1125." *Climate Dynamics* 41 (2013): 1685–1701.

Henninger, Joseph. "Beliefs in Spirits Among the Pre-Islamic Arabs." In *Magic and Divination in Early Islam*, edited by Emilie Savage-Smith, 1–53. Aldershot: Ashgate, 2004.

Heyberger, Bernard. *Les chrétiens du Proche-Orient au temps de la réforme catholique: Syrie, Liban, Palestine, XVIIe–XVIIIe siècles*. Rome: Ecole Française de Rome, 1994.

Heyworth-Dunne, James. *An Introduction to the History of Education in Modern Egypt*. London: Luzac, 1939.

——. "Printing and Translations under Muḥammad ʿAlī of Egypt: The Foundation of Modern Arabic." *Journal of the Royal Asiatic Society* 72 (1940): 325–49.

Hidalgo, Danielle and Kristen Barber, eds. *Narrating the Storm: Sociological Stories of Hurricane Katrina*. Newcastle: Cambridge Scholars, 2007.

Hippocrates. "The Sacred Disease." In *Hippocrates with an English Translation by W. H. S. Jones*. Cambridge, MA: Harvard University Press, 1923.

Hirsch, August. *Handbook of Geographical and Historical Pathology, 1: Acute Infective Diseases*. Translated by Charles Creighton. London: The New Sydenham Society, 1883.

——. "What Has Europe to Fear in the Future from Oriental Plague?" *The Practitioner: A Journal of Therapeutics and Public Health* 19 (1877): 223–40.

Hodge, Adam R. "'In Want of Nourishment for to Keep Them Alive': Climate Fluctuations, Bison Scarcity, and the Smallpox Epidemic of 1780–82 on the Northern Great Plains." *Environmental History* 17 (2012): 365–403.

Hoffman, Richard. "Frontier Food for Late Medieval Consumers: Culture, Economy, Ecology." *Environment and History* 7 (2001): 131–67.
Hoffmann, Irene. "Climate Change and the Characterization, Breeding and Conservation of Animal Genetic Resources." *Animal Genetics* 41, suppl. 1 (2010): 32–46.
Holtzman, Livnat. "Ibn Qayyim al-Jawziyyah (1292–1350)." In *Essays in Arabic Literary Biography 1350–1850*, edited by Joseph E. Lowry and Devin J. Stewart, 202–23. Wiesbaden: Harrassowitz Verlag, 2009.
Hopley, Russell. "Contagion in Islamic Lands: Responses from Medieval Andalusia and North Africa." *Journal for Early Modern Cultural Studies* 10 (2010): 45–64.
Howard-Jones, Norman. *The Scientific Backround of International Sanitary Conferences, 1851–1938*. Geneva: World Health Organization, 1975.
Huber, Valeska. "The Unification of the Globe by Disease? The International Sanitary Conferences on Cholera, 1851–1894." *The Historical Journal* 49, no. 2 (2006): 453–76.
Hünniger, Dominik. "Policing Epizootics: Legislation and Administration During Outbreaks of Cattle Plague in Eighteenth-Century Northern Germany as Continuous Crisis Management." In *Healing the Herds: Disease, Livestock Economies, and the Globalization of Veterinary Medicine*, edited by Karen Brown and Daniel Gilfoyle, 92–107. Athens, OH: Ohio University Press, 2010.
Hymes, Robert. "Epilogue: A Hypothesis on the East Asian Beginnings of the *Yersinia pestis* Polytomy." *The Medieval Globe* 1 (2014): 285–308.
Hyrapiet, Shireen. *Responding to a Tsunami: A Case Study from India*. Saarbrücken, Germany: VDM Verlag, 2007.
Ibn Kannān, Muḥammad. *Yawmiyyāt shāmiyya*. Damascus: Dār al-Ṭabbaʿ, 1994.
Ibn Kathīr. *Book of Evidences: The Miracles of the Prophet (P.B.U.H.)*. Translated by Ali Mwinyi Mziwa and Ibn R. Ramadhan. Al-Mansoura: Dār al-Gad, 2004.
Ibn Qayyim al-Jawziyya. *Medicine of the Prophet*. Translated by Penelope Johnstone. Cambridge: The Islamic Texts Society, 2004.
——. *Ṣaḥīḥ al-ṭibb al-nabawī fī ḍaw' al-maʿārif al-ṭibbīyah wa al-ʿilmīyah al-ḥadīthah*. ʿAjmān: Maktabat al-Furqān, 2003.
İbn-i Şerîf. *Yâdigâr*, edited by Ayten Altıntaş, Yahya Okutan, Doğan Koçer, and Mecit Yıldız. Istanbul: Yerküre, 2004.
Imber, Colin. "Frozen Legitimacy." In *Legitimizing the Order*, edited by Hakan T. Karateke and Maurus Reinkowski, 99–107. Leiden: Brill, 2005.
İshâk bin Murâd. *Edviye-i Müfrede*, edited by Mustafa Canpolat. Ankara: Türk Dil Kurumu, 2007.
İzzeddin, Kasım. *Mekke-i Mükerremede Kolera ve Hıfzıssıhha*. Istanbul: Mahmut Bey Matbaası, 1911.
al-Jabartī, ʿAbd al-Raḥmān. *ʿAjā'ib al-Āthār fī al-tarājim wa al-akhbār*. Cairo: Lajnat al-Bayān al-ʿArabī, 1958.

de Jaucourt, Louis. "Peste." In *Encyclopédie, ou dictionnaire raisonné des sciences, des arts et des métiers*, edited by Denis Diderot and Jean le Rond d'Alembert, 12: 452–58. Paris: Sociétés Typographiques, 1751–72.

Jennings, Ronald C. "Pious Foundations in the Society and Economy of Ottoman Trabzon, 1565–1640." *Journal of the Economic and Social History of the Orient* 33 (1990): 271–336.

——. "Plague in Trabzon and Reactions to It, According to Local Judicial Registers." In *Humanist and Scholar: Essays in Honor of Andreas Tietze*, edited by Heath W. Lowry and Donald Quataert, 27–36. Istanbul: Isis Press, 1993.

Jessopp, Augustus. "The Black Death in East Anglia." In *The Coming of the Friars and Other Historic Essays*, 166–261. London: T. Fisher Unwin, 1908.

——. "*A History of Epidemics in Britain, from A. D. 664 to the Extinction of the Plague* by Charles Creighton and *The Great Pestilence (1348–9), Now Commonly Known as the Black Death* by Francis Aidan Gasquet." *The English Historical Review*, 9, no. 35 (1894).

Jezernik, Bozidar. *Imagining "the Turk."* Newcastle upon Tyne: Cambridge Scholars, 2010.

Jones, Lori. "The Diseased Landscape: Medieval and Early Modern Plaguescapes." *Landscapes* 17, no. 2 (2016): 108–23.

Jones, P. D. and K. R. Briffa. "Unusual Climate in Northwest Europe During the Period 1730 to 1745 Based on Instrumental and Documentary Data." *Climatic Change* 79 (2006): 361–79.

Jones, Susan D. *Valuing Animals: Veterinarians and Their Patients in Modern America*. Baltimore: Johns Hopkins University Press, 2002.

Jordan, William C. *The Great Famine: Northern Europe in the Early Fourteenth Century*. Princeton, NJ: Princeton University Press, 1996.

al-Jumayʿī, ʿAbd al-Munʿim Ibrāhīm, ed. *Wathāʾiq al-Taʿlīm al-ʿĀlī fī Miṣr khilāl al-Qarn al-Tāsiʿ ʿAshar*. Cairo: Dār al-Kutub wa al-Wathāʾīq al-Qawmiyya, 2004.

Jütte, Robert. *Poverty and Deviance in Early Modern Europe*. Cambridge: Cambridge University Press, 1994.

"Kamaran'da Müessesat-ı Sıhhiye-i Osmaniye: Kamaran Adası." *Servet-i Fünun* 24, no. 603 (1902): 70–73.

"Kamaran'da Müessesat-ı Sıhhiye-i Osmaniye: Tahaffuzhâne ve Memurin." *Servet-i Fünun* 24, no. 604 (1902): 85–87.

"Kamaran'da Müessesat-ı Sıhhiye-i Osmaniye: Üçüncü Makale Tahaffuzhane ve Aksamı." *Servet-i Fünun* 24, no. 605 (1902): 103–06.

Kaniewski, D. et al. "The Medieval Climate Anomaly and the Little Ice Age in Coastal Syria Inferred from Pollen-Derived Palaeoclimatic Patterns." *Global and Planetary Change* 78 (2011): 178–87.

Kanold, Johann. *Historische Relation von der Pestilenz des Hornviehes welche anno 1711 und 1712 in Schlesien* [etc.]. Breslau: Ben Esaia Fellgiebels, 1713.

Karaçelebizade Abdülaziz. *Ravzatü'l-ebrār*. Bulaq: Al-Matbaʿa al-Amīriyya, 1832.

"Karantin i Gospitali v Smirn." *Zhurnal Ministerstva Vnutrennikh Del* 8 (1844): 295–312.

Karasszon, Dénes. *A Concise History of Veterinary Medicine*. Budapest: Akadémiai Kiadó, 1988.

Kashani-Sabet, Firoozeh. "'City of the Dead': The Frontier Polemics of Quarantines in the Ottoman Empire and Iran." *Comparative Studies of South Asia, Africa and the Middle East* 18 (1998): 51–58.

——. *Conceiving Citizens: Women and the Politics of Motherhood in Iran*. Oxford: Oxford University Press, 2011.

Kennedy, Hugh N. "Justinianic Plague in Syria and the Archaeological Evidence." In *Plague and the End of Antiquity: The Pandemic of 541–750*, edited by Lester K. Little, 87–95. Cambridge: Cambridge University Press, 2007.

Khalifa, Marwa A. "Redefining Slums in Egypt: Unplanned Versus Unsafe Areas." *Habitat International* 35, no. 1 (2011).

al-Khashshāb, Ismāʿīl. *Khulāṣat mā yurād min akhbār al-amīr Murād*. Cairo: Al-Maktaba al-Taʾrīkhiyya, 1992.

Khazeni, Arash. "Across the Black Sands and the Red: Travel Writing, Nature, and the Reclamation of the Eurasian Steppe circa 1850." *International Journal of Middle East Studies* 42, no. 4 (2010): 591–614.

——. *Tribes and Empire on the Margins of Nineteenth-Century Iran*. Seattle: University of Washington Press, 2009.

Kılıç, Orhan. *Genel Hatlarıyla Dünyada ve Osmanlı Devleti'nde Salgın Hastalıklar*. Elazığ: Fırat Üniversitesi Rektorlüğü, 2004.

Kim, Dong Jin, Han Sang Yoo, and Hang Lee. "Effects of the Periodical Spread of Rinderpest on Famine, Epidemic, and Tiger Disasters in the Late 17th Century." *Korean Journal of Medical History* 23 (2014): 1–56.

Kinglake, Alexander William. *Kinglake's Eothen*. London: Henry Frowde, 1906.

Kirkpatrick, Lee. *Attachment, Evolution, and the Psychology of Religion*. New York: Guilford Press, 2005.

Kishi, Hiroshi. "A Historical Study on Outbreaks of Rinderpest during the Yedo Era in Japan." *The Yamaguchi Journal of Veterinary Medicine* 3 (1976): 33–40.

Kjaegaard, Thorkild. *The Danish Revolution, 1500–1800: An Ecohistorical Interpretation*. Translated by David Hohnen. New York: Cambridge University Press, 1994.

Klimenko, Vladimir and Olga Solomina. "Climatic Variations in the East European Plain During the Last Millennium: State of the Art." In *The Polish Climate in the European Context: An Historical Overview*, edited by Rajmund Przybylak et al., 71–101. Berlin: Springer, 2010.

Knolles, Richard. *The Generall Historie of the Turkes.* Second edition. London: Adam Islip, 1610.

Koolmees, Peter A. "Epizootic Diseases in the Netherlands, 1713–2002." In *Healing the Herds: Disease, Livestock Economies, and the Globalization of Veterinary Medicine*, edited by Karen Brown and Daniel Gilfoyle, 19–41. Athens, OH: Ohio University Press, 2010.

Krech, Shepard. *The Ecological Indian: Myth and History*. New York: Norton, 1999.

Kuhnke, LaVerne. *Lives at Risk: Public Health in Nineteenth-Century Egypt.* Berkeley: University of California Press, 1990.

Kuletz, Valerie. *The Tainted Desert: Environmental Ruin in the American West.* New York: Routledge, 1998.

Kuneralp, Sinan. "Osmanlı Yönetimindeki (1831–1911) Hicaz'da Hac ve Kolera." *Osmanlı Tarihi Araştırma ve Uygulama Merkezi Dergisi* 7 (1996): 497–511.

Kunt, Metin. "A Prince Goes Forth (Perchance to Return)." In *Identity and Identity Formation in the Ottoman World: A Volume of Essays in Honor of Norman Itzkowitz*, edited by Baki Tezcan and Karl K. Barbir, 63–71. Madison: University of Wisconsin Press, 2007.

———. "Sultan, Dynasty and State in the Ottoman Empire: Political Institutions in the Sixteenth Century." *The Medieval History Journal* 6, no. 2 (2003): 217–30.

Kutluoğlu, Muhammad H. *The Egyptian Question (1831–1841): The Expansionist Policy of Mehmed Ali Paşa in Syria and Asia Minor and the Reaction of the Sublime Porte.* Istanbul: Eren, 1998.

Lâmiʿî Çelebi. *Nefehâtü'l-Üns: Evliyâ Menkıbeleri*, edited by Süleyman Uludağ and Mustafa Kara. Istanbul: Marifet Yayınları, 1998.

Lammel, Hans-Uwe. "Western European Perception and Representation of Plagues in Eastern Europe, the Ottoman Empire and the Near East, 1650–1800." In *Le interazioni fra economia e ambiente biologico nell'Europa preindustriale secc. XIII–XVIII*, edited by Simonetta Cavaciocchi, 399–421. Florence: Firenze University Press, 2010.

Lancisi, Giovanni Maria. *Dissertatio Historica de Bovilla Peste, Quae ex Campaniae Finibus Anno 1713 Latio Importata* [etc.]. Rome: G.M. Salvoni, 1715.

Leach, Melissa, and Robin Mearns. *The Lie of the Land: Challenging Received Wisdom on the African Environment.* Portsmouth, NH: Heinemann, 1996.

Le Bruyn, Corneille. *Voyage au Levant: c'est-à-dire, dans les principaux endroits de l'Asie Mineure, dans les isles de Chio, Rhodes, Chypre, &c.* Paris: Jean-Baptiste-Claude Bauche, 1725.

Leiser, Gary. "In Memoriam: Michael W. Dols." *Middle East Studies Association Bulletin* 24 (1990): 152–53.

Le Guyader, Hervé. *Étienne Geoffroy Saint-Hilaire, 1772–1844: A Visionary Naturalist.* Translated by Marjorie Grene. Chicago: University of Chicago Press, 2004.

Le Roy Ladurie, Emmanuel. "Un concept: l'unification microbienne du monde (XIVe–XVIIe siècles)." *Revue suisse d'histoire* 23, no. 4 (1973): 627–96.

——. *Histoire du climat depuis l'an mil.* Paris: Flammarion, 1967.

Levy, Jerrold E. "Epilepsy." In *The Cambridge World History of Human Disease*, edited by Kenneth F. Kiple, 713–18. Cambridge: Cambridge University Press, 1993.

Lewis, Martin W. and Kären E. Wigen. *The Myth of Continents: A Critique of Metageography.* Berkeley: University of California Press, 1997.

Li, Lillian. *Fighting Famine in North China: State, Market, and Environmental Decline, 1690s-1990s.* Stanford: Stanford University Press, 2007.

Little, Lester K. "Plague Historians in Lab Coats." *Past and Present* 213 (2011): 267–90.

Lockman, Zachary. *Contending Visions of the Middle East: The History and Politics of Orientalism.* Cambridge: Cambridge University Press, 2004.

Low, Michael Christopher. "Empire and the Hajj: Pilgrims, Plagues, and Pan-Islam under British Surveillance, 1865–1908." *International Journal of Middle East Studies* 40, no. 2 (2008): 269–90.

Lowry, Heath W. *The Nature of the Early Ottoman State.* Albany: SUNY Press, 2003.

——. "Pushing the Stone Uphill: The Impact of Bubonic Plague on Ottoman Urban Society in the Fifteenth and Sixteenth Centuries." *Journal of Ottoman Studies* 23 (2004): 93–132.

——. *The Shaping of the Ottoman Balkans, 1350–1550: The Conquest, Settlement and Infrastructural Development of Northern Greece.* Istanbul: Bahçeşehir University Publications, 2008.

Lubenau, Reinhold. *Beschreibung der Reisen des Reinhold Lubenau.* Königsberg: Beyer (Thomas and Oppermann), 1914–15.

Luterbacher, Jürg et al. "European Seasonal and Annual Temperature Variability, Trends, and Extremes Since 1500." *Science* 303 (2004): 1499–503.

——. et al. "Mediterranean Climate Variability over the Last Centuries: A Review." In *The Mediterranean Climate: An Overview of the Main Characteristics and Issues*, edited by P. Lionello, P. Malanotte-Rizzoli, and R. Boscolo, 27–148. Amsterdam: Elsevier, 2006.

——. et al. "A Review of 2000 Years of Paleoclimatic Evidence in the Mediterranean." In *The Climate of the Mediterranean Region*, edited by P. Lionello, 87–185. London: Elsevier, 2012.

Mackenzie, Mordach. "An Account of the Plague at Constantinople: In a Letter from Mordach Mackenzie, M. D. to Sir James Porter, His Majesty's Envoy Plenipotentiary at Brussels, and F. R. S." *Philosophical Transactions (1683–1775)* 54 (January 1, 1764): 69–82.

——. "Extracts of Several Letters of Mordach Mackenzie, M. D. Concerning the Plague at Constantinople." *Philosophical Transactions (1683–1775)* 47 (1751–52): 384–95.

MacMichael, William. *Journey from Moscow to Istanbul in the Years 1817, 1818.* London: John Murray, 1819.

MacLean, Gerald M. *The Rise of Oriental Travel: English Visitors to the Ottoman Empire, 1580–1720.* New York: Palgrave Macmillan, 2004.

Madzharski Pŭtepisi za Balkanite, XVI–XIX v. Sofia: Izdatelstvo "Nauka i Izkustvo," 1976.

Manolova-Nikolova, Nadia. *Chumavite Vremena (1700–1850).* Sofia: "IF-94," 2004.

Manoukian, Setrag. "Fatvas as Asymmetrical Dialogues: Muhammad Karim Khan Kirmani and his Questioners." In *Islamic Legal Interpretation: Muftis and their Fatwas,* edited by Muhammad Khalid Masud, Brinkley Messick, and David S. Powers, 162–72. Cambridge: Harvard College, 1996.

Mantran, Robert. *Istanbul au siècle de Soliman le Magnifique.* Paris: Hachette, 1994.

Marchand, Suzanne L. *German Orientalism in the Age of Empire: Religion, Race, and Scholarship.* Cambridge: Cambridge University Press, 2009.

Marcus, Abraham. *The Middle East on the Eve of Modernity: Aleppo in the Eighteenth Century.* New York: Columbia University Press, 1989.

Marei, Nasr. *The Arabian Horse of Egypt.* Cairo: American University in Cairo Press, 2010.

Marino, John. *Pastoral Economics in the Kingdom of Naples.* Baltimore: Johns Hopkins University Press, 1988.

Mariti, Giovanni. *Travels Through Cyprus, Syria and Palestine: with a General History of the Levant.* Dublin: Messrs. P. Byrne and A. Grueber, 1792.

Mascall, Leonard. *The First Booke of Cattell.* London: John Harison, 1610.

Masters, Bruce. *Christians and Jews in the Ottoman Arab World: The Roots of Sectarianism.* Cambridge: Cambridge University Press, 2001.

Maurand, Jérôme. *Itinéraire de Jérome Maurand d'Antibes à Constantinople (1544).* Paris: E. Leroux, 1901.

Mawson, Anthony. *Mass Panic and Social Attachment: The Dynamics of Human Behavior.* Aldershot: Ashgate, 2007.

Mazower, Mark. *Salonica: City of Ghosts: Christians, Muslims, and Jews, 1430–1950.* New York: Alfred A. Knopf, 2005.

McCann, James C. *Green Land, Brown Land, Black Land: An Environmental History of Africa, 1800–1990.* Portsmouth, NH: Heinemann, 1999.

——. "The Plow and the Forest: Narratives of Deforestation in Ethiopia, 1840–1992." *Environmental History* 2, no. 2 (1997): 138–59.

McGowan, Bruce. *Economic Life in Ottoman Europe: Taxation, Trade and the Struggle for Land, 1600–1800.* Cambridge: Cambridge University Press, 1981.

McGrew, Roderick. *Russia and the Cholera, 1823–1832.* Madison, WI: The University of Wisconsin Press, 1965.

McNeill, J. R. "Observations on the Nature and Culture of Environmental History." *History and Theory* 42, no. 4 (2003): 5–43.

——. "The State of the Field of Environmental History." *Annual Review of Environment and Resources* 35, no. 1 (2010): 345–74.

McNeill, William H. *Plagues and Peoples.* Garden City, NY: Anchor Press, 1976.

——. *The Pursuit of Truth: A Historian's Memoir.* Lexington: University Press of Kentucky, 2005.

Mead, Richard. *A Discourse on the Plague.* London: Printed for A. Millar, 1744.

Melchert, Christopher. "Marʿī b. Yûsuf." In *Essays in Arabic Literary Biography 1350–1850*, edited by Joseph E. Lowry and Devin J. Stewart. Wiesbaden: Harrassowitz Verlag, 2009.

Messick, Brinkley. *The Calligraphic State: Textual Domination and History in a Muslim Society.* Berkeley: University of California Press, 1993.

Meyerhof, Max. "The 'Book of Treasure,' an Early Arabic Treatise on Medicine." *Isis* 14 (1930): 55–76.

——. *Sharḥ asmāʾ al-ʿuqqār (L'explication des noms de drogues): un glossaire de matière médicale.* Cairo: Imprimerie de l'Institut français, 1940.

——. *Studies in Medieval Arabic Medicine.* London: Variorum Reprints, 1984.

——. ed. *The Book of the Ten Treatises on the Eye Ascribed to Hunain ibn Ishaq (809–877 A.D.).* Cairo: Government Press, 1928.

Mikhail, Alan. *The Animal in Ottoman Egypt.* Oxford: Oxford University Press, 2014.

——. "An Irrigated Empire: The View from Ottoman Fayyum." *International Journal of Middle East Studies* 42, no. 4 (2010): 569–90.

——. *Nature and Empire in Ottoman Egypt: An Environmental History.* Cambridge: Cambridge University Press, 2011.

——. "The Nature of Plague in Late Eighteenth-Century Egypt." *Bulletin of the History of Medicine* 82, no. 2 (2008): 249–75.

——. "Unleashing the Beast: Animals, Energy, and the Economy of Labor in Ottoman Egypt." *American Historical Review* 118 (2013): 317–48.

——. ed. *Water on Sand: Environmental Histories of the Middle East and North Africa.* Oxford: Oxford University Press, 2012.

Mikulincer, Mario and Phillip Shaver. *Attachment in Adulthood: Structure, Dynamics, and Change.* New York: Guilford Press, 2007.

Millán, Cristina Álvarez. "Graeco-Roman Case Histories and Their Influence on Medieval Islamic Clinical Accounts." *Social History of Medicine* 12 (1999): 19–43.

Miller, Joshua. *Psychosocial Capacity Building in Response to Disasters.* New York: Columbia University Press, 2012.

Milton, Shaun. "Western Veterinary Medicine in Colonial Africa: A Survey, 1902–1963." *Argos* 18 (1998): 313–22.

Minkin, Shane. "Simone's Funeral: Egyptian Lives, Jewish Deaths in Twenty-First-Century Cairo." *Rethinking History: The Journal of Theory and Practice* 16, no. 1 (2012): 71–89.

Miran, Jonathan. "Space, Mobility, and Translocal Connections Across the Red Sea Area since 1500." *Northeast African Studies* 12, no. 1 (2012): ix-xxvi.

Mishra, Saurabh. "Cattle, Dearth, and the Colonial State: Famines and Livestock in Colonial India, 1896–1900." *Journal of Social History* 46 (2013): 989–1012.

Mitchell, Timothy. *Rule of Experts: Egypt, Techno-Politics, Modernity.* Berkeley: The University of California Press, 2002.

Mollat, Michel. *The Poor in the Middle Ages: An Essay in Social History.* New Haven: Yale University Press, 1986.

Monahan, W. Gregory. *Year of Sorrows: The Great Famine of 1709 in Lyon.* Columbus: Ohio State University Press, 1993.

Moreh, Shmuel. "Reputed Autographs of ʿAbd Al-Raḥmān al-Jabartī and Related Problems." *Bulletin of the School of Oriental and African Studies* 28, no. 3 (1965): 524–40.

Morony, Michael G. "Economic Boundaries? Late Antiquity and Early Islam." *Journal of the Economic and Social History of the Orient* 47 (2004): 166–94.

——. "'For Whom Does the Writer Write?': The First Bubonic Plague Pandemic According to Syriac Sources." In *Plague and the End of Antiquity: The Pandemic of 541–750*, edited by Lester K. Little, 59–86. Cambridge: Cambridge University Press, 2007.

Morris, Colin. "Pilgrimage to Jerusalem in the Late Middle Ages." In *Pilgrimage: The English Experience from Becket to Bunyan*, edited by Colin Morris and Peter Roberts, 141–63. Cambridge: Cambridge University Press, 2002.

Moryson, Fynes. *An Itinerary Containing His Ten Yeeres Travell through the Twelve Dominions of Germany, Bohmerland, Sweitzerland, Netherland, Denmarke, Poland, Italy, Turky, France, England, Scotland and Ireland.* Glasgow: J. MacLehose and Sons, 1907.

Moulin, Anne Marie. "The Construction of Disease Transmission in Nineteenth-Century Egypt and the Dialectics of Modernity." In *The Development of Modern Medicine in Non-Western Countries: Historical Perspectives*, edited by Hormoz Ebrahimnejad, 42–58. London: Routledge, 2009.

Muḥyi-yi Gülşeni. *Menâkıb-i İbrâhîm-i Gülşeni ve Şemlelizâde Ahmed Efendi, Şîve-i Tarikat-ı Gülşeni*, edited by Tahsin Yazıcı. Ankara: Türk Tarih Kurumu, 1982.

Mustafa Âlî. *Gelibolulu Mustafa Âlî ve Künhü'l-ahbâr'ında II. Selim, III. Murat ve III. Mehmet Devirleri*, edited by Faris Çerçi. Kayseri: Erciyes University Press, 2000.

Nedoroscik, Jeffrey A. *The City of the Dead: A History of Cairo's Cemetery Communities.* Westport, CT: Greenwood Publishing, 1997.

Newfield, Tim. "A Cattle Panzootic in Early Fourteenth-Century Europe." *Agricultural History Review* 57 (2009): 155–90.

——. "A Great Carolingian Panzootic: The Probable Extent, Diagnosis and Impact of an Early Ninth-Century Cattle Pestilence." *Argos: Bulletin van het Veterinair Historisch Genootschap* 46 (2012): 200–10.

Noradounghian, Gabriel. *Recueil d'actes internationaux de l'empire ottoman, 1789–1856*. Paris: F. Pichon, 1900.

——. *Recueil des traités de l'empire ottoman, 1300–1789*. Paris: F. Pichon, 1897.

Noth, Albrecht and Lawrence I. Conrad. *The Early Arabic Historical Tradition: A Source-Critical Study*. Princeton, NJ: Darwin Press, 1994.

Nutton, Vivian. "The Reception of Fracastoro's Theory of Contagion: The Seed that Fell among Thorns?" *Osiris* 6 (1990): 196–234.

——. "The Seeds Of Disease: An Explanation of Contagion and Infection from the Greeks to the Renaissance." *Medical History* 27 (1983): 1–34.

"O Zemletriasenii." *Zhurnal Ministerstva Vnutrennikh Del* 1 (1829): 652 - 654.

Oman, Luke et al. "High-Latitude Eruptions Cast Shadow over the African Monsoon and the Flow of the Nile." *Geophysical Research Letters* 33 (2006): L18711.

Osborne, Michael A. "Zoos in the Family: The Geoffroy Saint-Hilaire Clan and the Three Zoos of Paris." In *New Worlds, New Animals: From Menagerie to Zoological Park in the Nineteenth Century*, edited by R. J. Hoage and William A. Deiss, 33–42. Baltimore: Johns Hopkins University Press, 1996.

Özcan, Abdülkadir, ed. *Kânûnnâme-i Âl-i Osman: Tahlil ve Karşılaştırmalı Metin*. Istanbul: Kitabevi, 2003.

Özdemir, Hikmet. *The Ottoman Army 1914–1918: Disease and Death on the Battlefield*. Translated by Saban Kardaş. Salt Lake City: University of Utah Press, 2008.

Özel, Oktay. "Osmanlı Anadolu'sunda Terkedilmiş/Kayıp Köyler Sorunu (17–19. Yüzyıllar." In *Ötekilerin Peşinde: Ahmet Yaşar Ocak'a Armağan*, edited by Mehmet Öz and Fatih Yeşil, 557–91. Istanbul: Timaş, 2015.

——. "Population Changes in Ottoman Anatolia During the 16th and 17th Centuries: The 'Demographic Crisis' Reconsidered." *International Journal of Middle East Studies* 36 (2004): 183–205.

——. "The Reign of Violence: The *celâlis*, *c*.1550–1700." In *The Ottoman World*, edited by Christine Woodhead, 184–202. London: Routledge, 2012.

Panzac, Daniel. *La peste dans l'empire ottoman, 1700–1850*. Leuven: Éditions Peeters, 1985.

——. "La peste dans les possessions insulaires du Grand Seigneur (XVIIe–XIXe siècles)." In *Insularités ottomanes*, edited by Nicolas Vatin and Gilles Veinstein, 223–40. Paris: Maisonneuve & Larose, 2004.

——. "Politique sanitaire et fixation des frontières: L'exemple ottoman (XVIIIe – XIXe siècles)." *Turcica* 31 (1999): 87–108.

——. *Quarantaines et lazarets: L'Europe et la peste d'Orient (XVIIe–XXe siècles)*. Aix-en-Provence: Édisud, 1986.

Paraskevas, Philippe. *Breeding the Arabian Horse*, vol. 1 of *The Egyptian Alternative*. Exeter: Obelisque Publications, 2010.

——. *In Search of the Identity of the Egyptian Arabian Bloodlines*, vol. 2 of *The Egyptian Alternative*. Exeter: Obelisque Publications, 2012.

Parker, Geoffrey. *Global Crisis: War, Climate Change and Catastrophe in the Seventeenth Century*. New Haven: Yale University Press, 2013.

Peçevi. *Tarih-i Peçevi*. [Istanbul: Matbaʿa-yi Āmire, 1866].

Pedani-Fabris, Maria, ed. *Relazioni di ambasciatori veneti al senato*, 14: *Costantinopoli, Relazioni inedite (1512–1789)*. Padua: Bottega d'Erasmo, 1996.

Peirce, Leslie. *The Imperial Harem: Women and Sovereignty in the Ottoman Empire*. Oxford: Oxford University Press, 1993.

Perry, Brian D., Delia Grace, and Keith Sones. "Current Drivers and Future Directions of Global Livestock Disease Dynamics." *Proceedings of the National Academy of Sciences* 110 (2013): 20871–77.

Pormann, Peter E. "Case Notes and Clinicians: Galen's *Commentary* on the Hippocratic *Epidemics* in the Arabic Tradition." *Arabic Sciences and Philosophy* 18 (2008): 247–84.

——. ed. *Epidemics in Contexts: Greek Commentaries on Hippocrates in the Arabic Tradition*. Berlin: de Gruyter, 2012.

——. and Emilie Savage-Smith. *Medieval Islamic Medicine*. Washington, DC: Georgetown University Press, 2007.

Post, John D. *The Last Great Subsistence Crisis in the Western World*. Baltimore: The Johns Hopkins University Press, 1977.

——. *Food Shortage, Climatic Variability, and Epidemic Disease in Preindustrial Europe*. Ithaca: Cornell University Press, 1985.

Potter, Henry Percy. "The Oriental Plague in Its Social, Economical, Political, and International Relations, Special Reference Being Made to the Labours of John Howard on the Subject." *Journal of the Statistical Society of London* 43, no. 4 (1880): 605–42.

Potter, Hillary, ed. *Racing the Storm: Racial Implications and Lessons Learned from Hurricane Katrina*. Lanham: Lexington Books, 2007.

Pouqueville, François-Charles-Hugues-Laurent. *Voyage en Morée, à Constantinople, en Albanie et dans plusieurs autres parties de l'empire ottoman pendant les années 1798, 1799, 1800 et 1801*. Paris: Gabon, 1805.

Prakash, Gyan and Kevin Michael Kruse, eds. *The Spaces of the Modern City: Imaginaries, Politics, and Everyday Life*. Princeton: Princeton University Press, 2008.

Proust, Achille Adrien. *La défense de l'Europe contre la peste et la Conférence de Venise de 1897.* Paris: Masson, 1897.

Rácz, Lajos. "The Price of Survival: Transformations in Environmental Conditions and Subsistence Systems in Hungary in the Age of Ottoman Occupation." *Hungarian Studies* 24 (2010): 21–39.

——. *The Steppe to Europe: An Environmental History of Hungary in the Traditional Age.* Cambridge: White Horse Press, 2013.

Radcliffe, J. Netten. "On the Prospect of a Reappearance of Plague in this Country and on the Continent of Europe." *Medical Times and Gazette* 1 (Jan 22, 1876): 83–85.

Radostits, O. M. and Stanley H. Done, eds. *Veterinary Medicine: A Textbook of the Diseases of Cattle, Sheep, Pigs, Goats, and Horses.* New York: Elsevier Saunders, 2007.

Raḍwān, Abū al-Futūḥ. *Tārīkh Maṭbaʿat Būlāq wa Lamḥa fī Tārīkh al-Ṭibāʿa fī Buldān al-Sharq al-Awsaṭ.* Cairo: al-Maṭbaʿa al-Amīriyya, 1953.

Ramazzini, Bernardino. *De Contagiosa Epidemia Quae in Patavino Agro, & Tota Fere Veneta Ditione in Boves Irrepsit Dissertatio.* Padua: Gio. Batt. Conzatti, 1712.

Raphael, Beverley. *When Disaster Strikes: How Individuals and Communities Cope with Catastrophe.* New York: Basic Books, 1986.

Raymond, André. "Les grands épidémies de peste au Caire aux XVIIe et XVIIIe siècles." *Bulletin d'études orientales* 25 (1972): 203–10.

al-Rāzī, Abū Bakr Muḥammad Ibn Zakārīyā. *al-Ḥāwī fī al-ṭibb.* Beirut: Dār al-Kutub al-ʿIlmiyya, 2002.

Reimer, Michael J. "Ottoman Alexandria: The Paradox of Decline and the Reconfiguration of Power in Eighteenth-Century Arab Provinces." *Journal of the Economic and Social History of the Orient* 37 (1994): 107–46.

Richards, Paul. *Fighting for the Rain Forest: War, Youth and Resources in Sierra Leone.* Portsmouth, NH: Heinemann, 1996.

Richardson, Harry et al., eds. *Natural Disaster Analysis After Hurricane Katrina: Risk Assessment, Economic Impacts and Social Implications.* Cheltenham, UK: Edward Elgar, 2008.

Robarts, Andrew. "Imperial Confrontations or Regional Cooperation? Bulgarian Migration and Ottoman-Russian Relations in the Black Sea Region, 1768–1830s." *Turkish Historical Review* 3, no. 2 (2012): 149–67.

——. *Migration and Disease in the Black Sea Region: Ottoman-Russian Relations in the Late Eighteenth and Early Nineteenth Centuries.* London: Bloomsbury Academic, 2017.

Roberts, Neil et al. "Palaeolimnological Evidence for an East–West Climate See-Saw in the Mediterranean Since AD 900." *Global and Planetary Change* 84–85 (2012): 23–34.

Roe, Thomas. *The Negotiations of Sir Thomas Roe, in His Embassy in the Ottoman Porte, from the Year 1621 to 1628 Inclusive.* London, 1740.

Rosenthal, Franz. "An Ancient Commentary on the Hippocratic Oath." *Bulletin of the History of Medicine* 30 (1956): 52–87.

——. "Bibliographical Notes on Medieval Muslim Dentistry." *Bulletin of the History of Medicine* 34 (1960): 52–60.

——. "The Defense of Medicine in the Medieval Muslim World." *Bulletin of the History of Medicine* 43 (1969): 519–32.

——. "Isḥāq b. Ḥunayn's *Ta'riḫ al-aṭibba'*." *Oriens* 7 (1954): 55–80.

——. "'Life is short, the art is long': Arabic Commentaries on the First Hippocratic Aphorism." *Bulletin of the History of Medicine* 40 (1966): 226–45.

——. "The Physician in Medieval Muslim Society." *Bulletin of the History of Medicine* 52 (1978): 475–91.

——. "ar-Rāzī on the Hidden Illness." *Bulletin of the History of Medicine* 52 (1978): 45–60.

Rothenberg, G. E. "The Austrian Sanitary Cordon and the Control of the Bubonic Plague: 1710–1871." *Journal of the History of Medicine and Allied Sciences* 28, no. 1 (1973): 15–23.

El-Rouayheb, Khaled. "Opening the Gate of Verification: The Forgotten Arab-Islamic Florescence of the 17th Century." *International Journal of Middle East Studies* 38 (2006), 263–81.

Russell, Alexander. *The Natural History of Aleppo.* London: G. G. & J. Robinson, 1794.

Russell, Patrick. *A Treatise of the Plague: Containing an Historical Journal, and Medical Account, of the Plague, at Aleppo, in the Years 1760, 1761, and 1762. Also, Remarks on Quarantines, Lazarettos, and the Administration of Police in Times of Pestilence. To Which Is Added, an Appendix, Containing Cases of the Plague; and an Account of the Weather, during the Pestilential Season.* London: Printed for G. G. J. and J. Robinson, 1791.

Rycaut, Paul. *The History of the Present State of the Ottoman Empire.* London: Charles Brome, 1686.

al-Ṣabbāgh, ʿAbd al-Laṭīf Muḥammad. "al-Ṭibb al-Bayṭarī fī Miṣr (1828–1849): Dirāsa Wathā'iqiyya." *Miṣr al-Ḥadītha* 8 (2009): 17–55.

Es-Sadrî, Musa. *Regâyibü'l-Menâkıb Sadreddin Konevî'nin Menkıbeleri,* edited by Emin Agar. Istanbul: Anka Yayınları, 2002.

Said, Edward. *Orientalism.* New York: Vintage Book, 1978.

Sajdi, Dana. *The Barber of Damascus: Nouveau Literacy in the Eighteenth-Century Ottoman Levant.* Stanford: Stanford University Press, 2013.

Sándor, Szilágyi, ed. *Szamosközi, István történeti maradványai (Chronicle of István Szamosközi).* Budapest, 1889.

Sandys, George. *A Relation of a Journey Begun An. Dom. 1610.* London: Ro. Allot, 1632.

Sarıyıldız, Gülden. *Hicaz Karantina Teşkilatı (1865–1914)*. Ankara: Türk Tarih Kurumu, 1996.

———. "Karantina Meclisi'nin Kuruluşu ve Faaliyetleri." *Belleten* 58, no. 222 (1994): 329–76.

Scambler, Graham. "Sociological Aspects of Epilepsy." In *Epilepsy*, edited by Anthony Hopkins, 497–510. London: Chapman and Hall, 1987.

Schacht, Joseph, and Max Meyerhof. *The Medico-Philosophical Controversy between Ibn Butlan of Baghdad and Ibn Ridwan of Cairo: A Contribution to the History of Greek Learning among the Arabs*. Cairo, 1937.

Schamiloglu, Uli. "Preliminary Remarks on the Role of Disease in the History of the Golden Horde." *Central Asian Survey* 12, no. 4 (1993): 447–57.

———. "The Rise of the Ottoman Empire: The Black Death in Medieval Anatolia and Its Turkish Civilization." In *Views from the Edge: Essays in Honor of Richard W. Bulliet*, edited by Neguin Yavari, Lawrence G. Porter, Jean-Marc Ran Oppenheim, 255–79. New York: Columbia University Press, 2004.

Schönig, Hanne. "Reflections on the Use of Animal Drugs in Yemen." *Quaderni di Studi Arabi* 20–21 (2002–3): 157–84.

Schweigger, Salomon. *Sultanlar Kentine Yolculuk, 1578–1581*. Translated by S. Türkis Noyan. Istanbul: Kitap Yayınevi, 2004.

Searight, Sarah. "A Waghorn Letter Book for 1840." *Journal of the Royal Asiatic Society* 7, no. 2 (1997): 229–48.

Sechel, Teodora Daniela, ed. *Medicine Within and Between the Habsburg and Ottoman Empires, 18th–19th Centuries*. Bochum: Dieter Winkler, 2011.

Şehsuvaroğlu, Bedi N. *Tarihi Kolera Salgınları ve Osmanlı Türkleri*. Istanbul: İsmail Akgün Matbaası, 1954.

———. "Türkiye Karantina Tarihine Giriş: Türkiye'de Karantina Tesis ve Teşkilleri." *İstanbul Tıp Fakültesi Mecmuası* 3 (1957): 319–39.

Selânikî Mustafa Efendi. *Tarih-i Selânikî*, edited by Mehmet İpşirli. 2 vols. Ankara: Türk Tarih Kurumu, 1999.

Sharrer, G. Terry. "The Great Glanders Epizootic, 1861–1866: A Civil War Legacy." *Agricultural History* 69 (1995): 79–97.

Shatzmiller, Maya. "Economic Performance and Economic Growth in the Early Islamic World." *Journal of the Economic and Social History of the Orient* 54 (2011): 132–84.

Shaw, Stanford J. *Between Old and New: The Ottoman Empire under Sultan Selim III, 1789–1807*. Cambridge, MA: Harvard University Press, 1971.

Shefer-Mossensohn, Miri. "Communicable Disease in Ottoman Palestine: Local Thoughts and Actions." *Korot* 21 (2011–12): 19–49.

———. *Ottoman Medicine: Healing and Medical Institutions 1500–1700*. Albany, NY: State University of New York Press, 2009.

Shehada, Housni Alkhateeb. *Mamluks and Animals: Veterinary Medicine in Medieval Islam*. Leiden: Brill, 2013.

Silvera, Alain. "The First Egyptian Student Mission to France under Muhammad Ali." *Middle Eastern Studies* 16 (1980): 1–22.

Simonsohn, Uriel. *A Common Justice: the Legal Allegiances of Christians and Jews under Early Islam*. Philadelphia: University of Pennsylvania Press, 2011.

Sims, D. *Understanding Cairo: The Logic of a City Out of Control*. Oxford: Oxford University Press, 2011.

Sirohi, Smita and Axel Michaelowa. "Sufferer and Cause: Indian Livestock and Climate Change." *Climatic Change* 85 (2007): 285–98.

Slavin, Philip. "The Fifth Rider of the Apocalypse: The Great Cattle Plague in England and Wales and Its Economic Consequences, 1319–1350." In *Le interazioni fra economia e ambiente biologico nell'Europa preindustriale secc. XIII–XVIII*, edited by Simonetta Cavaciocchi, 165–79. Florence: Firenze University Press, 2010.

——. "The Great Bovine Pestilence and Its Economic and Environmental Consequences in England and Wales, 1318–51." *The Economic History Review* 65 (2012): 1239–66.

——. "Warfare and Ecological Destruction in Early Fourteenth-Century British Isles." *Environmental History* 19 (2014): 528–50.

Smith, Jane I. and Yvonne Yazbeck Haddad. *The Islamic Understanding of Death and Resurrection*. Oxford: Oxford University Press, 2002.

"Some Turkish Lazarets and Other Sanitary Institutions in the Near East, I." *The Lancet* 169, no. 4365 (Apr. 27, 1907): 1188–89.

"Some Turkish Lazarets and Other Sanitary Institutions in the Near East, III." *The Lancet* 169, no. 4367 (May 11, 1907): 1317–20.

Sonbol, Amira el-Azhary. *The Creation of a Medical Profession in Egypt, 1800–1922*. Syracuse, NY: Syracuse University Press, 1991.

Spinage, Clive A. *Cattle Plague: A History*. New York: Kluwer, 2003.

Stallings, Robert. "Weberian Political Sociology and Sociological Disaster Studies." *Sociological Forum* 17, no. 2 (2002): 281–305.

Stearns, Justin. "Contagion in Theology and Law: Ethical Considerations in the Writings of Two 14th Century Scholars of Nasrid Granada." *Islamic Law and Society* 14 (2007): 109–29.

——. "Enduring the Plague: Ethical Behavior in the Fatwas of an 8th/14th Century Mufti and Theologian." In *Muslim Medical Ethics: From Theory to Practice*, edited by Jonathan Brockopp and Thomas Eich, 38–54. Columbia, SC: University of South Carolina Press, 2008.

——. *Infectious Ideas: Contagion in Premodern Islamic and Christian Thought in the Western Mediterranean*. Baltimore, MD: Johns Hopkins University Press, 2011.

——. "New Directions in the Study of Religious Responses to the Black Death." *History Compass* 7, no. 5 (2009): 1363–75.

Steinberg, Philip and Rob Shields, eds. *What Is a City?: Rethinking the Urban After Hurricane Katrina*. Athens, GA: University of Georgia Press, 2008.

Stühring, Carsten. "Managing Epizootic Diseases in 18th-Century Bavaria." In *Le interazioni fra economia e ambiente biologico nell'Europa preindustriale secc. XIII–XVIII*, edited by Simonetta Cavaciocchi, 473–80. Florence: Firenze University Press, 2010.

Sublet, Jacqueline. "La peste prise aux rêts de la jurisprudence: le traité d'Ibn Ḥağar al-ʿAsqalānī sur la peste." *Studia Islamica* 33 (1971): 141–49.

Sufian, Sandra. "Colonial Malariology, Medical Borders, and Sharing Scientific Knowledge in Mandatory Palestine." *Science in Context* 19 (2006): 381–400.

——. *Healing the Land and the Nation: Malaria and the Zionist Project in Palestine, 1920–1947*. Chicago: University of Chicago Press, 2007.

Sugimoto, Seiko et al. "Sociocultural Frame, Religious Networks, Miracles: Experiences from Tsunami Disaster Management in South India." In *The Indian Ocean Tsunami: The Global Response to a Natural Disaster*, edited by Pradyumna Karan et al., 213–35. Lexington: University Press of Kentucky, 2011.

Summers, William. *The Great Manchurian Plague of 1910–1911: The Geopolitics of an Epidemic Disease*. New Haven: Yale University Press, 2012.

Sussman, George D. "Was the Black Death in India and China?" *Bulletin of the History of Medicine* 85, no. 3 (2011): 319–55.

Swabe, Joanna. *Animals, Disease, and Human Society: Human-Animal Relations and the Rise of Veterinary Medicine*. London: Routledge, 1999.

Takeda, Junko Thérèse. *Between Crown and Commerce: Marseille and the Early Modern Mediterranean*. Baltimore: Johns Hopkins University Press, 2011.

Tatcı, Mustafa. *Üsküdarlı Muhammed Nasûhî ve Divanı*. Istanbul: Kaknüs Yayınları, 2004.

Tawtal, Ferdinan. *Wathāʾiq taʾrīkhiyya ʿan ḥalab*. 4 vols. Beirut: al-Maṭbaʿa al-Kathulikiyya, 1958–63.

Taylor, Christopher S. *In the Vicinity of the Righteous: Ziyāra and the Veneration of Muslim Saints in Late Medieval Egypt*. Leiden: Brill, 1999.

Tedrus, G. M., L. C. Fonseca, F. De Pietro Magri, and P. H. Mendes. "Spiritual/Religious Coping in Patients with Epilepsy: Relationship with Sociodemographic and Clinical Aspects and Quality of Life." *Epilepsy and Behavior* 28 (2013): 386–90.

Temkin, Owsei. *The Falling Sickness A History of Epilepsy from the Greeks to the Beginnings of Modern Neurology*. Baltimore: Johns Hopkins University Press, 1979.

Terzioğlu, Derin. "Sufi and Dissident in the Ottoman Empire: Niyazî-i Mısrî (1618–1694)." Unpublished PhD dissertation, Harvard University, 1999.

Tetsuya, Ohtoshi. "Cairene Cemeteries as Public Loci in Mamluk Egypt." *Bulletin de l'Institut français d'archéologie orientale* 57 (1958): 25–79.

Tezcan, Baki. "The Debut of Kösem Sultan's Political Career." *Turcica* 40 (2008): 347–35.

——. "The Question of Regency in the Ottoman Dynasty: The Case of the Early Reign of Ahmed I." *Archivum Ottomanicum* 25 (2008): 185–98.

——. *The Second Ottoman Empire: Political and Social Transformation in the Early Modern World.* Cambridge: Cambridge University Press, 2010.

Tingley, Martin P. and Peter Huybers. "Recent Temperature Extremes at High Northern Latitudes Unprecedented in the Past 600 Years." *Nature* 496 (2013): 201–5.

Tolan, John Victor. *Saracens Islam in the Medieval European Imagination.* New York: Columbia University Press, 2002.

Topçular Kâtibi ʿAbdülkâdir Efendi Tarihi, edited by Ziya Yılmazer. Ankara: Türk Tarih Kurumu, 2003.

Touchan, Ramzi et al. "Reconstructions of Spring/Summer Precipitation for the Eastern Mediterranean from Tree-Ring Widths and Its Connection to Large-Scale Atmospheric Circulation." *Climate Dynamics* 25 (2005): 75–98.

"Tri Miesiatsa za Dunavaem." *Syn Otechetsva* 1, no. 5 (1833): 273–85.

Trouillot, Michel-Rolph. *Silencing the Past: Power and the Production of History.* Boston: Beacon Press, 1995.

Tucker, William F. "Natural Disasters and the Peasantry in Mamlûk Egypt." *Journal of the Economic and Social History of the Orient* 24 (1981): 215–22.

Turna, Nalan. "İstanbul'un Veba ile İmtihanı: 1811–1812 Veba Salgını Bağlamında Toplum ve Ekonomi." *Studies of the Ottoman Domain* 1, no. 1 (2011): 23–58.

Tytler, James. *A Treatise on the Plague and Yellow Fever.* Salem: Printed by Joshua Cushing, for B. B. Macanulty, 1799.

Ullmann, Manfred. *Islamic Medicine.* Edinburg: Edinburg University Press, 1978.

——. *Die Natur- und Geheimwissenschaften im Islam.* Leiden: Brill, 1972.

Ünver, Ahmet Süheyl. "About the History of the Leproseries in Turkey." In Emanuel Berghoff, ed., *Festschrift zum 80. Geburtstag Max Neuburgers*, 447–50. Vienna: Maudrich, 1948.

——. "Les épidémies de choléra dans les terres balkaniques aux XVIIIe et XIXe siècles." *Etudes Balkaniques* 4 (1973): 89–97.

——. "Sur l'histoire de la peste en Turquie." In *Neuvième Congrès international d'histoire de la médecine, Bucureşti (România) 10-18 septembre 1932; comptes-rendus*, edited by Victor Gomoiu and Victoria Gomoiu, 479–83. Bucharest, 1932.

——. "Taun Nedir? Veba Nedir?" *Dirim* 3–4 (1978): 363–66.

——. and Bedi N. Şehsuvaroğlu. *Türkiye'de Cüzam Tarihi Üzerine Araştırma.* Istanbul: İsmail Akgün Matbaası, 1961.

van den Boogert, Maurits. *Aleppo Observed: Ottoman Syria through the Eyes of Two Scottish Doctors, Alexander and Patrick Russell.* Oxford: Oxford University Press, 2010.

van Ess, Josef. *Der Fehltritt des Gelehrten: die "Pest von Emmaus" und ihre theologischen Nachspiele.* Heidelberg: Universitätsverlag C. Winter, 2001.

——. "Texts and Contexts: Heroes of the Plague." In *Text and Context in Islamic Societies,* edited by Irene A. Bierman, 13–22. Reading: Ithaca, 2004.

Varlık, Nükhet. "Conquest, Urbanization and Plague Networks in the Ottoman Empire, 1453–1600." In *The Ottoman World,* edited by Christine Woodhead, 251–63. London: Routledge, 2012.

——. "From '*Bête Noire*' to '*le Mal de* Constantinople': Plagues, Medicine, and the Early Modern Ottoman State." *Journal of World History* 24, no. 4 (2013): 741–70.

——. "New Science and Old Sources: Why the Ottoman Experience of Plague Matters." *The Medieval Globe* 1 (2014): 193–227.

——. *Plague and Empire in the Early Modern Mediterranean World: The Ottoman Experience, 1347–1600.* Cambridge: Cambridge University Press, 2015.

——. "Plague, Conflict, and Negotiation: The Jewish Broadcloth Weavers of Salonica and the Ottoman Central Administration in the Late Sixteenth Century." *Jewish History* 28 (2014): 261–88.

Vatin, Nicolas and Stephane Yerasimos. *Les cimetières dans la ville: status, choix et organisation des lieux d'inhumation dans Istanbul intra muros.* Istanbul: Institut français d'études anatoliennes Georges Dumézil, 2001.

Verdery, Richard N. "The Publications of the Būlāq Press under Muḥammad ʿAlī of Egypt." *Journal of the American Oriental Society* 91, no. 1 (1971): 129–32.

Vitkus, Daniel J. "Early Modern Orientalism: Representations of Islam in Sixteenth- and Seventeenth-Century Europe." In *Western Views of Islam in Medieval and Early Modern Europe: Perception of Other,* edited by David R. Blanks and Michael Frasetto, 207–30. New York: St. Martin's Press, 1999.

von Moltke, Helmuth. *Unter dem Halbmond: Erlebnisse in der alten Türkei, 1835–1839.* Tübingen: Erdmann, 1979.

"Vospominaniia Doktora Zeidlitsa o Turetskom Pokhod 1829 Goda." *Russkii Arkhiv* 1–4 (1878): 412–35.

Waller, Richard. "'Clean' and 'Dirty': Cattle Disease and Control Policy in Colonial Kenya, 1900–40." *Journal of African History* 45 (2004): 45–80.

Walløe, Lars. "Medieval and Modern Bubonic Plague: Some Clinical Continuities." In *Pestilential Complexities: Understanding Medieval Plague,* edited by Vivian Nutton, 59–73. London: Wellcome Trust Centre for the History of Medicine at University College London, 2008.

Watts, Sheldon. "Cholera Politics in Britain in 1879: John Netten Radcliffe's Confidential Memo on 'Qurantine in the Red Sea'." *The Journal of the Historical Society* 7, no. 3 (2007): 291–347.

Weeber, Stanley. *Post-Rita Reflections: a Sociological Journey*. Lanham: Hamilton Books, 2009.

Westermann, Ekkehard, ed. *Internationaler Ochsenhandel (1350–1750)*. Stuttgart: Klett-Cotta, 1979.

Whalen, Brett Edward, ed. *Pilgrimage in the Middle Ages: A Reader*. Toronto: University of Toronto Press, 2011.

Whetton, Peter, Ian Rutherford, and Robert Allan. "Historical ENSO Teleconnections in the Eastern Hemisphere." *Climatic Change* 28 (1994): 221–53.

White, Sam. *The Climate of Rebellion in the Early Modern Ottoman Empire*. Cambridge: Cambridge University Press, 2011.

——. "Rethinking Disease in Ottoman Society." *International Journal of Middle East Studies* 42 (2010): 549–67.

Wiet, Gaston. "La grande peste noire en Syrie et en Égypt." In *Études d'Orientalisme dédiées à la mémoire de Lévi-Provençal*, 1: 367–84. Paris: Maisonneuve et Larose, 1962.

Wilkinson, Lise. *Animals and Disease: An Introduction to the History of Comparative Medicine*. Cambridge: Cambridge University Press, 1992.

Winter, Michael. "A Seventeenth-Century Arabic Panegyric of the Ottoman Dynasty." *Asian and African Studies* 13 (1979): 130–56.

Wockoeck, Ursula. *German Orientalism: The Study of the Middle East and Islam from 1800–1945*. London: Routledge, 2009.

Wunder, Amanda. "Western Travelers, Eastern Antiquities, and the Image of the Turk in Early Modern Europe." *Journal of Early Modern History* 7, no. 1–2 (2003): 89–119.

Yaylagül, Özen. *Ebvâb-ı şifâ*. Ankara: KÖKSAV, 2010.

Yerasimos, Stefanos. *Les voyageurs dans l'empire ottoman, XIVe–XVIe siècles: Bibliographie, itinéraires et inventaire des lieux habités*. Ankara: Türk Tarih Kurumu, 1991.

Yıldırım, Nuran and Hakan Ertin, "European Physicians/Specialists during the Cholera Epidemic in Istanbul 1893–1895 and their Contribution to the Modernization of Healthcare in the Ottoman State." In *Health, Culture and the Human Body: Epidemiology, Ethics and History of Medicine; Perspectives from Turkey and Central Europe*, edited by İlhan İlkılıç, Hakan Ertin, Rainer Brömer and Hajo Zeeb, 189–215. Istanbul: BETIM Center Press, 2014.

Yıldız, Sara Nur. "From Cairo to Ayasuluk: Hacı Paşa and the Transmission of Islamic Learning to Western Anatolia in the Late Fourteenth Century." *Journal of Islamic Studies* 25, no. 3 (2014): 263–97.

Yılmaz, Coşkun and Necdet Yılmaz, eds. *Osmanlılarda Sağlık*, 2 vols. Istanbul: Biofarma, 2006.

Yünal, Abdurrahman, ed. *Menâkıb-ı Hazret-i Üftâde*. Bursa: Celvet Yayınları, 1996.

Zablotskii-Desiatovskii, A. P. *Graf P.D. Kiselev i ego vremia*. Saint Petersburg: Tip. M. M. Stasiulevicha 1882.

Zaman, Muhammad Qasim. "Death, Funeral Processions, and the Articulation of Religious Authority in Early Islam." *Studia Islamica* 93 (2001): 27–58.

"Zapisnaia Knizhka Grafa P. Kh. Grabbe." *Russkii Arkhiv* 4 (1888): 1–46.

Zell, Roland. "Global Climate Change and the Emergence/Re-emergence of Infectious Diseases." *International Journal of Medical Microbiology* 293, suppl. 37 (2004): 16–26.

Zhou, Xun. *The Great Famine in China, 1958–1962: A Documentary History*. New Haven: Yale University Press, 2012.

Zilfi, Madeline C. "The Kadizadelis: Discordant Revivalism in Seventeenth-Century Istanbul." *Journal of Near Eastern Studies* 45, no. 4 (1986): 251–269.

——. *The Politics of Piety: The Ottoman Ulema in the Postclassical Age (1600–1800)*. Minneapolis: Bibliotheca Islamica, 1988.

Zylberman, Patrick. "Civilizing the State: Borders, Weak States and International Health in Modern Europe." In *Medicine at the Border: Disease, Globalization and Security, 1850 to the Present*, edited by Alison Bashford, 21–40. New York: Palgrave Macmillan, 2006.

INDEX